Hartman's Complete Guide for the EKG Technician

Wilma Lynne Clarke, EdD, RN

SECOND EDITION

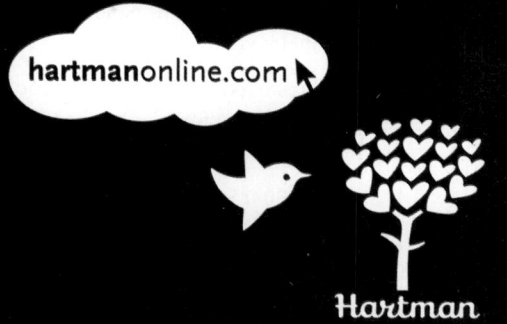

Credits

Managing Editor
Susan Alvare Hedman

Developmental Editor
Kristin Calderon

Designer
Kirsten Browne

Production
Anika Steppe

Illustration
Tracy Kopsachilis and Tess Marhofer

Proofreaders
Sylvie Althoff
Pamela Juarez
Holly Trimble

Editorial Assistant
Angela Storey

Sales/Marketing
Deborah Rinker-Wildey
Kendra Robertson
Erika Walker
Col Foley
Caroyl Scott
Erin Kleymann

Customer Service
Fran Desmond
Thomas Noble
Brian Fejer
Hank Bullis
Della Torres

Information Technology
Eliza Martin

Warehouse Coordinator
Chris Midyette

Copyright Information

© 2023 by Hartman Publishing, Inc.
1313 Iron Ave SW
Albuquerque, New Mexico 87102
(505) 291-1274
web: hartmanonline.com
e-mail: orders@hartmanonline.com
Twitter: @HartmanPub

All rights reserved. No part of this book may be reproduced, in any form or by any means, without permission in writing from the publisher.

ISBN 978-1-60425-151-7

PRINTED IN CANADA

Notice to Readers

Though the guidelines and procedures contained in this text are based on consultations with healthcare professionals, they should not be considered absolute recommendations. The instructor and readers should follow employer, local, state, and federal guidelines concerning healthcare practices. These guidelines change, and it is the reader's responsibility to be aware of these changes and of the policies and procedures of her or his healthcare facility.

The publisher, author, editors, and reviewers cannot accept any responsibility for errors or omissions or for any consequences from application of the information in this book and make no warranty, express or implied, with respect to the contents of the book. The publisher does not warrant or guarantee any of the products described herein or perform any analysis in connection with any of the product information contained herein.

Special Thanks

A very warm thank you goes to our insightful reviewers, listed in alphabetical order:

Michele Knorrp, LVN
Elkhart, TX

Dennis Leahy, MD, FACC
San Diego, CA

Eppie Rivas, PhD, MAEd, BSN, RN
Las Cruces, NM

Carolyn Stewart, MSN, RN, CPP
Anderson, SC

We are very appreciative of the many sources who shared their informative images with us:

- Alamy
- Dreamstime
- Hill-Rom Services, Inc.
- Medline Industries, LP
- Philips
- Statewide Program for Infection Control and Epidemiology (SPICE), UNC, Chapel Hill
- Ben Taylor, PhD, PA-C, DFAAPA
- 3M
- ZOLL Medical Corporation

Gender Usage

This textbook uses gender pronouns interchangeably to denote healthcare team members and patients.

Contents

Page

1 The Role of the EKG Technician

1. Describe the role of the EKG technician and identify healthcare settings in which EKG technicians work   1
2. Identify soft skills and personal traits needed for success as an EKG technician   3
3. Describe the certification process for the EKG technician   6
4. Describe the importance of continuing education and recertification   7
5. Demonstrate proper communication with other members of the healthcare team   7
6. Discuss the chain of command and understand the importance of following a facility's policies and procedures   8
7. Discuss outside organizations important to the function of healthcare facilities   9

2 Basic Patient Care Skills

1. Explain the importance of monitoring vital signs   12
2. Discuss the role of the EKG technician in infection prevention and control   13
3. List guidelines for measuring body temperature and observing skin condition   19
4. Define *pulse* and list guidelines for counting pulse   21
5. Define *respirations* and list guidelines for counting respirations   23
6. Define *blood pressure* and list guidelines for measuring blood pressure   24
7. Describe normal vital sign ranges for pediatric patients   27
8. Obtain pulse oximetry readings and identify normal ranges for pulse oximetry   27
9. Describe the importance of assessing and reporting pain and level of consciousness   28
10. Describe patient body positions commonly used during EKG testing   30

Learning Objective

Page

3 Anatomy and Physiology

1. Discuss key concepts of anatomy and physiology and define anatomical terms   31
2. Describe the parts of the cardiovascular system and their functions   33
3. Describe the parts of the respiratory system and their functions   34
4. Describe the relationship between the nervous system and the cardiovascular system   35
5. Identify the three layers of the heart   35
6. Describe the major vessels that enter and leave the heart, including the coronary arteries   36
7. Describe the chambers and valves of the heart and the movement of blood through the heart   36
8. Describe two circulatory paths: pulmonary and systemic   38
9. Discuss the relationship between the cardiovascular system and the respiratory system   39

4 Common Cardiovascular Diseases and Disorders

1. Describe coronary artery disease   41
2. Describe ischemia and myocardial infarction   41
3. Describe cardiomyopathy   43
4. Describe congestive heart failure   43
5. Describe heart valve disease   44
6. Describe blood clots and possible complications   45
7. Describe hypertension   46

5 Introduction to EKG Technology and Applications

1. Describe the electrical activity of the heart and how it is recorded by EKG machines   48
2. Discuss the portable EKG machine   49
3. Describe the types of EKG-based tests and discuss the indications for each   50

Learning Objective	Page
4. Identify EKG leads and lead groups	51
5. Describe electrode placement and the use of different leads	53
6. Demonstrate proper setup of the EKG machine	55

6 Basic EKG Procedures

Learning Objective	Page
1. Describe patient identification, patient preparation, and response to emergency situations during EKG testing	58
2. Demonstrate the performance of the 12-lead EKG test	59
3. Explain patient preparation and monitoring for telemetry	61
4. Demonstrate the performance of a stress test	62
5. Discuss Holter and other ambulatory monitoring	65
6. Discuss the importance of accurate record-keeping and patient confidentiality	66

7 EKG Adaptations and Troubleshooting

Learning Objective	Page
1. Discuss artifact and identify situations that require adaptations during EKG testing	68
2. Demonstrate solutions to different types of EKG artifact	69
3. Demonstrate adaptations to electrode placement and patient positioning	72
4. Identify sources of information for EKG machine troubleshooting and maintenance	75

8 The Cardiac Conduction System and EKG Tracings

Learning Objective	Page
1. Explain the difference between the mechanical and electrical activity of the heart	77
2. Explain the electrical conduction system of the heart	78
3. Understand the features of an EKG tracing	79
4. Identify important intervals and segments on the EKG tracing and list normal measurements	81
5. Demonstrate the measurement of time on the EKG tracing using small and large blocks	82
6. List the 6 steps used to analyze an EKG tracing	82
7. Discuss the first step in analyzing heart rhythms: three methods to determine heart rate from the EKG tracing	83
8. Discuss the second step in analyzing heart rhythms: how to examine an EKG tracing for regularity	84
9. Discuss the third step in analyzing heart rhythms: examining the P wave on an EKG tracing	86
10. Discuss the fourth step in analyzing heart rhythms: measuring the PR interval on an EKG tracing	87
11. Discuss the fifth step in analyzing heart rhythms: measuring the QRS complex on an EKG tracing	88
12. Discuss the importance of following each step when analyzing an EKG tracing	91

9 Overview of Rhythm Interpretation

Learning Objective	Page
1. Explain how EKG rhythms are named and discuss the importance of recognizing cardiac rhythms	94
2. Identify sinus rhythms	96
3. Discuss what sinus rhythms mean for the patient	98
4. Identify atrial rhythms	101
5. Discuss what atrial rhythms mean for the patient	106
6. Identify junctional rhythms	111
7. Discuss what junctional rhythms mean for the patient	114
8. Identify ventricular rhythms	118
9. Discuss what ventricular rhythms mean for the patient	125
10. Identify heart block rhythms	132
11. Discuss what heart block rhythms mean for the patient	135
12. Recognize artificially paced rhythms on EKG tracings	142
13. Discuss possible complications with artificial pacemakers	143
14. Discuss ST segment changes and other signs of injury on the EKG tracing	145

Learning Objective	Page

10 Emergency Situations

1. Recognize emergency situations during cardiac testing	152
2. Discuss proper notification of supervisor and 911 in a medical emergency	153
3. Explain the care of a conscious patient experiencing a cardiac emergency	156
4. Demonstrate the care of an unconscious patient experiencing a cardiac emergency	156
5. Describe cardiopulmonary resuscitation (CPR) and defibrillation using an automated external defibrillator (AED)	158
6. Describe the care of a patient experiencing a stroke	159
7. Discuss drugs that may be used in a cardiac emergency	159
8. Describe response to nonmedical emergencies	160

Glossary 163

Index 175

Procedure	Page

Procedures

Washing hands (hand hygiene)	14
Putting on (donning) gloves	16
Removing (doffing) gloves	16
Donning a full set of PPE	17
Doffing a full set of PPE	17
Measuring and recording an oral temperature	20
Measuring and recording a temporal temperature	20
Counting and recording pulse by palpation	22
Counting and recording apical pulse by auscultation	23
Counting and recording radial pulse and counting and recording respirations	24
Measuring and recording blood pressure manually	25
Measuring and recording blood pressure electronically	26
Measuring and recording a pulse oximetry reading	28
Obtaining a 12-lead EKG	60
Applying a telemetry pack	61
Conducting an exercise stress test	64
Applying an ambulatory monitor	66

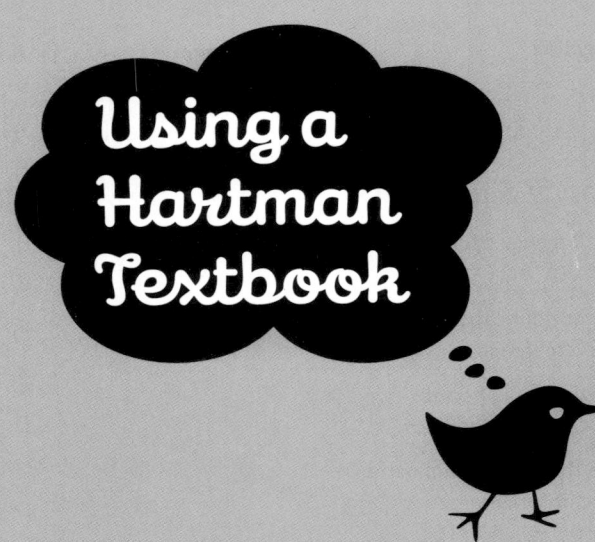

Using a Hartman Textbook

Understanding how this book is organized and what its special features are will help you make the most of this resource!

We have assigned each chapter its own colored tab. Each colored tab contains the chapter number and title, and is located on the side of every page.

1. Describe the role of the EKG technician and identify healthcare settings in which EKG technicians work

Everything in this book and the instructor's teaching material is organized around **learning objectives.** A learning objective is a very specific piece of knowledge or a very specific skill. After reading the text, you will know you have mastered the material if you can do what the learning objective says.

myocardial infarction

Bold key terms are located throughout the text, followed by their definitions. They are also listed in the glossary at the back of this book.

Obtaining a 12-lead EKG

All **care procedures** are highlighted by the same black bar for easy recognition.

Quick Reference

Quick Reference charts are a summary of the most vital information in this book.

Tip
Snooping is Illegal

Tip boxes contain extra information that will help you be an even better EKG technician.

Take Action Now!

Take Action Now! boxes will help you recognize situations that require an immediate response.

Chapter Review

Chapter-ending bulleted lists reinforce your knowledge of the information found in the chapter. If you have trouble recalling the material in the summary, you can return to the text and reread the material.

1

The Role of the EKG Technician

1. Describe the role of the EKG technician and identify healthcare settings in which EKG technicians work

Information from **electrocardiograms** (**EKGs**) plays an important part in the **diagnosis**, or determination of medical condition, and treatment of patients. The EKG, sometimes called *ECG*, is a quick, painless test that records the electrical activity of the heart. (Chapters 5 and 6 explain in more detail how this works.) Along with blood tests, physical examinations, X-rays, and other medical tests, doctors use the EKG to diagnose and treat conditions and diseases of the heart and circulatory system.

Cardiologists are doctors who specialize in the health of the heart. Cardiologists often use an EKG as their first tool of investigation. Pharmacists, nurses, paramedics, sports medicine professionals, and physical therapists also use this information to assess and treat patients based on the doctor's diagnosis.

Working with a team of medical professionals, the **EKG technician** performs or assists with EKG tests (Fig. 1-1). Different EKG tests are used to get specific kinds of information about the heart. Types of EKGs include 3-lead, 12-lead, ambulatory monitor (such as Holter), and stress tests. Chapter 5 describes each one in detail.

EKGs are performed in many different settings. An EKG may be ordered as part of a routine exam in an ambulatory care setting such as a doctor's office or primary care clinic (Fig. 1-2). **Ambulatory care** refers to any setting where medical care is given without the patient being admitted to a hospital. This is also called **outpatient treatment**.

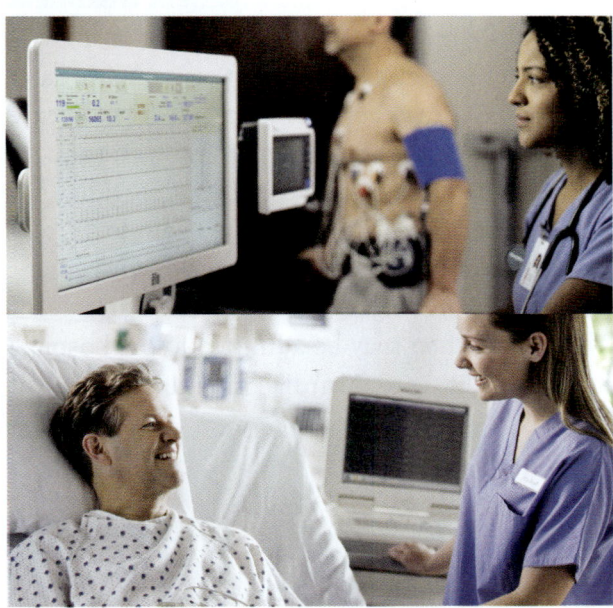

Fig. 1-1. *Depending on doctors' orders the EKG technician may conduct different tests on patients.* (TOP PHOTO: WELCH ALLYN™ IS A TRADEMARK OF HILL-ROM SERVICES, INC. © 2022 HILL-ROM SERVICES, INC. REPRINTED WITH PERMISSION - ALL RIGHTS RESERVED; BOTTOM PHOTO: COURTESY OF ROYAL PHILIPS)

The following are examples of ambulatory care facilities where EKGs might be conducted:

- Doctor's office
- Urgent care center
- Free-standing emergency department
- Occupational health clinic
- Primary care clinic

- Cardiology specialty clinic
- Outpatient surgery center
- Rehabilitation or physical therapy clinic

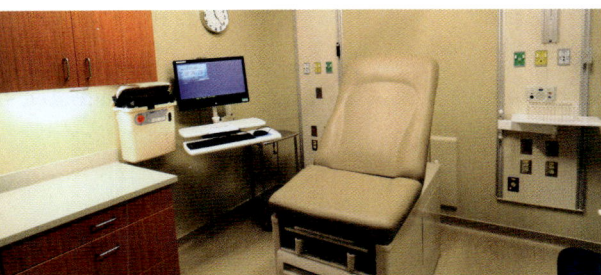

Fig. 1-2. EKGs are conducted in doctors' offices, urgent care centers, and other ambulatory care settings.

EKG technicians may also work in **acute care**, which refers to treatment given when the patient is admitted to the hospital. Acute care is included in the broad category called **inpatient treatment** (Fig. 1-3). In an acute care setting such as a hospital emergency department or intensive care unit, an EKG may be ordered to help a healthcare provider diagnose a **myocardial infarction (MI), or heart attack**, that requires emergency intervention. The patient may be taken to a hospital's cardiac catheterization lab, which is a special laboratory for diagnosing heart disease. The patient then may be admitted to the hospital for further EKGs and cardiac monitoring.

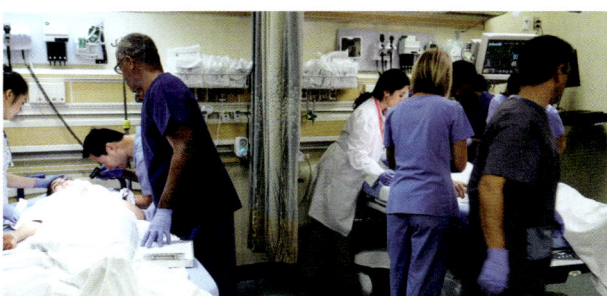

Fig. 1-3. Different types of care facilities might employ EKG technicians.

The following are examples of inpatient treatment facilities where EKGs might be ordered or conducted:

- Hospital
- Specialty hospital (for example, a hospital specializing in cardiac care)
- Long-term care facility
- Inpatient rehabilitation facility

A correct, readable copy of the EKG is essential to patient care. EKG technicians must make sure that EKG tracings are clear and accurate. The EKG technician must be able to perform several types of EKGs. She must explain the procedure to the patient in a calm, reassuring manner and answer any questions the patient may have. The EKG technician may also obtain vital signs and medical history before performing the EKG (Fig. 1-4). Healthcare facilities should have a detailed job description that includes the EKG technician's **scope of practice**. This outlines the duties she is expected and legally allowed to perform.

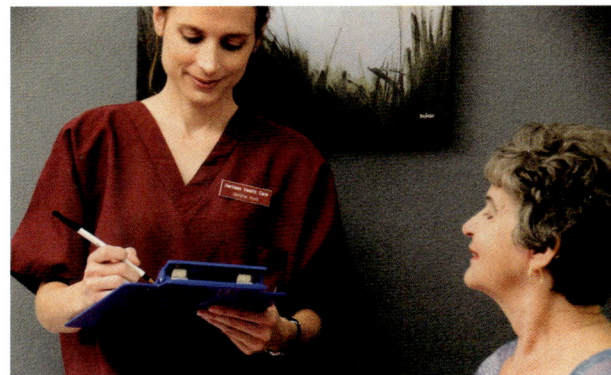

Fig. 1-4. EKG technicians may take or confirm a patient's medical history before conducting tests.

Tip

History-Taking

Healthcare workers may gather several different types of information about a patient during an appointment. Important information includes symptoms or issues the patient is experiencing and medications the patient takes. *Past medical history* includes any medical issues, concerns, or complications in the patient's past. A previous heart attack or a congenital heart defect are examples of past medical history. *Family history* includes any significant health problems in the patient's close relatives. Both of the patient's parents having had high blood pressure is an example of family history. *Social history* relates to behaviors that could affect the patient's health; smoking, drinking, and exercise habits are examples.

2. Identify soft skills and personal traits needed for success as an EKG technician

EKG technicians work with patients, family members, and other healthcare workers, sometimes under stressful conditions (Fig. 1-5). Often EKG technicians may receive on-the-job training for additional duties or attend school to gain additional credentials (such as a diploma, degree, or certificate) to advance their careers. Employers value certifications and other credentials, but they also consider personal traits when hiring and promoting employees.

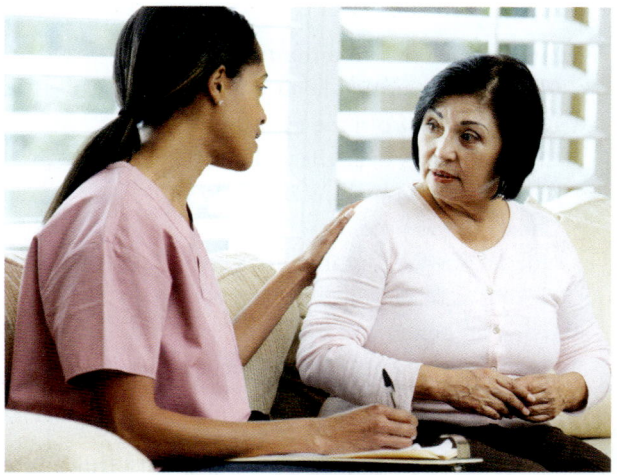

Fig. 1-5. Working well with patients and family members is an important part of an EKG technician's job.

The personal traits employers look for are often called **soft skills** (as opposed to **hard skills** such as measuring blood pressure). Soft skills are important in seeking and keeping an EKG technician job. Careful attention to these skills can help build a network of contacts and references. Soft skills may come naturally to some, but they often take practice. Many employers report that employees with good soft skills are harder to find than employees with good hard skills. Many firings are the direct result of poor soft skills.

The following soft skills are essential to an EKG technician's job:

Acceptance of constructive feedback: Constructive feedback (sometimes called *constructive criticism*) involves giving opinions about a person's work and making helpful suggestions for change. It is different from hostile criticism, which is angry, negative, and never appropriate in the workplace. An EKG technician should listen and respond to constructive feedback given by a coworker or supervisor. This feedback is intended to help her improve skills or grow professionally.

Care for personal appearance: EKG technicians should follow facility policy for dress and personal appearance. The policy may be quite detailed. It may address the color of scrubs, type of shoes, piercings and other jewelry, tattoos, use of nail polish, etc.

Regular grooming and proper hygiene are key to a professional appearance. These practices include daily baths or showers; regular dental care; clean, neat hairstyles; and clean, short nails. Clothing or scrubs should fit properly and be clean and free of stains and wrinkles (Fig. 1-6). Many facilities assign certain colors of scrubs to employees according to their jobs. Scrubs should be chosen based on quality rather than fashion. Makeup should be used in moderation. Most facilities do not allow the use of perfumes and colognes due to possible allergic reactions or sensitivities.

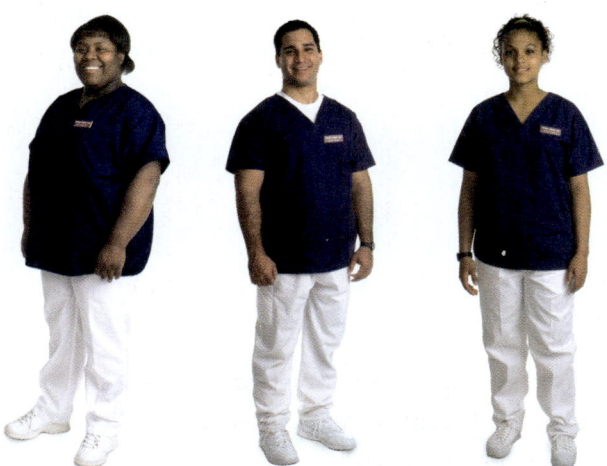

Fig. 1-6. Wearing a clean, wrinkle-free uniform, keeping long hair tied back, and wearing clean, closed-toe shoes are all parts of proper grooming.

Reliable attendance: Most employers have policies about attendance and arriving late. Being late or absent often is unprofessional and can even lead to job loss. Absences and late arrivals can affect patient care. Employees who are late or absent may delay medical care for patients or delay the departure of coworkers. This may cause an entire day or shift to run behind schedule. This creates stress that can reduce the quality of care provided.

Attention to detail: The ability to identify and focus on important information is essential. Always checking identification before treating a patient, for example, is very important. The EKG technician must also pay close attention when setting up testing and checking the finished EKG tracing to be sure it is clear and readable. Correctly noting, or documenting, all care provided is another detail-oriented task (Fig. 1-7).

Communication skills: EKG technicians must have excellent communication skills. They must be able to listen carefully. They have to relay information both orally and in writing. EKG technicians must be able to give instructions and information to patients in words they can understand, using a calm, reassuring manner. They must also be able to use the proper medical terminology when communicating information to the other care team members. Good communication skills helps EKG technicians avoid misunderstandings and errors.

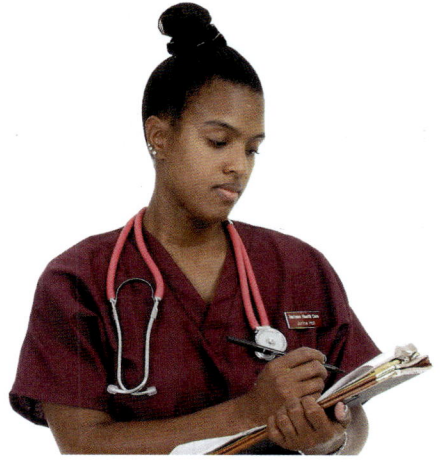

Fig. 1-7. Careful attention to detail is an essential skill for EKG technicians.

> **Tip**
>
> **Nonverbal Communication**
>
> Nonverbal communication such as body language can change the message that the EKG technician is trying to send. Here are some examples of positive and negative body language.
>
> **Positive Nonverbal Communication**
> - Standing up straight with arms relaxed
> - Leaning toward the speaker
> - Making eye contact
> - Nodding or smiling
> - Offering a handshake or greeting
> - Taking notes
> - Using a cheerful tone of voice
> - Smiling
>
> **Negative Nonverbal Communication**
> - Slouching or resting head in hands
> - Leaning back from the speaker
> - Crossing arms over chest
> - Avoiding eye contact, looking down
> - Checking the time
> - Not acknowledging the other person
> - Picking at or playing with something
> - Using an angry tone of voice
> - Frowning, wincing, rolling eyes

Acceptance of cultural diversity: A culture is a system of learned beliefs and behaviors that is practiced by a group of people. *Cultural diversity refers to different groups of people with varied backgrounds and experiences living together in the world.* The EKG technician may encounter patients and family members from different cultural groups, with different knowledge, behaviors, beliefs, values, attitudes, religions, and customs. Healthcare workers must provide culturally sensitive care. Practices that may differ from one culture to another include how close to stand, whether to touch another person during conversation, and whether to make eye contact. When a facility has many patients from a specific cultural group, management often provides training to the staff. Not being culturally sensitive may be seen as **prejudice** (an unfavorable opinion of a person or group of people based on race, religion, etc. that is without basis) and can result in legal action against the facility.

Compassion: Working with people in healthcare settings requires a genuine sense of concern for others, known as *compassion*. Compassion is often shown through nonverbal communication such as holding a patient's hand or gently touching his shoulder (Fig. 1-8). The EKG technician should consider the patient's cultural background before using touch. Some cultures find touch too personal for strangers. **Empathy**, or the ability to understand and share in the feelings of another person, is part of compassion. True empathy is nonjudgmental. It focuses on acceptance of the other person's feelings. **Sympathy**, the expression of concern for a person's feelings or situation, is another part of compassion.

Flexibility: Healthcare providers and insurers often look for ways to control costs. Employers value employees who are able to be flexible within their scope of practice. If there are no EKGs to be conducted at a given time, the technician might be asked to help with tasks such as scheduling patients, making follow-up calls, filing, or stocking supplies.

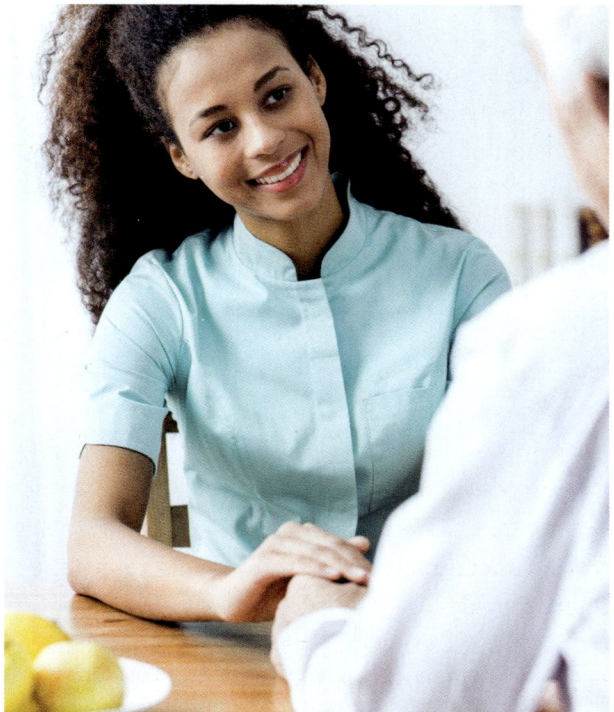

***Fig. 1-8.** Touch can communicate compassion.*

Initiative: Employees who can recognize and complete tasks that need to be done are showing *initiative*. There is likely always something to do in a healthcare setting. Stocking, straightening, and cleaning are just a few examples. Employers appreciate workers who are willing to seek out and perform work without waiting to be asked.

Integrity: *Integrity* is the quality of having strong moral principles and being honest. Patients and their families are often under extreme stress when they are in a healthcare facility. This stress, along with illness, may make them vulnerable, or more likely to be harmed in some way. Patients may also be vulnerable due to a physical or mental disability. Healthcare workers must always be honest and trustworthy when dealing with patients and family members. Some healthcare organizations have a **code of ethics** that employees must follow. This describes what is considered morally right or wrong behavior on the job. A person of integrity has his own internal code of ethics and lives by it.

Problem-solving ability: The EKG technician must be able to obtain clear, readable EKGs on a variety of patients. This is not always easy. It often requires the ability to identify and solve problems. Problem-solving skills may be needed when working with patients who need alternate electrode placement, patients with language barriers, or pediatric patients. The EKG technician must work with other members of the healthcare team to develop solutions to any challenges that arise (Fig. 1-9).

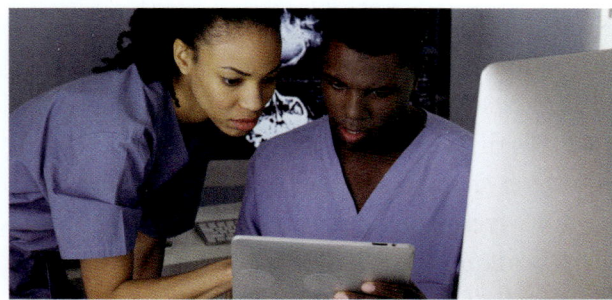

***Fig. 1-9.** EKG technicians are part of a team. Together with other healthcare workers, they can identify problems and find solutions.*

Timeliness: Both employers and patients appreciate a healthcare worker who promptly does his assigned tasks. This communicates respect for the employer's and the patient's time.

Tact: *Tact* is the ability to say something without causing offense. The first thing that comes to mind in a difficult situation is not always the most tactful thing to say. Patients and their families may not always be tactful, but the EKG technician must always respond tactfully. Carefully choosing words can help calm a tense situation.

Understanding of teamwork: Working with others with different personalities, backgrounds, or skills to achieve a desired outcome is called *teamwork*. Good team players can function in the role of team leader or team member. Teams function best when all members of the team, no matter their roles, strive to do their best.

3. Describe the certification process for the EKG technician

Many healthcare workers are required to have a certificate or license in the state where they practice. **Certification** is a process used in health care to show that skills are mastered for some positions. A school or organization offers a training program to meet certain standards in that healthcare field. The school, organization, or a state government agency may maintain a registry that can be checked by potential employers to verify certification.

Nursing assistants (NAs), patient care technicians (PCTs), and EKG technicians are examples of healthcare workers who may need to be certified. Certification laws vary from state to state. While no state currently requires certification for EKG technicians, many facilities require it. Certification is definitely an advantage when looking for a job.

Licensure is a legal process that must be completed to practice a medical profession in a state. It involves completing an approved course, passing an exam, and, in some cases, passing a skills test. Licensed practical nurses (LPNs), registered nurses (RNs), and doctors (MDs) are examples of licensed healthcare professionals.

Healthcare workers who are not licensed generally do their jobs under the authority of a licensed professional. A healthcare worker may lose certification if he is convicted of a crime, commits malpractice, or fails to complete required continuing education.

The National Healthcareer Association (nhanow.com) and the National Center for Competency Testing (ncctinc.com) are two organizations that certify EKG technicians. Community colleges and employers sometimes offer their own EKG technician certificates. In most cases, students must complete an approved training class before taking a certification test. Some organizations certify tehcnicians who do not take a course if they have on-the-job experience and pass the certification test.

Most EKG technician training programs include **clinical experience** to give students actual hands-on practice with patients. *Clinicals*, as this training is sometimes called, may be arranged by the instructor and take place under the supervision of healthcare professionals (Fig. 1-10). If it is not possible to do clinicals at a healthcare facility, the instructor may set up a lab area for volunteers to have EKGs performed.

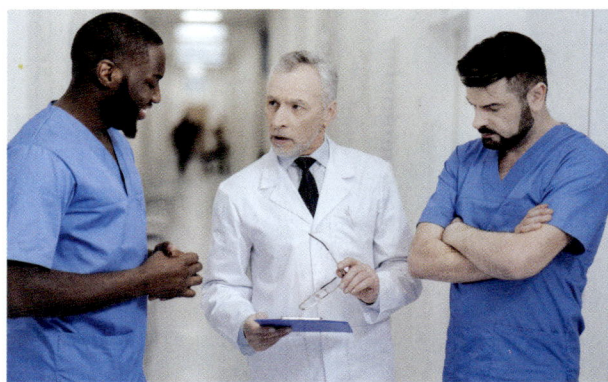

Fig. 1-10. EKG technicians in training may gain clinical experience at hospitals or other healthcare facilities.

An EKG technician student should check the certifying agency's website at the beginning of training and during training. The website has the latest information about testing requirements and fees, as well as study and review materials available for purchase. In most cases certification tests are computer-based and timed. Results are received immediately after testing is complete. The tests are given at special testing centers and must be scheduled in advance.

Tip

Researching Certification Agencies

In addition to the certification agencies listed in this book, other organizations offer EKG technician certification. Many of them are online. Since no federal guidelines address the training and certification of EKG technicians, it can be difficult to know which organizations offer a recognized certificate. Potential employers and EKG technician instructors can help with this issue. Before paying for a certification program, it is important to check that the agency is legitimate.

An EKG technician must receive a high school diploma before she can be certified. Most testing agencies award temporary certificates to high school students until they submit copies of their high school diplomas.

4. Describe the importance of continuing education and recertification

Every healthcare position requires continuing education to help keep employees up-to-date on changes in medicine that affect their jobs. Continuing education (also called *in-service education* or *continuing education units* [CEUs]) may also address new equipment procedures or an employer's policy changes. Continuing education may be required by state or federal guidelines, by the certifying agency, or by the employer. For EKG technicians, continuing education requirements are set by the certifying agency and the employer.

Most healthcare employers require **cardiopulmonary resuscitation (CPR)** certification for all employees who work with patients. The American Heart Association (AHA, heart.org) sets the standards for CPR instruction and certification. EKG technicians are usually required to maintain AHA Basic Life Support (BLS) certification, which must be renewed every two years. Many employers offer free courses to employees and will only accept CPR certifications from the American Heart Association (Fig. 1-11).

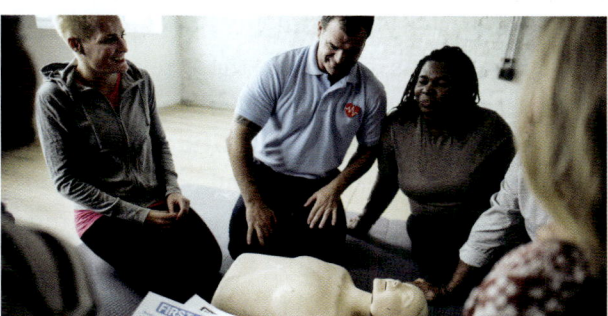

Fig. 1-11. *Employers may provide CPR training to EKG technicians at no cost.*

Most healthcare certifications require renewal every few years. This usually involves providing proof of active practice and continuing education and paying a fee. The EKG technician is responsible for meeting deadlines and completing requirements for renewal. This can be done by checking the certifying agency's website regularly for information. For example, the NHA currently requires 10 continuing education credits every two years. The requirement increases to 15 credits if the certification has lapsed for more than 30 days. The NHA offers activities that qualify as continuing education. Proof of completed training offered by an employer can also satisfy the requirement. Agencies charge a fee for renewal. The EKG technician is usually responsible for this fee, but some employers reimburse it.

5. Demonstrate proper communication with other members of the healthcare team

EKG technicians communicate regularly with many medical professionals, including doctors, nurses, physical therapists, and pharmacists.

They may also work with emergency responders such as emergency medical technicians or volunteer ambulance crews. Professional and accurate oral and written communication are critical since this information is used by the medical team to make treatment decisions. Poor communication can result in medical errors that may cause patient harm.

The EKG technician must be able to use correct abbreviations, medical terminology, and anatomical terms, especially those related to the cardiovascular system. The EKG technician may also be required to learn a specific medical computer program for documenting patient care in electronic health records (Fig. 1-12). Upcoming chapters cover this material in detail.

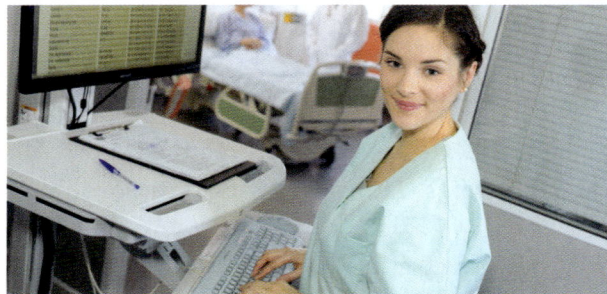

Fig. 1-12. *EKG technicians may need to learn specialized software to document patient care.*

Quick Reference
Common abbreviations for the EKG technician

AED	automated external defibrillator
bid	twice a day
BP	blood pressure
BSI	body substance isolation
CAD	coronary artery disease
CCU	cardiac care unit
CEU	continuing education unit
CHF	congestive heart failure
CNA	certified nursing assistant
COPD	chronic obstructive pulmonary disease
CPR	cardiopulmonary resuscitation
CVA	cerebrovascular accident (stroke)
DOB	date of birth
Dx	diagnosis
ECG, EKG	electrocardiogram
ED	emergency department
ER	emergency room
Hx	history
ICU	intensive care unit
K	potassium
LPN	licensed practical nurse
MD	doctor of medicine
MI	myocardial infarction
NP	nurse practitioner
NPO	nothing by mouth
NSR	normal sinus rhythm
O_2	oxygen
OR	operating room
PA	physician assistant
PCT	patient care technician
PRN	as needed
PT	physical therapist
$\bar{q}$	every
qd	once a day
qid	four times a day
R/O	rule out
RN	registered nurse
Rx	prescription
SA	sinoatrial
SOB	shortness of breath
SOBE	shortness of breath on exertion
Stat	immediately
tid	three times a day
TPR	temperature, pulse, respiration
VS	vital signs

6. Discuss the chain of command and understand the importance of following a facility's policies and procedures

Every medical facility has a **chain of command**. The chain of command shows the line of authority in a facility. It helps employees know who can assign work to them. It also shows the correct path for expressing concerns or needs. The chain of command protects employers and employees from liability. **Liability** is a legal term that means a person can be held responsible for his actions if he harms someone else.

Licensed healthcare professionals such as registered nurses usually direct the actions of EKG technicians. Next up the chain is the department director or unit supervisor, who reports to the clinic or medical director, or to the chief executive officer (CEO).

If an employee has a concern or complaint, it is important to document emails and meetings with supervisors. If the employee does not feel the issue was properly handled she can go to the next person up the chain of command (Fig. 1-13). The employee should remain professional at all times. Depending on the complaint, the human resources department might be able to assist with the problem. The chain of command is designed to help both the employee and the organization. It is a very effective tool when properly used.

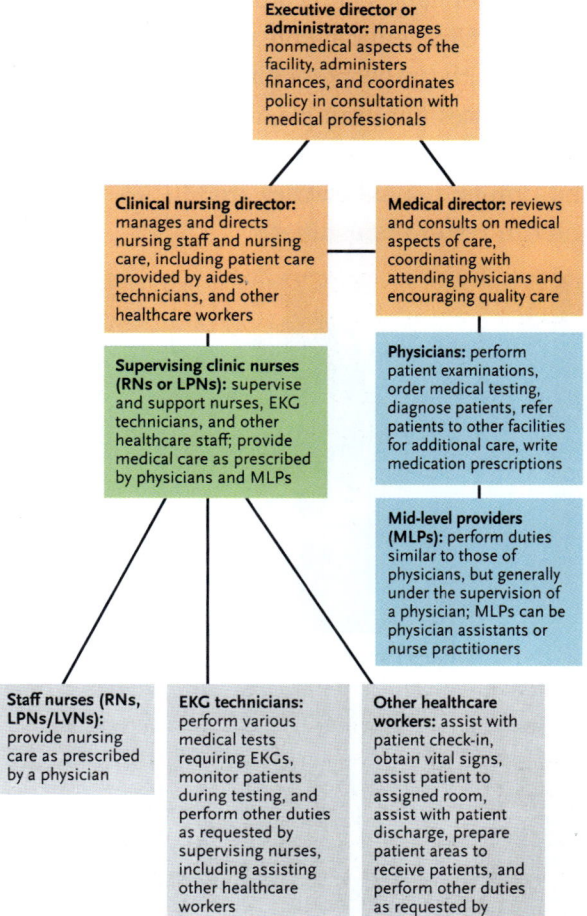

Fig. 1-13. *This is a simplified example of a facility chain of command. It is important for the EKG technician to understand her facility's specific chain of command.*

Each healthcare facility also has written **policies** and **procedures** that guide employees in their duties. A policy is a course of action that should be taken every time a certain situation occurs. A procedure is a set of steps used to do a task. Policies and procedures are regularly revised to reflect changes in law or advances in medical knowledge. New employee orientation typically includes an introduction to these documents and where they can be found. Policies and procedures may be kept in a book or binder in a central area, or they may be available online. Failure to follow policies and procedures can result in disciplinary action or job loss.

> **Tip**
>
> **Legal and Ethical Behavior**
> Part of behaving professionally at work is following the facility's policies and procedures. In addition, EKG technicians should always do their jobs in a way that is both *legal* and *ethical*. This means not breaking laws and not doing things that are dishonest, deceptive, or known to be morally wrong. Learning Objective 7, below, describes legal issues regarding patient **confidentiality**, or the legal and ethical principle of keeping information private.
>
> EKG technicians should understand what *slander* and *libel* are. Spoken untruths or defamatory (insulting) comments about a person are considered slander. When this type of comment is written, it is called libel. These are not crimes but are considered civil offenses. They can result in lawsuits. Healthcare workers who speak or write untrue comments are guilty of slander or libel. Such comments should never be documented in a patient's chart or spoken to coworkers, patients, or family members. This is unethical and healthcare workers can be taken to court for such actions.

7. Discuss outside organizations important to the function of healthcare facilities

Many organizations separate from employers and facilities may affect the actions of healthcare workers. Government agencies, insurance companies, and professional organizations influence or control various parts of patient care.

This affects the way workers are expected to do their jobs.

The federal government has created protections for healthcare information that affect healthcare workers. Congress passed the Health Insurance Portability and Accountability Act, also known as HIPAA, in 1996. HIPAA protects the confidentiality, or privacy, of a person's health information and includes strict guidelines for the handling and sharing of **protected health information** (**PHI**). HIPAA identifies 18 types of information considered to be PHI:

- Name
- Postal address
- All elements of dates associated with an individual (birth date, hospital admission date, etc.) except year
- Telephone number
- Fax number
- Email address
- URL (website) address
- IP address (a number that identifies a device connected to a computer network)
- Social security number
- Account numbers of any kind
- License or certificate numbers of any kind
- Medical records number
- Health plan beneficiary number
- Device identifiers and their serial numbers
- Vehicle identifiers such as license plate numbers and serial numbers
- Biometric identifiers (fingerprints, voiceprints, etc.)
- Full-face photos and other comparable images
- Any other unique identifying number, code, password, or characteristic

HIPAA also has serious penalties for misuse or mishandling of PHI. The penalties include civil (noncriminal) charges that may involve fines and criminal charges that may involve fines and/or jail time. Healthcare workers may also lose their certification or license if convicted of a HIPAA violation.

It is important for all members of the healthcare team to protect PHI at all times. Breaches of confidentiality can happen intentionally or unintentionally. Intentional breaches can happen when a healthcare worker shares medical information with another healthcare worker who is not involved in the care of the patient. Unintentional breaches can happen when healthcare records are left in unsecured locations, when workers do not properly log out of electronic health records, or when paper copies of records are not discarded properly. Unintentional breaches can also happen when healthcare workers discuss patient care in public places (for example, in the hospital cafeteria or in an elevator) (Fig. 1-14). Both intentional and unintentional breaches are HIPAA violations and can result in penalties.

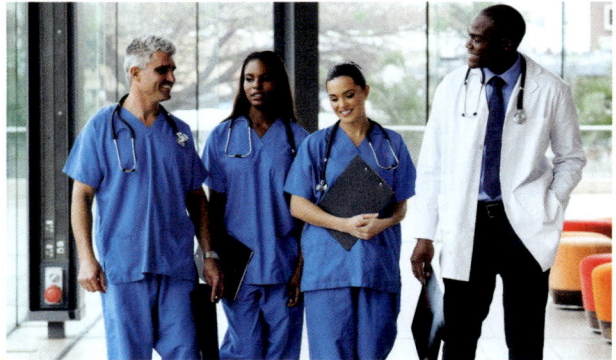

Fig. 1-14. Patient care should be discussed in private settings and not in lobbies or other areas open to the public.

Tip

Snooping Is Illegal

It is a HIPAA violation for an EKG technician to view a patient's medical record if she is not involved in that patient's care. Viewing medical records without a valid reason is called *snooping* and may result in

> disciplinary action. Most facilities also prohibit employees from accessing their own medical records. While this is not a HIPAA violation, this rule helps ensure that employees access their own records in the same way patients can access theirs.

Congress passed the Health Information Technology for Economic and Clinical Health (HI-TECH) Act in 2009. This requires healthcare facilities to convert to electronic health records (EHR) to more easily coordinate care among providers. This law also increased protections over PHI in electronic health records. Healthcare facilities protect electronic records by giving individual usernames and passwords to each employee. Computer systems can record information about who has logged on to the system and the files they opened. It is important that all healthcare professionals guard their usernames and passwords carefully. They will be held responsible for records accessed on their accounts. Healthcare professionals can also be penalized if they log in to view charts of patients whose care they are not directly involved in.

The Joint Commission (jointcommission.org) is a nonprofit organization that evaluates and accredits healthcare facilities. Evaluations are conducted every three years to assess the quality and safety of patient care. The Joint Commission offers accreditation to healthcare facilities on a voluntary basis. The accreditation process involves inspections, called *surveys*, by a team of healthcare professionals, called *surveyors*. The data collected is used for ongoing improvement of the facility. Information on accredited facilities is also shared with the public at qualitycheck.org.

The American Heart Association conducts research and sets the standards of treatment for Basic Life Support (BLS) and Advanced Cardiovascular Life Support (ACLS). Most healthcare providers require and pay for annual AHA training and certifications for employees based on their scope of practice (Learning Objective 4).

Chapter Review

- Electrocardiograms are important diagnostic tools, and EKG technicians play an important role in providing quality health care.

- EKG technicians may work in a variety of settings, including ambulatory or acute care facilities.

- Hard skills, such as measuring vital signs and conducting EKGs, are important, but soft skills, such as compassion and tact, are also very important.

- Working as an EKG technician requires training and continuing education. National organizations such as the National Healthcareer Association and the National Center for Competency Testing offer certification for EKG technicians.

- EKG technicians must understand and respect their facility's chain of command and their own scope of practice. This means they must only perform tasks they are trained and allowed to perform.

- In addition to individual organizations, various agencies control and influence how health care is provided and what healthcare workers do on the job. It is important for EKG technicians to understand the policies, procedures, and laws that apply to the work they do.

2

Basic Patient Care Skills

1. Explain the importance of monitoring vital signs

Vital signs give important information about a patient's cardiovascular system, especially the function of the heart. Vital signs are usually measured before patients are seen by a doctor or other healhcare provider. These measurements are considered the patient's **baseline** measurements. If the patient is having many tests, has a new complaint or a complaint that gets worse, or has a change in level of consciousness (for example, loses consciousness), vital signs may be measured again.

> **Tip**
>
> **Identification**
>
> An EKG technician should wear a name tag that shows her name and job title. Federal law requires that patients be informed of the identity and position of the healthcare workers who care for them. During any encounter with patients or family members, the EKG technician must follow facility rules about identification. The technician should also introduce herself and state her title before beginning any procedure.

Vital signs include body temperature, pulse rate, respiration rate, and blood pressure. Blood oxygen level (measured by pulse oximetry) and pain level may also be included in the initial assessment. Information gathered in this process is a combination of **objective information** (signs) and **subjective information** (symptoms). *Signs* are considered objective because they are measurements that can be verified by a medical professional. *Symptoms* are subjective because they are based on the personal experience or feelings of the patient.

> **Quick Reference**
>
> **Ranges for Adult Vital Signs**
>
> | Temp. Site | Fahrenheit | Celsius |
> |---|---|---|
> | Mouth (oral) | 97.6°–99.6° | 36.5°–37.5° |
> | Rectum (rectal) | 98.6°–100.6° | 37.0°–38.1° |
> | Armpit (axillary) | 96.6°–98.6° | 35.9°–37.0° |
> | Ear (tympanic) | 96.6°–99.7° | 35.9°–37.6° |
> | Temporal Artery (forehead) | 97.2°–100.1° | 36.2°–37.8° |
>
> **Normal Pulse Rate:** 60–100 beats per minute
> **Normal Respiratory Rate:** 12–20 respirations per minute
>
> **Blood Pressure Ranges**
>
> | | | |
> |---|---|---|
> | Normal | Systolic
Diastolic | 90–119 mm Hg *and*
60–79 mm Hg |
> | Low (hypotensive) | Systolic
Diastolic | Below 90 mm Hg *or*
Below 60 mm Hg |
> | Elevated | Systolic
Diastolic | 120–129 mm Hg *and*
less than 80 mm Hg |
> | Stage 1 hypertension | Systolic
Diastolic | 130–139 mm Hg *or*
80–89 mm Hg |
> | Stage 2 hypertension | Systolic
Diastolic | At or over 140 mm Hg *or*
At or over 90 mm Hg |
> | Hypertensive crisis | Systolic
Diastolic | Over 180 mm Hg *and/or*
Over 120 mm Hg |

2. Discuss the role of the EKG technician in infection prevention and control

A **microorganism** is a living thing that is so small it is only visible under a microscope. Microorganisms are always present in the environment. Infections occur when harmful microorganisms, called **pathogens**, invade the body and multiply. **Infection prevention**, also referred to as *infection control*, is the set of practices used to prevent the spread of harmful microorganisms and control the spread of disease. An EKG technician must understand how to protect against infection.

There are two main types of infections: localized and systemic. A localized infection is an infection that is limited to a specific location in the body. It has local symptoms, which means the symptoms are near the site of infection. For example, if a wound becomes infected, the area around it may become red, swollen, warm, and painful. A systemic infection affects the entire body. This type of infection travels through the bloodstream and is spread throughout the body. It causes general symptoms, such as fever, chills, or mental confusion.

A healthcare-associated infection (HAI), formerly called *nosocomial infection*, is an infection acquired in a healthcare setting during the delivery of medical care. It can be either localized or systemic. HAIs can be transmitted to a patient from healthcare workers or through equipment at the facility.

The chain of infection is a way of describing how disease is transmitted from one human being to another (Fig. 2-1). Definitions and examples of each of the six links in the chain of infection follow.

Link 1: The causative agent is a pathogenic microorganism that causes disease. Microorganisms are everywhere—on skin, in food, in the air, and in water. Causative agents include bacteria, viruses, fungi, and parasites.

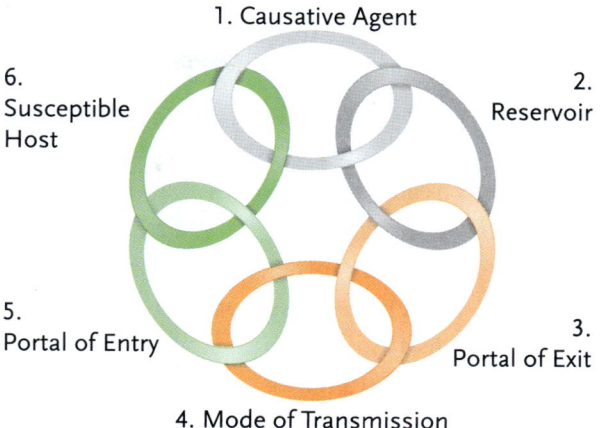

Fig. 2-1. *The chain of infection.*

Link 2: A reservoir is where the pathogen lives and multiplies. A reservoir can be a human, animal, plant, soil, or substance. Warm, dark, and moist places are the ideal environments for microorganisms to live, grow, and multiply. Some microorganisms need oxygen to survive, while others do not. Examples of reservoirs include the lungs, blood, and the large intestine.

Link 3: The portal of exit is any body opening on an infected person that allows pathogens to leave. These include the nose, mouth, eyes, or nonintact skin.

Link 4: The mode of transmission describes how the pathogen travels. Transmission can occur through the air or through direct or indirect contact. Direct contact happens by touching the infected person or his secretions. Indirect contact results from touching an object contaminated by the infected person, such as a needle, dressing, tissue, or bed linen. The primary route of disease transmission within the healthcare setting is via the hands of healthcare workers.

Link 5: The portal of entry is any body opening on an uninfected person that allows pathogens to enter. These include the nose, mouth, eyes, other mucous membranes, cuts in the skin, and cracked skin. Mucous membranes are the membranes that line body cavities that open to the outside of the body. These include the linings of the mouth, nose, eyes, rectum, and genitals.

Link 6: A susceptible host is an uninfected person who could become ill. Examples include all healthcare workers and anyone in their care who is not already infected with that particular disease. If one of the links in the chain of infection is broken, then the spread of infection is stopped. Infection prevention practices help stop pathogens from traveling (Link 4) and from getting on a person's hands, nose, eyes, mouth, skin, etc. (Link 5). Immunizations (Link 6) reduce a person's chances of getting sick from diseases such as hepatitis B and influenza.

Transmission (passage or transfer) of most infectious diseases can be blocked by using proper infection prevention practices, such as handwashing. Handwashing, also called **hand hygiene**, is the most important way to stop the spread of infection. All caregivers should wash their hands often.

Washing hands (hand hygiene)

Equipment: soap, paper towels

1. Turn on the water at the sink. Keep your clothes dry because moisture breeds bacteria. Do not let your clothing touch the outside portion of the sink or counter.

2. Wet your hands and wrists thoroughly (Fig. 2-2).

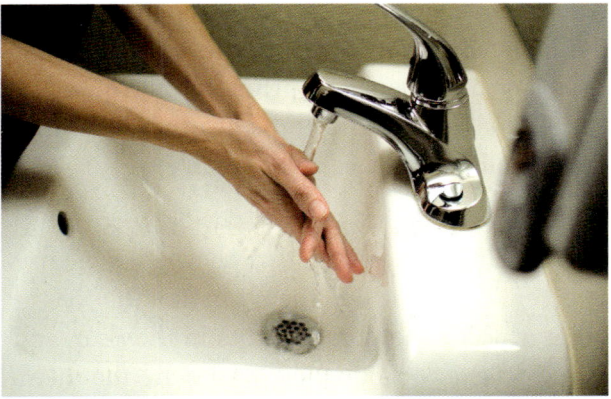

Fig. 2-2. *Keeping arms angled downward, wet hands and wrists thoroughly.*

3. Apply soap to your hands.

4. Keep your hands lower than your elbows and your fingertips down. Rub your hands together and fingers between each other to create a lather. Lather all surfaces of your wrists, fingers, and hands, using friction for at least 20 seconds. Friction helps clean (Fig. 2-3).

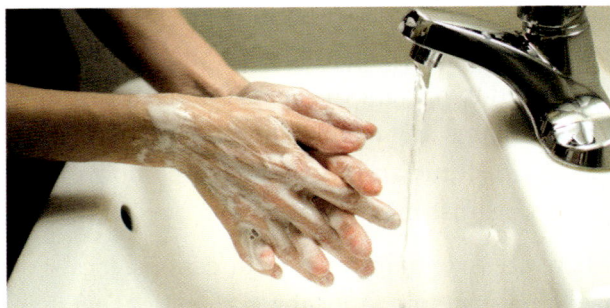

Fig. 2-3. *Using friction for at least 20 seconds, lather all surfaces of your wrists, fingers, and hands.*

5. Clean your fingernails by rubbing them in the palm of your other hand.

6. Keep your hands lower than your elbows and your fingertips down. Being careful not to touch the sink, rinse thoroughly under running water. Rinse all surfaces of your hands and wrists. Run water down from wrists to fingertips (Fig. 2-4). Do not run water over unwashed arms down to clean hands.

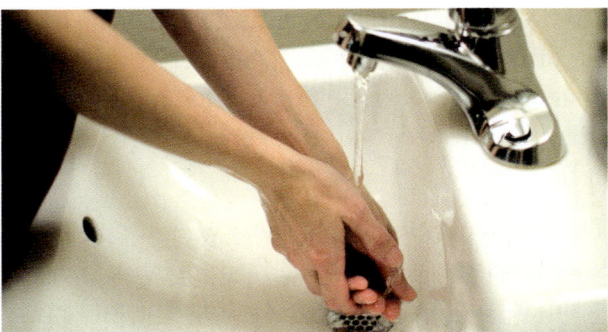

Fig. 2-4. *Rinse wrists and hands thoroughly without touching the sink. Let water run down from wrists to fingertips.*

7. Use a clean, dry paper towel to dry all surfaces of your fingers, hands, and wrists. Do not wipe the towel on unwashed forearms and then wipe your clean hands. Dispose

of the paper towel in the waste container without touching the container. If your hands touch the sink or wastebasket, start over.

8. Use a clean, dry paper towel to turn off the faucet (Fig. 2-5). Dispose of the paper towel in the waste container. Do not contaminate your hands by touching the surface of the sink or faucet.

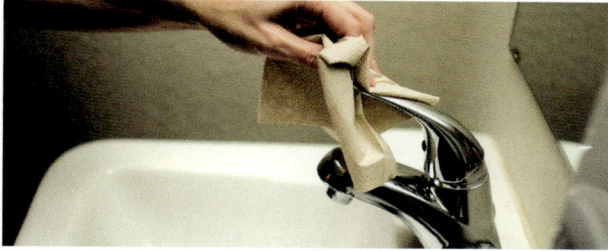

Fig. 2-5. Use a clean, dry paper towel to turn off the faucet so that you do not contaminate your hands.

Quick Reference
When to wash hands
- At the beginning of a shift
- Whenever hands are visibly soiled
- Before and after any patient contact
- After contact with any body fluids
- Before and after wearing personal protective equipment (PPE)
- Before and after eating or smoking
- Before and after using the toilet
- After touching garbage or trash
- Before and after applying makeup
- After any contact with pets
- At the end of a shift

Two key federal government agencies issue the infection prevention and safety regulations and recommendations used in developing the policies and procedures of healthcare facilities. The **Occupational Safety and Health Administration** (**OSHA**, osha.gov) sets standards to protect workers, provides safety education, inspects worksites, investigates workplace accidents, and sets fines for safety violations. The **Centers for Disease Control and Prevention** (**CDC**, cdc.gov) conducts research, promotes public health, investigates disease outbreaks, and makes recommendations for infection prevention and control.

The CDC's infection prevention recommendations include two levels: **Standard Precautions** and **Transmission-Based Precautions**. Standard Precautions are used with every patient for every interaction. These precautions treat all blood, body fluids, nonintact skin, and mucous membranes as if they were infected. *Mucous membranes* include the linings of the mouth, nose, eyes, rectum, and genitals. Often there are no visible signs or symptoms when a patient has a communicable disease (an illness that can be passed from person to person). An EKG technician should never assume a patient is healthy.

Standard Precautions and Transmission-Based Precautions are ways to stop the spread of infection by interrupting the mode of transmission. In other words, these guidelines do not stop an infected person from spreading pathogens. However, by following these guidelines, the EKG technician helps prevent those pathogens from infecting her or her patients.

Guidelines: Standard Precautions

G **Wash your hands** before putting on gloves. Wash your hands immediately after removing your gloves. Be careful not to touch clean objects with your used gloves.

G **Wear gloves** if you may come into contact with blood; body fluids or secretions; broken or open skin, such as abrasions, acne, cuts, stitches, or staples; or mucous membranes.

G **Remove gloves** immediately when finished with a procedure and wash or sanitize your hands using an alcohol-based hand rub.

G **Immediately wash all skin surfaces that have been contaminated** with blood and body fluids.

G **Wear a disposable gown** that is resistant to body fluids if you may come into contact with blood, body fluids, secretions, or excretions, or when splashing or spraying of blood or body fluids is likely. If a patient has a contagious illness, wear a gown even if it is not likely you will come into contact with blood or body fluids. Follow policy regarding gown use.

G **Wear a mask and protective goggles and/or a face shield** if you may come into contact with blood, body fluids, secretions, or excretions, or when splashing or spraying of blood or body fluids is likely. A mask and face shield may also be required as a precaution against some illnesses (such as COVID-19).

Standard Precautions require the use of gloves whenever contact with body fluids or nonintact skin is possible. Gloves, along with gowns, masks, goggles, and face shields are part of **personal protective equipment (PPE).**

Putting on (donning) gloves

1. Wash your hands.

2. If you are right-handed, slide one glove on your left hand (reverse if left-handed).

3. Using your gloved hand, slide the other hand into the second glove.

4. Interlace your fingers to smooth out folds and create a comfortable fit.

5. Carefully look for tears, holes, or discolored spots. Replace the glove if needed.

6. Adjust your gloves until they are pulled up over your wrist and fit correctly. If wearing a gown, pull the cuffs of the gloves over the sleeves of the gown (Fig. 2-6).

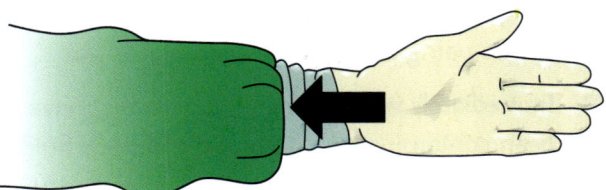

Fig. 2-6. Adjust gloves until they are pulled up over the sleeves of the gown, if a gown is worn.

Removing (doffing) gloves

1. Touch only the outside of one glove. With one gloved hand, grasp the other glove at the palm and pull the glove off (Fig. 2-7).

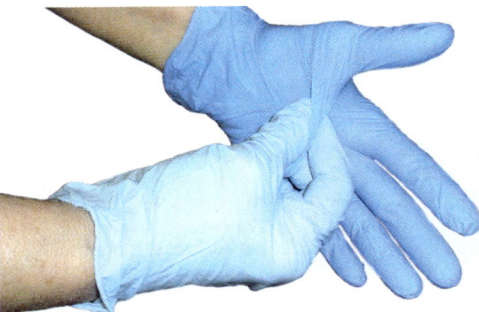

Fig. 2-7. Grasp the glove at the palm and pull it off.

2. With the fingertips of your gloved hand, hold the glove you just removed. With your ungloved hand, slip two fingers underneath the cuff of the remaining glove at the wrist. Do not touch any part of the outside of the glove (Fig. 2-8).

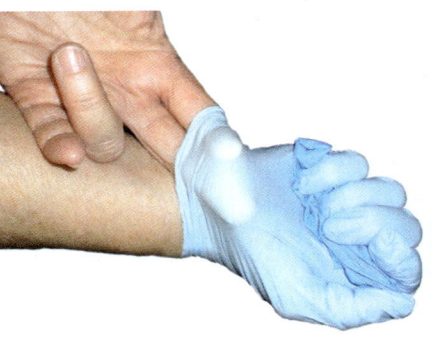

Fig. 2-8. Reach inside the glove at the wrist, without touching any part of the outside of the glove.

3. Pull down, turning this glove inside out and over the first glove as you remove it.

4. You should now be holding one glove from its clean inner side and the other glove should be inside it.

5. Drop both gloves into the proper container without contaminating yourself.

6. Wash your hands.

Standard Precautions also require a gown, mask, and goggles if exposure to blood or body fluids may occur. PPE should be removed properly to avoid contaminating the healthcare worker.

The EKG technician may need to don a full set of PPE when working with certain patients in acute care settings. This helps protect the technician and others from the spread of illness. It may also be necessary when a patient has a chest injury that could expose the technician to blood.

Donning a full set of PPE

1. Wash your hands.
2. Put on your gown.
3. Put on your mask.
4. Put on your goggles or face shield.
5. Put on your gloves.

Most PPE is removed and discarded before exiting a patient's room. Masks are an exception. During times of high virus transmission, masks may be worn at all times in a facility. Special masks called respirators are always removed after leaving the room and closing the door.

Doffing a full set of PPE

1. Remove and discard your gloves.
2. Remove and discard your goggles and faceshield.
3. Remove and discard your gown.
4. Remove and discard your mask.
5. Wash your hands. Washing hands is always the final step after removing and disposing of PPE.

The next level of infection prevention beyond Standard Precautions is Transmission-Based Precautions. There are three categories of Transmission-Based Precautions:

- Airborne Precautions
- Droplet Precautions
- Contact Precautions

The use of these precautions is based on the illness the patient has and how it is spread to others. The precautions may be used separately or in combination, but they are always used *in addition to* Standard Precautions. Some facilities use the word *isolation* to refer to a patient who is under Transmission-Based Precautions.

Airborne Precautions are used for patients with diseases or suspected diseases that are spread through the air after a person coughs or sneezes. These very small pathogens attach to particles in the air and can remain floating for some time. Precautions include wearing special masks, such as N95 or HEPA respirators, to avoid being infected. Federal regulations require that healthcare facilities have policies for the use of respirators. They must address medical evaluation, training, and fit testing.

No respiratory protection can filter out all pathogens, and respiration is not the only way to be exposed to airborne pathogens. This is why it is very important to follow Standard Precautions as well. Handwashing should be done before and after donning a respirator. Facilities have specific guidelines for working with patients under Airborne Precautions (Fig. 2-9). Common airborne diseases include tuberculosis, measles, COVID-19, and chickenpox.

Droplet Precautions are used for patients with diseases or suspected diseases that are spread by droplets when a person coughs, sneezes, or is suctioned. (*Suctioning* is a process that removes mucus and secretions from the lungs.) Unlike airborne pathogens, droplet-carried pathogens do not travel more than 6 feet. A regular face mask is used to care for patients under Droplet Precautions. Handwashing should be performed before and after donning a mask. A patient under Droplet Precautions should be given a mask if she is being moved from room to room.

Influenza (flu) is an example of a disease that is spread by droplets (Fig. 2-10).

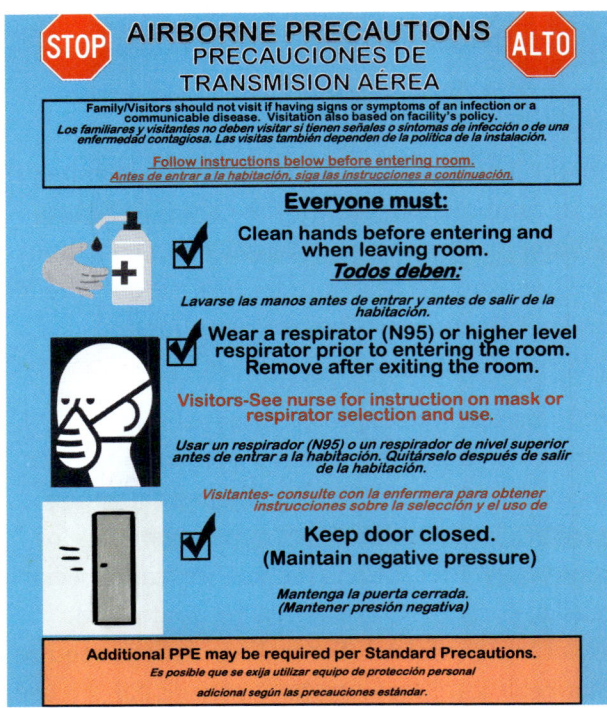

Fig. 2-9. Infection prevention guidelines will often be posted on the door for patients under Transmission-Based Precautions. (IMAGE COURTESY OF THE NORTH CAROLINA STATEWIDE PROGRAM FOR INFECTION CONTROL AND EPIDEMIOLOGY (SPICE), UNC, CHAPEL HILL, SPICE.UNC.EDU.)

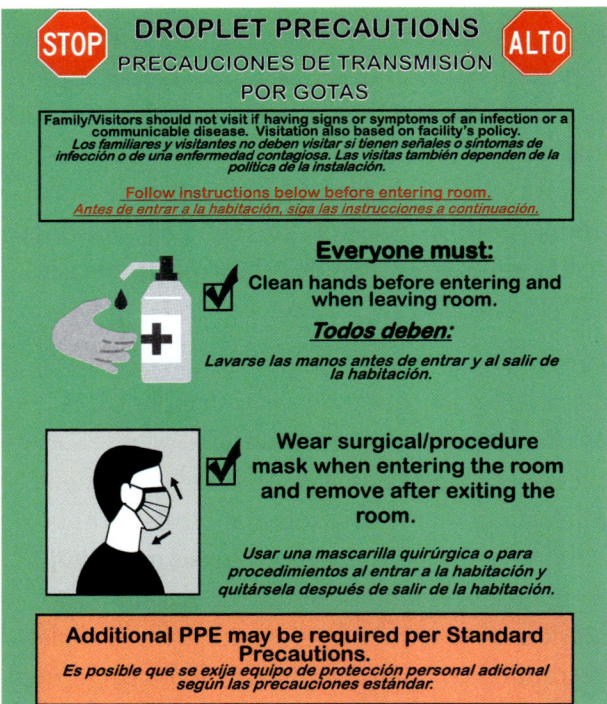

Fig. 2-10. Droplet Precautions may be in place for some patients with diseases such as influenza. (IMAGE COURTESY OF THE NORTH CAROLINA STATEWIDE PROGRAM FOR INFECTION CONTROL AND EPIDEMIOLOGY (SPICE), UNC, CHAPEL HILL, SPICE.UNC.EDU.)

Contact Precautions are used for patients with diseases or suspected diseases that are spread by touch. This includes touching an infected person or touching a contaminated object (an object touched by an infected person). A healthcare worker is at risk for these diseases any time she has skin-to-skin contact with an infected patient. For these precautions, the EKG technician should use a gown, gloves, mask, and eye protection when measuring vital signs and conducting tests (Fig. 2-11). Examples of diseases spread by contact include **methicillin-resistant *Staphylococcus aureus* (MRSA)**, conjunctivitis (pink eye), and *Clostridium difficile* (often called *C. diff*). These illnesses can spread quickly and can be hard to control.

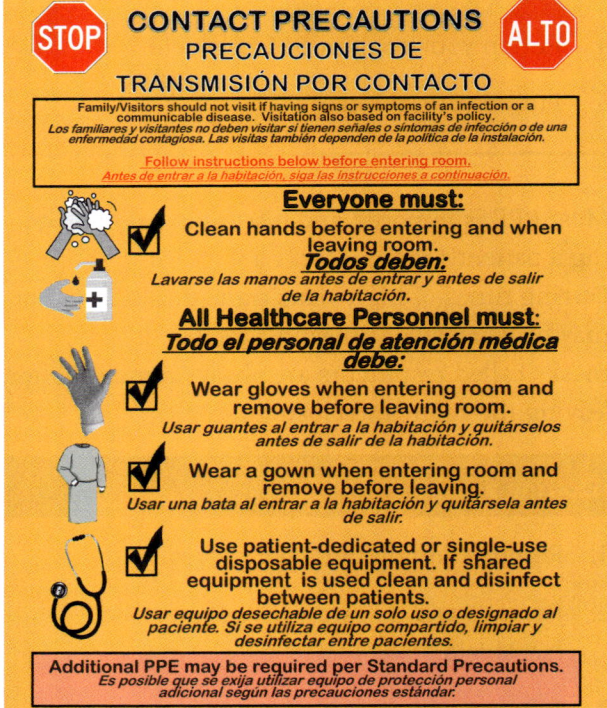

Fig. 2-11. Contact Precautions can help prevent the spread of very dangerous illnesses that can be transmitted by touch. (IMAGE COURTESY OF THE NORTH CAROLINA STATEWIDE PROGRAM FOR INFECTION CONTROL AND EPIDEMIOLOGY (SPICE), UNC, CHAPEL HILL, SPICE.UNC.EDU.)

The EKG technician should also be familiar with OSHA's Bloodborne Pathogens Standard. This standard requires employers to protect healthcare workers from exposure to bloodborne hazards. Bloodborne pathogens are infectious microorganisms found in the blood that can cause infection and disease. Blood that cannot be seen may be present in body fluids or secretions even though the patient appears healthy. Human immunodeficiency virus (HIV) and hepatitis are bloodborne diseases. OSHA bloodborne pathogens requirements for employers include the following:

- A written exposure control plan
- Readily available personal protective equipment in proper sizes
- Biohazard disposal containers
- Free hepatitis B vaccination
- Ongoing training

Employers must also maintain a log of contaminated sharps injuries. *Sharps* are needles and other sharp objects. Healthcare workers should immediately report injuries. They must undergo testing and follow-up care as directed in the exposure control plan.

General infection prevention guidelines that apply to all patients include the following:

- Don any necessary PPE outside a patient's room and remove it before exiting the patient's room (leaving a mask or respirator on as required).
- Never reuse disposable equipment or share it among patients.
- Clean and disinfect reusable (nondisposable) equipment after use. Follow the manufacturer's instructions and facility policy. Failure to do so could result in equipment not working properly or patient contamination.
- Never place patient equipment on contaminated surfaces, such as a chair or a counter that has not been disinfected.
- Be familiar with the types of available PPE.
- Follow directions listed on any signs on the patient's door.

> **Tip**
>
> **Compassion and Infection Prevention**
> Treat patients with dignity and respect while using infection prevention precautions. Patients with Transmission-Based Precautions in place may feel isolated. It is important to be compassionate when working with them.

3. List guidelines for measuring body temperature and observing skin condition

Body temperature is normally very close to 98.6 degrees Fahrenheit (F) or 37 degrees Celsius (C). Body temperature reflects a balance between heat created by the body and heat lost to the environment. Temperature varies throughout the day and can be affected by age, illness, exercise, and the environment.

Different thermometers are used to measure body temperature at different sites (Fig. 2-12). Which site is used will depend on the patient's age and condition, and on the facility's policy. Each site can result in a slightly different reading.

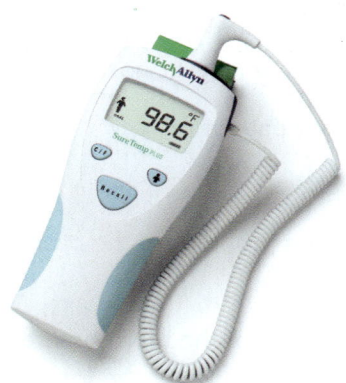

Fig. 2-12. *An electronic thermometer.* (WELCH ALLYN™ IS A TRADEMARK OF HILL-ROM SERVICES, INC. © 2022 HILL-ROM SERVICES, INC. REPRINTED WITH PERMISSION - ALL RIGHTS RESERVED;)

In medical settings, electronic (oral) and temporal (forehead-scanning) thermometers are most commonly used. Oral temperatures may not be accurate if the patient has eaten, smoked, drunk fluids, chewed gum, or exercised within the last 10–20 minutes.

NOTE: Patient care procedures in this textbook all begin with "Identify yourself by name. Identify the patient according to facility policy." In many settings, healthcare workers must state their titles when introducing themselves. Patients are usually asked to state their full name and date of birth. EKG technicians must always follow facility policy for identifying themselves and patients. The *provider* mentioned in closing steps is the healthcare professional the EKG technician reports to.

Measuring and recording an oral temperature

Equipment: electronic thermometer, gloves, disposable sheath/cover for thermometer, tissues, pen and paper

Do not take an oral temperature if the patient has smoked, eaten, drunk fluids, chewed gum, or exercised in the last 10–20 minutes.

1. Identify yourself by name. Identify the patient according to facility policy.
2. Wash your hands.
3. Explain the procedure to the patient. Speak clearly, slowly, and directly. Maintain face-to-face contact whenever possible.
4. Provide for patient privacy.
5. Put on gloves.
6. Remove the probe from the base unit. Put on the probe cover.
7. Insert the end of the thermometer into the patient's mouth, under the tongue and to one side.
8. Tell the patient to hold the thermometer in her mouth with her lips closed. Assist as necessary. The patient should breathe through her nose. Ask the patient not to bite down or talk. Leave in place until you hear a tone or see a flashing or steady light.
9. Read the temperature on the display screen. Remember the temperature reading. Remove the probe.
10. Press the eject button to discard the cover. Return the probe to the holder.
11. Remove and discard your gloves. Wash your hands.
12. Immediately record the temperature, date, time, and method used (oral).
13. Report any changes in the patient to the provider.

Measuring and recording a temporal temperature

Equipment: temporal thermometer, gloves, pen and paper

1. Identify yourself by name. Identify the patient according to facility policy.
2. Wash your hands.
3. Explain the procedure to the patient. Speak clearly, slowly, and directly. Maintain face-to-face contact whenever possible.
4. Provide for patient privacy.
5. Put on gloves.
6. Remove the cover from the end of the thermometer.
7. Press and hold the button on the thermometer while you slide the thermometer straight across the forehead parallel to the eyebrows, halfway between the hairline and the eyebrows.
8. Observe for the beep and/or flashing light. This means that the thermometer has registered a temperature.
9. Release the button and read the display. Remember the temperature reading.
10. Remove and discard your gloves. Wash your hands.
11. Immediately record the temperature, date, time, and method used (temporal).

12. Report any changes in the patient to the provider.

> **Tip**
>
> **Temperatures at Different Sites**
>
> Normal temperature range varies for each temperature site. The normal reading for oral temperature measurement is 97.7°F–99°F (36.5°C–37.2°C). Temporal and tympanic readings will be slightly higher, while axillary readings will be lower. A rectal thermometer provides the most accurate measurement. EKG technicians will typically use oral and temporal thermometers.

The look and feel of a patient's skin may indicate a medical concern. As an EKG technician measures a patient's temperature, she can also observe the skin. Normally skin is warm and dry. The areas inside the mouth and nose are pink. Abnormalities in temperature and skin condition should be reported to the nurse or healthcare provider immediately.

Quick Reference

Skin Variations

Skin abnormality	Description	Significance
Hot and dry	Skin is hot to the touch, and the patient is not sweating.	May indicate fever or heat-related emergency. Patient needs to be cooled immediately.
Diaphoresis	Excessive sweating; skin may feel cool (also called clammy)	Patient may have fever, be in severe pain, or be in an environment that is too hot. Diaphoresis can also be a sign of myocardial infarction (heart attack).
Cyanosis	Blue color of nail beds, around mouth, inside nose or mouth	Patient has decreased oxygen in the blood.
Pallor (pale skin)	Skin is lighter than normal for the patient's natural skin tone. Assess nail beds and lining of mouth and nose in patients with dark complexions.	Patient has decreased circulation.
Flushing (redness)	Skin is red.	Patient may have fever, be in severe pain, or be in an environment that is too hot.

4. Define *pulse* and list guidelines for counting pulse

Pulse is the beat that is felt at different points in the body called pulse points (Fig. 2-13). Pulse is generated when the heart contracts and pumps blood through the arteries. Pulse rate is the number of heartbeats per minute and can be measured by **palpation** (feeling with the fingers) or **auscultation** (listening with a stethoscope).

Pulse rate can be checked at different places on the body. The most common pulse point that is checked is the **radial pulse** at the inside of the wrist, where the radial artery runs just beneath the skin. Other common pulse points are the **carotid pulse** on the side of the neck and the **brachial pulse** on the inside of the upper arm above the elbow.

> **Tip**
>
> **Pulse Points**
>
> In nonemergency settings the radial pulse is most commonly used to check an adult's or child's heart rate. Because the radial pulse may be difficult to find if the patient's blood pressure is low (due to blood loss, for instance), the carotid pulse is checked first in emergency situations. It can be difficult to find some pulse points on an infant. The best pulse point for counting an infant's heart rate by palpation is the brachial artery, on the inside of the upper arm. This pulse point is close to the skin and easy to find.

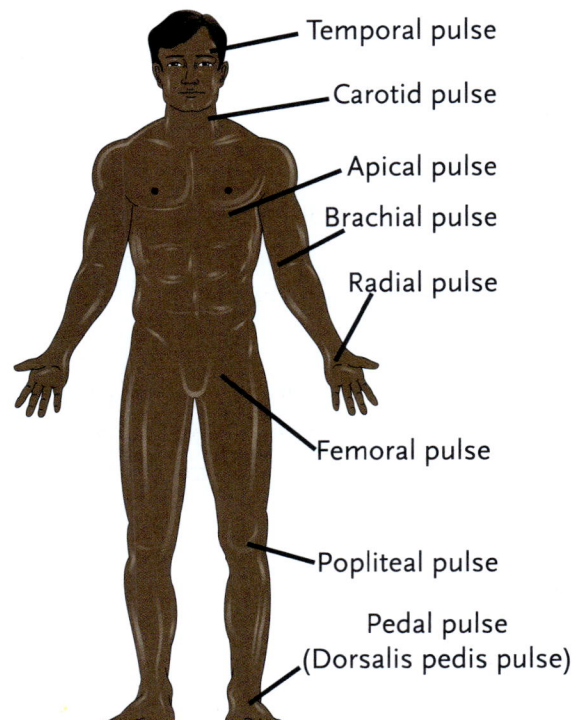

Fig. 2-13. *Common pulse points.*

A patient's pulse should be easy to feel (easily palpable) and should be regular. A normal adult pulse rate is 60–100 beats per minute (BPM). A rate of less than 60 BPM may be normal in an athlete. Slow rates may also indicate a heart problem (Chapters 4 and 9 contain more information about heart conditions and related heart rhythms). Heart rates over 100 BPM can indicate dehydration, blood loss, stress, or fever. Very rapid heart rates (over 130–140 BPM) may result from cardiac muscle disease and can be fatal if not treated promptly. The faster the heart rate, the less blood gets into the coronary arteries that supply the heart muscle. (Chapter 10 details actions necessary in an emergency situation like this.)

Using a stethoscope to listen to the heartbeat is called *auscultation*. The stethoscope is placed on the left side of the chest, below and to the left of the nipple, between the fifth and sixth ribs (Fig. 2-14). This location is called the *fifth intercostal space in the left midclavicular line*. (More information on medical terms for the body—called *anatomical terms*—will be given in Chapter 3.) Pulse is easily auscultated here because the **apex**, or tip, of the heart lies under this area. This is called the **apical pulse**. When measured at the same time, the palpated and auscultated pulse rates should be equal and regular. A difference of more than 8–10 beats per minute should be reported immediately.

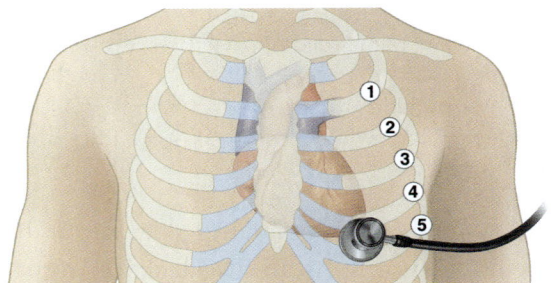

Fig. 2-14. *Proper placement of the stethoscope for counting apical pulse.*

Counting and recording pulse by palpation

Equipment: watch with a second hand or readout for seconds, pen and paper

1. Identify yourself by name. Identify the patient according to facility policy.

2. Wash your hands.

3. Explain the procedure to the patient. Speak clearly, slowly, and directly. Maintain face-to-face contact whenever possible.

4. Provide for patient privacy.

5. Locate the pulse at the pulse point you will be using. For the radial pulse, place the tips of your index finger and middle finger on the thumb side of the patient's wrist. If the patient is an infant, palpate the brachial pulse on the inside of the upper arm.

6. Using your watch, count the beats for 1 full minute.

7. Wash your hands.

8. Immediately record the pulse rate, including the site where the reading was taken and any irregularity, according to facility policy.

9. Report to the provider if the pulse is less than 60 beats per minute, over 100 beats per minute, or if the rhythm is irregular.

Counting and recording apical pulse by auscultation

Equipment: stethoscope, watch with second hand or readout for seconds, alcohol wipes, pen and paper

1. Identify yourself by name. Identify the patient according to facility policy.

2. Wash your hands.

3. Explain the procedure to the patient. Speak clearly, slowly, and directly. Maintain face-to-face contact whenever possible.

4. Provide for patient privacy.

5. Before using the stethoscope, wipe the diaphragm (the part that touches the patient's chest) and earpieces with alcohol wipes.

6. Locate the pulse at the pulse point you will be using (apical).

7. Put on the stethoscope and place the diaphragm at the patient's left fifth intercostal space in the midclavicular line (on the left side of the chest, just below the nipple). Listen for the heartbeat (Fig. 2-15).

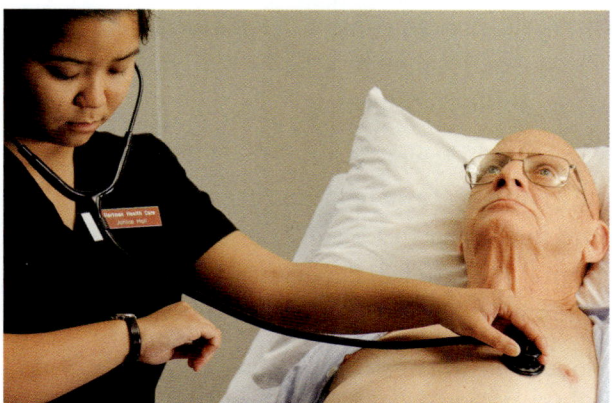

Fig. 2-15. Count the heartbeats for one full minute to measure the apical pulse.

8. Using your watch, count the beats for 1 full minute. Each *lubdub* that you hear is counted as one beat.

9. Wash your hands.

10. Immediately record the pulse rate, including the site where the reading was taken (apical) and any irregularity, according to facility policy.

11. Report to the provider if the pulse is less than 60 beats per minute, over 100 beats per minute, or if the rhythm is irregular.

The normal pulse rate for an adult is 60–100 beats per minute. The pulse should be regular and easily palpated or auscultated. Vital signs can be considerably different for children. Learning Objective 7 contains information on normal ranges for pediatric patients.

5. Define *respirations* and list guidelines for counting respirations *watching for respiration for min.*

Respiration is the process of inhaling air into the lungs and exhaling air out of the lungs. One inhalation and one exhalation together are counted as one respiration. Respiration should be unlabored and quiet. A person who requires effort to breathe, uses the neck and chest muscles to inhale, and makes noises with each breath has *labored breathing*. Labored breathing or any other abnormal breathing should be reported to the nurse or provider immediately.

The following terms describe abnormal respirations:

- **Apnea**: the absence of breathing
- **Dyspnea**: difficulty breathing
- **Orthopnea**: difficulty breathing when lying down, which may be relieved by sitting up
- **Tachypnea**: rapid breathing

- **Cheyne-Stokes**: alternating periods of slow, irregular breathing and rapid, shallow breathing, along with short periods of apnea

Many medical professionals recommend counting the pulse and then counting respirations without letting go of the patient's wrist or removing the stethoscope from the patient's chest. People may breathe more quickly when they are aware of being observed. Counting respirations immediately after counting the pulse rate may provide more accurate results.

Counting and recording radial pulse and counting and recording respirations

Equipment: stethoscope (if measuring pulse by auscultation), watch with second hand or readout for seconds, alcohol wipes, pen and paper

1. Identify yourself by name. Identify the patient according to facility policy.
2. Wash your hands.
3. Explain the procedure to the patient. Speak clearly, slowly, and directly. Maintain face-to-face contact whenever possible.
4. Provide for patient privacy.
5. Locate the pulse at the pulse point you are using.
6. Using your watch, count the beats for 1 full minute.
7. While keeping your fingertips on the wrist or the stethoscope on the chest, count the patient's respirations for 1 full minute by observing the rise and fall of his chest (Fig. 2-16).
8. Wash your hands.
9. Immediately record the pulse and respiratory rates, including the site where the pulse was taken and any irregularity, according to facility policy.

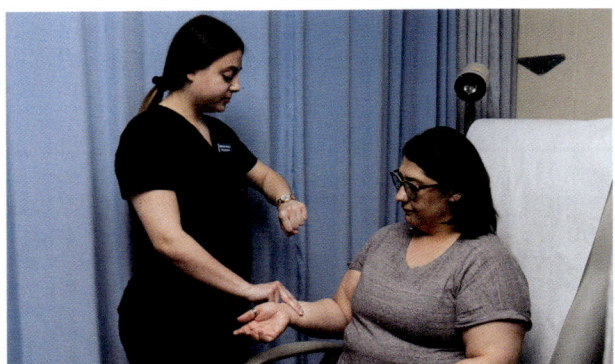

Fig. 2-16. *Count the respiratory rate directly after counting the radial pulse rate. Do not make it obvious that you are watching the patient's breathing.*

10. Report to the provider if the pulse or respiratory rate is abnormal or significantly different from a previous reading.

6. Define *blood pressure* and list guidelines for measuring blood pressure

Blood pressure is an important indicator of how the heart is working and should be checked regularly. High blood pressure (**hypertension**) often occurs without noticeable symptoms. Blood pressure is measured in millimeters of mercury (mm Hg) and is recorded as a fraction, for example, 110/70.

The top, larger number is the systolic reading. The **systolic** reading measures the pressure on the walls of the arteries when the ventricles are contracting and pushing blood from the heart. The normal range for systolic blood pressure for adults is 90–119 mm Hg.

The bottom, lower number is the diastolic reading. The **diastolic** reading measures the pressure in the arteries when the heart is at rest. The normal range for diastolic blood pressure for adults is 60–79 mm Hg.

Blood pressure can be measured manually or electronically using a **sphygmomanometer**. An aneroid sphygmomanometer is a manual device that requires the use of a stethoscope to determine the reading (Fig. 2-17). It consists of an inflatable cuff with a pressure gauge and a bulb to control inflation. The cuffs come in various sizes to accommodate patients of all ages and weights (Fig. 2-18). It is very important to use the correct size and perform the procedure properly to get an accurate reading. Most sphygmomanometers have markings inside the cuff to help judge the fit. When the cuff is placed on the patient's upper arm, the mark on the outside of the cuff should fall within these range markings. This means the fit is correct.

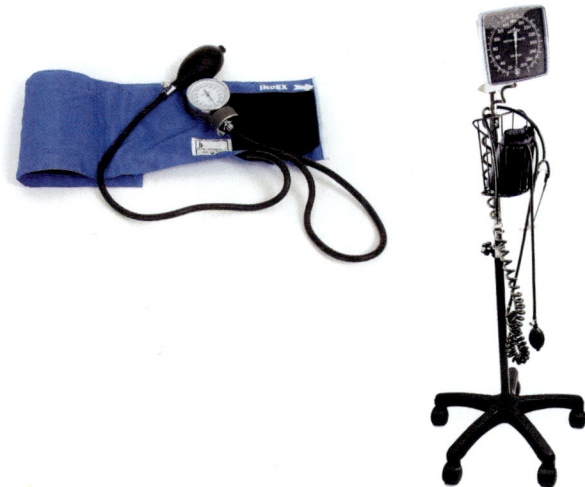

Fig. 2-17. *Two types of aneroid sphygmomanometers.*

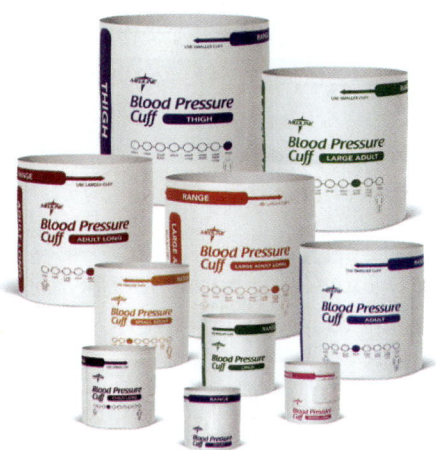

Fig. 2-18. *Cuffs come in a range of sizes. Using the correct size helps ensure an accurate reading.* (IMAGE COURTESY OF MEDLINE INDUSTRIES, LP. USED WITH PERMISSION.)

The patient should be seated or lying down with her arm at the level of the heart and her legs uncrossed (crossed legs can result in higher blood pressure readings). If the patient has had a mastectomy or has paralysis from a stroke or accident, blood pressure should not be measured on the affected side. Blood pressure should also not be measured on an arm with a dialysis shunt or IV.

Measuring and recording blood pressure manually

Equipment: sphygmomanometer, stethoscope, alcohol wipes, pen and paper

1. Identify yourself by name. Identify the patient according to facility policy.

2. Wash your hands.

3. Explain the procedure to the patient. Speak clearly, slowly, and directly. Maintain face-to-face contact whenever possible.

4. Provide for patient privacy.

5. Before using the stethoscope, wipe the diaphragm and earpieces with alcohol wipes.

6. Ask the patient to roll up his sleeve so that the upper arm is exposed. Do not measure blood pressure over clothing.

7. Position the patient's arm with their palm up. The arm should be level with the heart.

8. With the valve open, squeeze the cuff. Make sure it is completely deflated.

9. Place the blood pressure cuff snugly on the patient's upper arm. The center of the cuff with the sensor/arrow is placed over the brachial artery (1–1½ inches above the elbow, toward the inside of the elbow) (Fig. 2-19).

10. Ask the patient to remain still and quiet during the measurement.

11. Locate the brachial pulse with your fingertips.

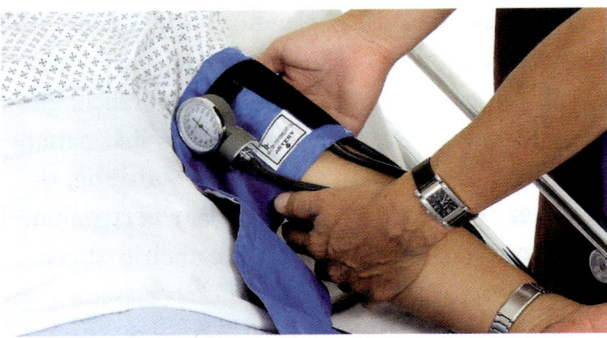

Fig. 2-19. Place the center of the cuff over the brachial artery.

12. Place the earpieces of the stethoscope in your ears.

13. Place the diaphragm of the stethoscope over the brachial artery.

14. Close the valve (clockwise) until it stops. Do not overtighten it (Fig. 2-20).

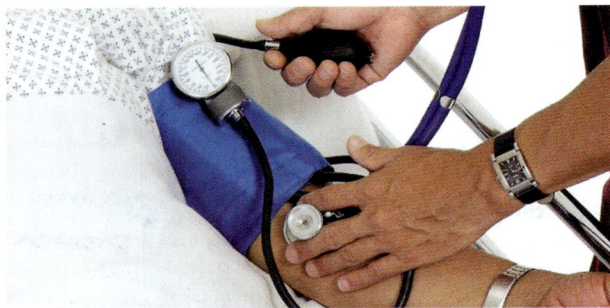

Fig. 2-20. Close the valve by turning it clockwise until it stops. Do not overtighten it.

15. Inflate the cuff to between 160 mm Hg and 180 mm Hg. If a beat is heard immediately upon cuff deflation, completely deflate the cuff. Reinflate the cuff to no more than 200 mm Hg.

16. Open the valve slightly with the thumb and index finger. Deflate the cuff slowly. Releasing the valve slowly allows you to hear beats accurately.

17. Watch the gauge. Listen for the sound of the pulse.

18. Remember the reading at which the first pulse sound is heard. This is the systolic pressure.

19. Continue listening for a change or muffling of pulse sound. The point of a change or the point at which the sound disappears is the diastolic pressure. Remember this reading.

20. Open the valve. Deflate the cuff completely. Remove the cuff.

21. Wash your hands.

22. Immediately record both the systolic and diastolic pressures. Record the numbers like a fraction, with the systolic reading on top and the diastolic reading on the bottom (for example, 110/70). Note which arm was used. Use RA for right arm and LA for left arm.

23. Clean the earpieces and diaphragm of the stethoscope with alcohol wipes. Store equipment.

24. Wash your hands.

25. Report any changes in the patient to the provider.

Blood pressure can also be measured electronically. Electronic blood pressure machines are generally reliable if the patient's blood pressure is in or near normal range. If the reading is abnormal, the EKG technician should repeat the procedure manually and note the results on the patient's chart as a manual reading.

Measuring and recording blood pressure electronically

Equipment: electronic sphygmomanometer, pen and paper

1. Identify yourself by name. Identify the patient according to facility policy.

2. Wash your hands.

3. Explain the procedure to the patient. Speak clearly, slowly, and directly. Maintain face-to-face contact whenever possible.

4. Provide for patient privacy.

5. Ask the patient to roll up his sleeve so that the upper arm is exposed. Do not measure blood pressure over clothing.

6. Position the patient's arm with their palm up. The arm should be level with the heart.

7. Make sure the cuff is completely deflated. Place the blood pressure cuff snugly on the patient's upper arm. The center of the cuff with the sensor/arrow is placed over the brachial artery (1–1½ inches above the elbow, toward the inside of the elbow).

8. Ask the patient to remain still and quiet during measurement.

9. Turn on the blood pressure device and press the start button.

10. When the measurement is complete the reading will be displayed on the screen and the machine may beep. The cuff should deflate.

11. Remove the cuff.

12. Wash your hands.

13. Immediately record both the systolic and diastolic pressures that are displayed on the screen. Note which arm was used. Use RA for right arm and LA for left arm.

14. Clean and store equipment.

15. Wash your hands.

16. Report any changes in the patient to the provider.

A blood pressure measurement can be described as *normotensive* (normal), *hypotensive* (low), or *hypertensive* (high). Adult blood pressure ranges are listed on page 13. Hypotension, or low blood pressure, can occur when a patient is dehydrated due to vomiting or diarrhea, or when someone is bleeding excessively. Hypotension can also be normal in some patients. A person with hypotension may not have any symptoms. The nurse or provider should be notified immediately if the patient has a low blood pressure reading and weakness, dizziness, or **tachycardia** (rapid heart rate). The technician should also immediately report a low blood pressure reading if the patient mentions recent bleeding, nausea, vomiting, or diarrhea. High blood pressure, or hypertension, can occur due to stress, smoking, kidney disease, or a diet high in sodium or fat. Hypertension can also be hereditary and unrelated to lifestyle.

7. Describe normal vital sign ranges for pediatric patients

Vital sign ranges are different for children than they are for adults. Normal ranges for pediatric vital signs vary depending on the age of the patient. Most facilities use adult vital sign ranges for children aged 12 and older. Pulse and respiratory rates decrease as children age, and blood pressure increases as children age. Normal body temperature range does not change with age.

Quick Reference

Pediatric Vital Signs

Age	Heart Rate	Systolic BP	Diastolic BP	Respiratory Rate
0–3 mo.	110–160	65–85	45–55	30–60
3–12 mo.	90–150	70–100	50–65	25–45
12–24 mo.	90–150	90–105	55–70	20–30
Preschool	80–120	90–110	55–75	20–30
School-age	70–100	90–119	60–75	14–22
Adolescent	60–100	90–119	70–80	12–20

8. Obtain pulse oximetry readings and identify normal ranges for pulse oximetry

A **pulse oximeter** is used to measure **oxygen saturation**, or the amount of oxygen in the blood. The part of the pulse oximeter that is placed on the patient is called a sensor. Sensors may be reusable or disposable (Fig. 2-21). Disposable sensors are generally used for pediatric patients, but they may also be used when the reusable sensor is not working well on adult patients. The sensor is placed on the patient's finger, toe, or earlobe.

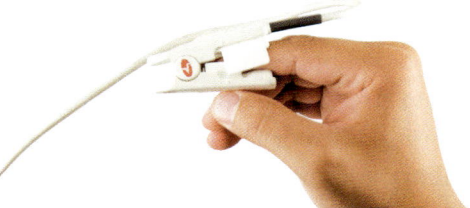

Fig. 2-21. *A pulse oximeter sensor is usually clipped on a patient's finger.*

If the patient's blood oxygen has dramatically decreased (severe **hypoxia**) it will be difficult to get an accurate reading. Getting an accurate reading may also be hard if the patient is very cold, has poor circulation, or is wearing dark fingernail polish. The EKG technician may need to remove dark nail polish.

Oxygen saturation and blood pressure are often monitored continuously in a hospital. In this case, the sensor should not be placed on the same side of the patient as the automatic blood pressure monitor. This will cause the pulse oximeter alarm to sound every time the blood pressure cuff inflates.

A normal pulse oximetry reading for adult and pediatric patients is 95%–100%. When recording the reading, the technician should also note if the patient is receiving supplemental oxygen. Pulse oximetry is not always accurate in patients with dark skin. If a reading does not match a patient's condition (e.g., the reading is normal but the patient says they do not feel they are getting enough oxygen), report the situation to a provider.

Measuring and recording a pulse oximetry reading

Equipment: Pulse oximeter, proper sensor type, nail polish remover if needed, pen and paper

1. Identify yourself by name. Identify the patient according to facility policy.

2. Wash your hands.

3. Explain the procedure to the patient. Speak clearly, slowly, and directly. Maintain face-to-face contact whenever possible.

4. Provide for patient privacy.

5. Choose the sensor. Most machines have a reusable sensor that works for most adult patients. Disposable probes are generally used for pediatric patients.

6. Identify the site for the sensor—finger, earlobe, or toe. Remove nail polish if needed.

7. Place the sensor on the proper site.

8. Instruct the patient to keep the sensor in place until a reading is displayed. If oxygen saturation will be monitored continuously, instruct the patient to leave the sensor on until a healthcare worker removes it.

9. Wash your hands.

10. Record the pulse oximetry reading.

11. Report the reading to the provider if the reading is abnormal or significantly different from a previous reading.

9. Describe the importance of assessing and reporting pain and level of consciousness

Pain is not a vital sign, but it is very important to monitor and manage. Pain levels may be difficult to assess since pain is a subjective experience. This means that pain is not something that can be measured like pulse or blood pressure, although it can affect vital signs. It must be reported by the patient, and people experience and talk about pain differently. The patient's description of pain can be very important in cardiovascular assessment. The EKG technician can use the following questions to get specific information about a patient's pain:

- Where is the pain?
- When did the pain start?
- What were you doing when the pain started?
- What makes the pain better or worse?
- Can you describe the pain? For example, is it sharp or dull? Is it constant or does it come and go?
- Can you rate the pain on a scale of 0 to 10, with 0 being no pain and 10 being the worst pain you can imagine?
- Does the pain radiate or move to any other part of the body?

A pain scale with faces may be used for pediatric patients, as shown below (Fig. 2-22).

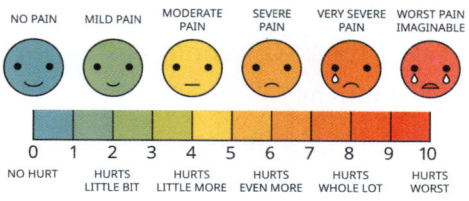

Fig. 2-22. *It may be easier for some patients, especially children, to use an illustrated pain scale to describe their pain.*

Cultural beliefs and practices and even the patient's personality or mood can affect a patient's report of pain. These factors may make patients less or more likely to freely discuss their pain. The EKG technician should report these signs which may be related to pain:

- Increased pulse, respirations, blood pressure
- Sweating
- Nausea, vomiting
- Tightening of the jaw
- Squeezing the eyes shut
- Holding or guarding a body part
- Frowning
- Grinding teeth
- Increased restlessness
- Agitation or irritability
- Change in behavior
- Crying
- Groaning, sighing
- Pacing
- Repetitive movements

Repositioning may reduce or relieve pain. It is important to be caring, gentle, empathetic, and responsive to patients who are in pain. The EKG technician should document the patient's description of pain and report changes to the nurse or provider immediately. Reports of pain should never be ignored or dismissed.

Like pain, level of consciousness is not a vital sign but is important to assess and document. Most of the EKG technician's patients will be alert and oriented. *Alert* means that the patient's eyes are open and he responds to questions readily. The EKG technician should notify the nurse or provider if the patient requires touch or physical stimulation to respond. *Oriented* means that a patient is able to state his name, the date, and where he is. Some patients may be confused and have difficulty with this. It important to establish the patient's baseline, or how the patient normally responds and acts. Confusion may be normal for some patients. The nurse or provider should be notified immediately if there is a change in the patient's baseline level of consciousness.

Take Action Now!

The EKG technician should get help immediately if a patient's level of consciousness changes noticeably. If an initially alert and oriented patient suddenly seems confused or is not responding appropriately, it could be a sign of a developing medical emergency. A patient who loses consciousness or is struggling to stay conscious also needs help right away. If in doubt, call for help.

10. Describe patient body positions commonly used during EKG testing

EKG technicians assist patients into different positions for EKG testing. Some patients require special positioning due to conditions or circumstances. Those situations are addressed in Chapter 7. The positions used for routine EKG testing are described here.

Many routine EKGs are conducted with the patient in a **supine** position. This means the patient is lying flat on his back (Fig. 2-23).

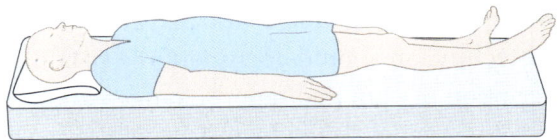

Fig. 2-23. *This patient is in the supine position.*

The EKG technician should also be familiar with Fowler's and semi-Fowler's positions. In **Fowler's position**, the patient's head is elevated 45–60 degrees. This position is often used in a hospital setting (Fig. 2-24).

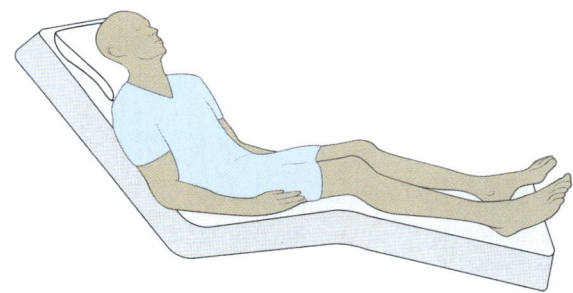

Fig. 2-24. *In Fowler's position the patient's head is elevated.*

The patient's head is elevated 45 degrees or less in semi-Fowler's position. This position is used in certain EKG adaptations, as described in Chapter 7.

Chapter Review

- In addition to their work with EKG machines, EKG technicians have a role in the basic care of patients.
- This role often involves measuring and recording vital signs, which include body temperature, pulse, respirations, and blood pressure.
- EKG technicians may also measure and record patients' blood oxygen saturation levels with a pulse oximeter.
- EKG technicians are expected to document any pain a patient might be experiencing. This can be challenging since people experience and express pain differently.
- Level of consciousness is also important to monitor. If a patient becomes disoriented or less alert, the EKG technician should report this to a nurse or provider.
- Patient care must be performed using infection prevention and control practices. EKG technicians use Standard Precautions during every interaction with every patient. All blood, body fluids, nonintact skin, and mucous membranes are treated as if they carry an infectious disease. Additional Transmission-Based Precautions may be used for patients with certain diagnoses.

3
Anatomy and Physiology

1. Discuss key concepts of anatomy and physiology and define anatomical terms

The human body can be broken down into 10 systems. These systems are often described in terms of **anatomy**, or the parts of the system, and **physiology**, or how the system functions. Body systems are made up of organs. Organs are organized groups of tissues with specific functions. Tissues are composed of cells, which are the basic units of the body.

Body systems have specific functions that work together to maintain **homeostasis**, a state of balance and stability. Homeostasis is the ongoing, complex interaction of body systems that must occur in order for the body to function at its best. For example, the nervous system regulates breathing to ensure that the respiratory system receives enough oxygen for the body to function properly.

Quick Reference

Body system	Main function
Integumentary	Protects internal organs, provides barrier against harmful microorganisms, retains body fluids, helps maintain body temperature
Musculoskeletal	Provides framework for the body, protects internal organs, allows for body movement and stability, stores minerals, produces blood cells
Cardiovascular	Circulates blood, gases, and nutrients to all cells and transports waste products away from the cells
Respiratory	Provides oxygen to all cells and rids body of carbon dioxide
Nervous	Sends, receives, and interprets information from all over the body; coordinates internal body functions in response to environmental conditions
Gastrointestinal	Takes in, digests, and absorbs nutrients to nourish cells; eliminates waste products
Urinary	Processes and eliminates waste products from filtered blood
Endocrine	Regulates body functions by producing and releasing hormones
Lymphatic/Immune	Removes excess fluids and waste products from the body's tissues; transports white blood cells throughout the body/fights infection
Reproductive	Produces hormones and male and female sex cells to make reproduction possible

Metabolism is the name for physical and chemical processes carried out by the body systems to maintain homeostasis. Changes in metabolism due to disease or injury can result in loss of homeostasis. Changes in metabolism also produce the signs and symptoms that are observed or measured when assessing a patient (Chapter 2).

Knowledge of anatomical terms is key to understanding body systems. Medical professionals use anatomical terms to describe parts of the body (Fig. 3-1). They use special directional terms to describe and document positions and locations on the body (Figs. 3-2 and 3-3).

Anatomical terms for parts of the body include the following:

- Axilla: armpit
- Thorax: chest
- Thoracic cavity: area inside the chest
- Mediastinum: central compartment of the thoracic cavity where the heart is located
- Clavicle: collarbone
- Sternum: breastbone

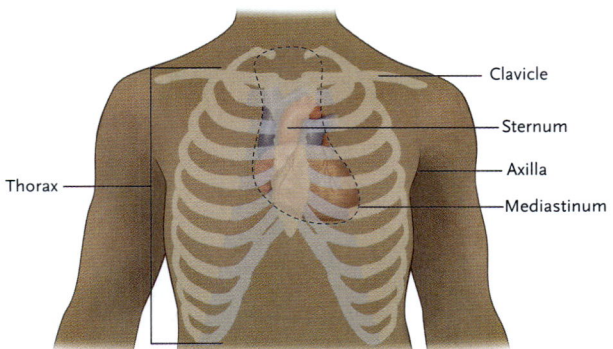

Fig. 3-1. *These anatomical terms describe parts of the body near the heart and lungs.*

Anatomical terms of location and direction include the following:

- Anterior or ventral: the front of the body or body part
- Posterior or dorsal: the back of the body or body part
- Superior: toward the head
- Inferior: away from the head
- Medial: toward the midline of the body
- Lateral: to the side, away from the midline of the body
- Proximal: closer to the torso
- Distal: farther away from the torso
- Intercostal: between the ribs

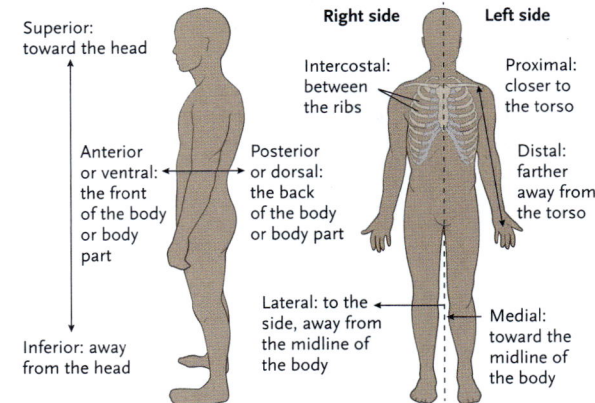

Fig. 3-2. *Instructions or doctors' orders for conducting EKGs may include terms of location or direction.*

Anatomical lines of reference include the following:

- Midline: imaginary line through the middle of the body
- Midclavicular line: imaginary line parallel to the midline and passing through the midpoint of the clavicle on the anterior (front) surface of the body
- Anterior axillary line: imaginary line parallel to the midclavicular line beginning at the anterior axillary fold
- Midaxillary line: imaginary line parallel to the anterior axillary line beginning at the midpoint of the axillary fold under the arm

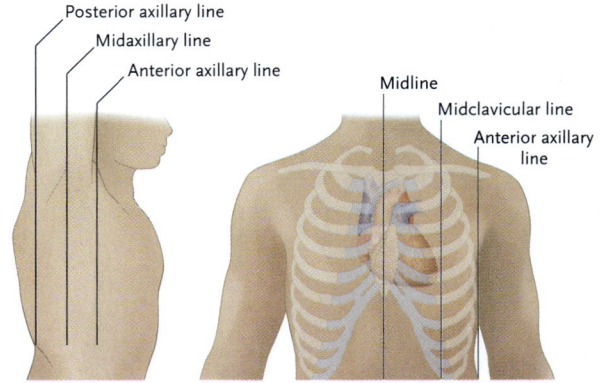

Fig. 3-3. *In order to understand the proper use of an EKG machine technicians need to be familiar with these anatomical lines of reference.*

> **Tip**
>
> **Using Medical Terms**
> Anatomical terms can help EKG technicians communicate accurately with other care team members. However, patients and their families may not be familiar with these and other medical or scientific terms. Technicians should use words that are likely to be understood when speaking to patients and family members.

2. Describe the parts of the cardiovascular system and their functions

The cardiovascular, or circulatory, system is made up of the heart, blood vessels, and blood. A healthy cardiovascular system is essential for life. EKG technicians perform or assist with medical tests that give information about how well the cardiovascular system is functioning. It is important that they understand basic facts about how the system works.

The heart is located in the chest, also known as the thorax or thoracic cavity, between the lungs in the mediastinum (Fig. 3-4). The center of the heart lies just to the left of the midline of the body between the second rib and the fifth intercostal space. The heart is slightly tilted so the base—or wide, superior end—points toward the right shoulder. The apex, or narrow, inferior end points toward the left hip.

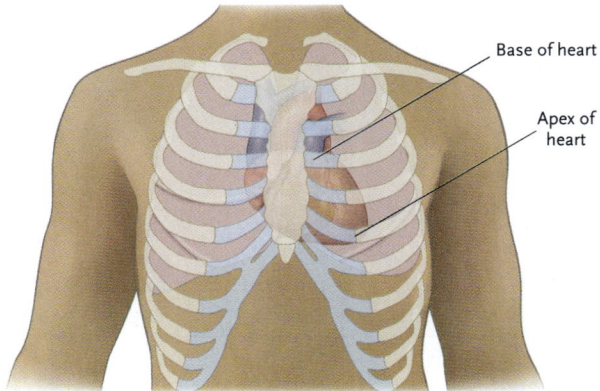

Fig. 3-4. Location of the heart within the chest.

The function of the heart is to pump blood through the blood vessels to all cells of the body.

The heart's interior is divided into four chambers. The two upper chambers, or left atrium and right atrium, receive blood. The two lower chambers, or ventricles, pump blood. (Learning Objective 7 has more detailed information about the structure and action of the heart.)

The average healthy adult's body contains five to six liters of blood. Blood is composed of a liquid portion called **plasma** and a solid portion called **formed elements** (Fig. 3-5). Blood transports gases, nutrients, wastes, and hormones throughout the body. It also protects against infections, forms clots to stop blood loss in the case of injury, regulates body temperature, and helps the body maintain homeostasis.

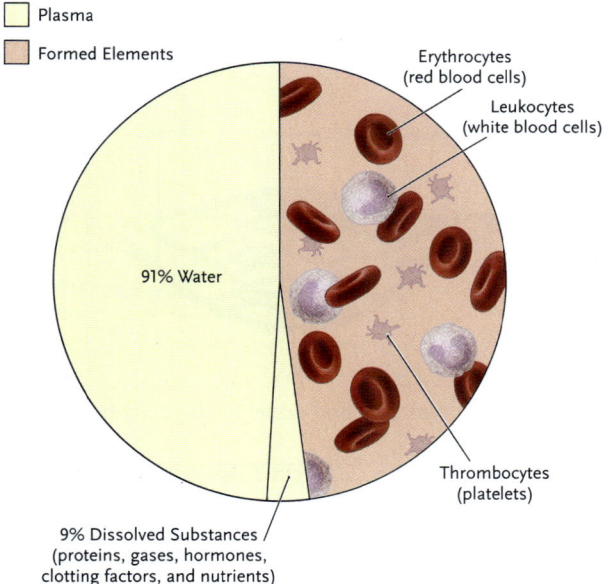

Fig. 3-5. Blood is made up of liquid and solid components.

About 55% of the total blood volume is made up of plasma, which is a clear, straw-colored fluid. Plasma is about 91% water and 9% dissolved substances, including proteins, gases, hormones, and nutrients. Some of the proteins in the plasma are important for proper blood clotting.

Formed elements make up about 45% of the blood volume. They include red blood cells, or **erythrocytes**, white blood cells, or **leukocytes**, and platelets, or **thrombocytes**. Erythrocytes contain **hemoglobin**, a protein that transports oxygen and carbon dioxide. Leukocytes protect the body against foreign substances such as bacteria and viruses. Thrombocytes play a role in blood clotting.

There are three types of blood vessels found in the body: arteries, capillaries, and veins (Fig. 3-6). **Arteries** carry **oxygen-rich blood** (also called *oxygenated blood*) away from the heart to all cells, including the cells of the heart. The special arteries that carry oxygenated blood to the tissues of the heart itself are called *coronary arteries*. The aorta is the largest artery in the body. It receives blood from the left ventricle when the heart contracts. Arteries become smaller and connect with arterioles, or small arteries, before connecting with capillaries.

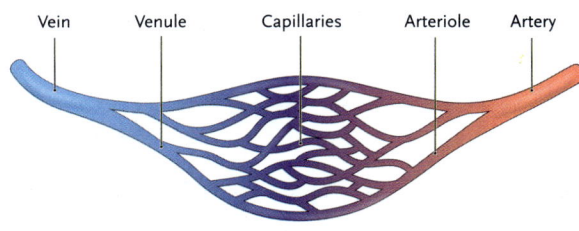

Fig. 3-6. *Each type of blood vessel in the body has its own name.*

The **capillaries** are very small blood vessels where exchanges are made. Exchanges of oxygen and carbon dioxide, and of nutrients and waste products, take place between the blood and the cells. The capillaries connect to venules, or small veins, which then connect to larger **veins**. The veins carry blood containing waste products and carbon dioxide back to the heart. This blood is called **oxygen-depleted blood** or *deoxygenated blood*.

3. Describe the parts of the respiratory system and their functions

The cardiovascular system and the respiratory system work together to provide the body with the oxygen it needs and to remove carbon dioxide from the body. Breathing, or respiration, allows the body to take in oxygen and remove carbon dioxide. Each respiration has two parts: inhalation and exhalation. During inhalation, the intercostal muscles contract, pulling the ribs up and out. The **diaphragm**, a muscle that divides the thoracic cavity from the abdomen, contracts or flattens. This contraction creates a larger space in the thoracic cavity and draws air in through the mouth and nose. Air then passes through the **pharynx**, an area of the throat behind the mouth and nasal cavity, into the **larynx**, or voice box.

The larynx is located at the top of the **trachea**, or windpipe. The bottom of the trachea divides into two branches, the right and left **bronchi** (singular: *bronchus*). Each bronchus leads to a lung and then subdivides into smaller airways called **bronchioles**. At the end of the respiratory tract are the **alveoli**, which are tiny, elastic sacs surrounded by capillaries. Oxygen and carbon dioxide are exchanged between the alveoli and capillaries (Fig. 3-7).

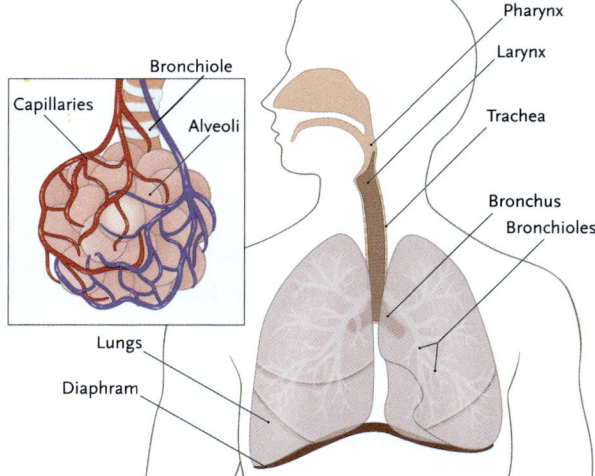

Fig. 3-7. *The process of respiration brings oxygen into the body and removes carbon dioxide from the body.*

Oxygenated blood flows from the pulmonary capillaries to venules and to the pulmonary veins before arriving at the left atrium. The blood is then pumped to the left ventricle and through the aorta to all cells.

4. Describe the relationship between the nervous system and the cardiovascular system

The nervous system is another system with close connections to the cardiovascular system. It controls and coordinates all body functions. It also senses and interprets information from outside the body. Information from outside the body is called **stimuli**. The nervous system prompts the body to respond to stimuli by sending electrical impulses through nerve tissue.

There are two major parts of the nervous system: the **central nervous system** and the **peripheral nervous system**. The brain and spinal cord make up the central nervous system. The peripheral nervous system is composed of nerves that branch off the brain and spinal cord and go to all parts of the body.

The peripheral nervous system has one part that controls voluntary actions—actions a person chooses to make—called the **somatic nervous system**. It has another part that controls involuntary actions—actions that happen without choice or effort—called the **autonomic nervous system (ANS)**. The autonomic nervous system controls the heart by sending electrical impulses through special nerve pathways in the heart. These impulses cause the heart muscle to contract, or beat.

The ANS includes the **sympathetic nervous system** and the **parasympathetic nervous system**. The sympathetic and parasympathetic nervous systems work opposite one another to maintain homeostasis (Fig. 3-8). The sympathetic nervous system is stimulated when a person experiences stress, fear, or a threat. This stimulation increases heart rate, respiratory rate, blood pressure, and muscle tension. It also slows digestion and waste elimination. This is called the *fight-or-flight response*. These changes give the body energy to fight or run away from a threat.

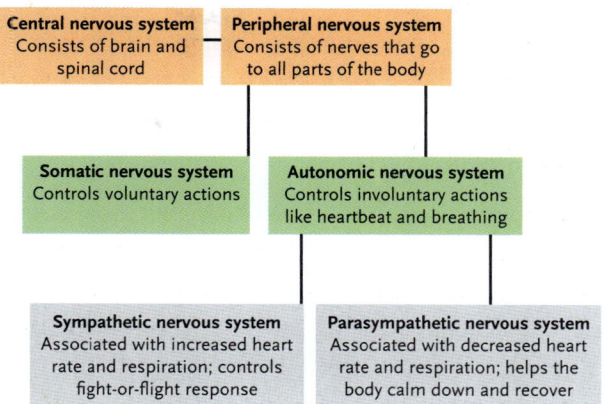

Fig. 3-8. The nervous system is the control center of the body. It has many different divisions to manage different body functions.

Stimulation of the parasympathetic nervous system decreases heart rate, blood pressure, and respiration. It increases digestion and resumes waste elimination. It helps the body to recover after stimulation of the sympathetic nervous system. If the parasympathetic nervous system overresponds, a patient may feel weak or faint due to low heart rate and low blood pressure.

Modern medical therapies use ANS stimulation to treat abnormal heart rhythms. More information on different heart rhythms can be found in Chapter 9.

5. Identify the three layers of the heart

The walls of the heart have three layers, each with a special function (Fig. 3-9). The outermost layer is the **epicardium**. This thin layer of connective tissue and fat protects the heart and also contains the coronary arteries that supply oxygen and nutrients to the heart. The middle layer of the heart is the **myocardium**. The myocardium is the thickest layer of the heart. It is composed of special muscle cells that can continually contract. The **endocardium** is the thin, innermost layer of the heart. This lining forms a smooth, elastic surface that makes it possible for blood to flow without stopping or clotting.

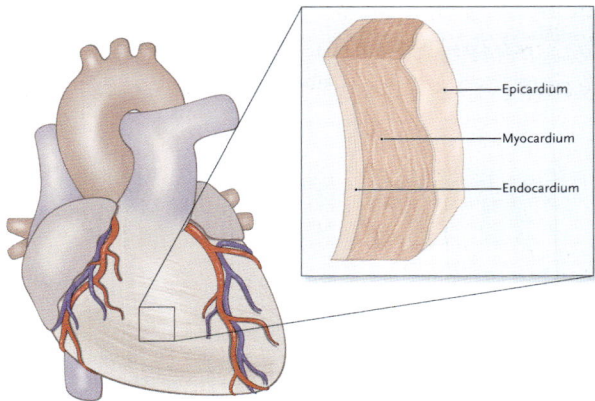

Fig. 3-9. *Each layer of the heart has a specific function.*

6. Describe the major vessels that enter and leave the heart, including the coronary arteries

As described in Learning Objective 2, major blood vessels enter and leave the heart chambers. This works to circulate blood to the heart and throughout the body. Veins carry blood toward the heart. Arteries carry blood away from the heart (Fig. 3-10). Two large veins called the **superior vena cava** and the **inferior vena cava** join together to return oxygen-depleted blood to the right atrium. This blood is pumped to the right ventricle and leaves the heart via the pulmonary arteries to go to the lungs. Most arteries, since they are carrying blood away from the heart, carry oxygen-rich blood. The pulmonary arteries are the only arteries that carry deoxygenated blood.

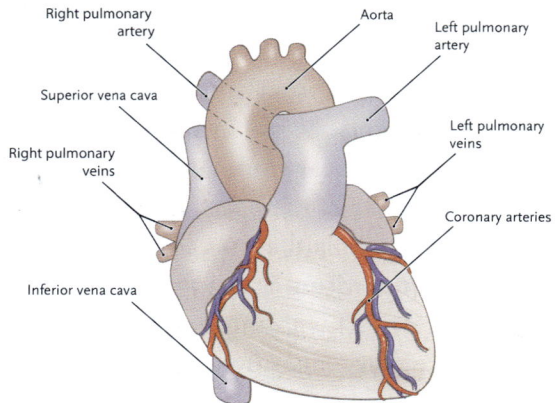

Fig. 3-10. *Veins carry blood toward the heart. Arteries carry the blood away from the heart.*

The pulmonary veins bring oxygenated blood back to the left atrium. Most veins, since they are carrying blood toward the heart, carry oxygen-depleted blood. Pulmonary veins are the only veins that carry oxygenated blood.

The **aorta** is the largest artery in the body. It carries oxygenated blood from the left ventricle. It then branches into smaller arteries that carry blood throughout the body. These branches include the **coronary arteries**. The heart muscle does not receive oxygen or nutrients from the blood that moves through its chambers. It is the coronary arteries that provide oxygen and nutrients to the heart itself (Fig. 3-11). The right and left coronary arteries branch into smaller arteries that flow to different areas of the heart.

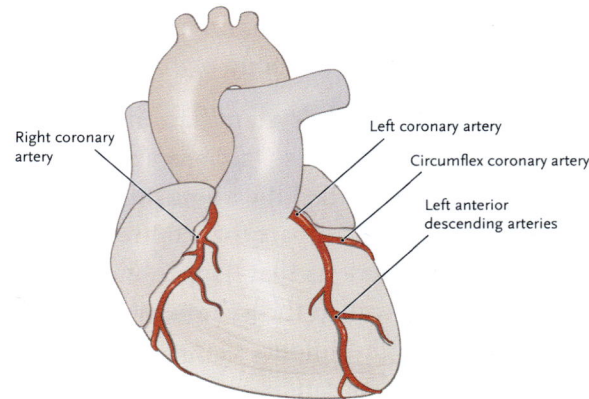

Fig. 3-11. *The coronary arteries supply oxygen and nutrients to the heart muscle itself.*

7. Describe the chambers and valves of the heart and the movement of blood through the heart

The heart can be described as a double pump. It pumps oxygen-depleted blood into the lungs and pumps oxygen-rich blood to the body. The right side of the heart receives oxygen-depleted blood from the veins and pumps it to the lungs. In the lungs the blood receives oxygen again, becoming oxygen-rich. The left side of the heart receives the oxygen-rich blood from the lungs and pumps it out to the body through the arteries.

The right and left sides of the heart are separated by a wall called a **septum**. The heart has two upper chambers called **atria** (singular: *atrium*) and two lower chambers called **ventricles**. The part of the septum between the atria is the *interatrial septum*. The part between the ventricles is the *interventricular septum*. The chambers contract and relax in a rhythmic pattern to produce blood flow.

The contraction phase of this pattern is called **systole**. The relaxation phase is called **diastole**. When the heart is functioning normally, the atria contract (systole) while the ventricles relax (diastole). Then the atria relax (diastole) while the ventricles contract (systole). This back-and-forth action between the upper and lower chambers allows the chambers to fill with blood before they contract to pump the blood. The systolic (top number) and diastolic (bottom number) measurements of blood pressure relate to the contraction and relaxation of the ventricles.

The chambers of the heart work together to move deoxygenated blood to the lungs and then deliver oxygenated blood to the rest of the body. First, the right atrium receives deoxygenated blood from the body and pumps it to the right ventricle. The right ventricle pumps the deoxygenated blood to the lungs through the pulmonary arteries. The lungs oxygenate the blood, which then returns to the heart through the pulmonary veins.

The left atrium receives blood from the pulmonary veins and pumps it to the left ventricle. The left ventricle pumps oxygenated blood to the aorta. Blood is then pumped to the body through smaller arteries that branch off from the aorta. These include the coronary arteries that supply oxygen and nutrients to the heart muscle. The left ventricle has the thickest and most muscular wall of any of the heart's chambers. This is because it must pump blood throughout the body.

A series of valves ensures that blood flows in the correct direction as it is pumped through the heart. The four major valves of the heart are the **tricuspid valve**, the **pulmonary valve**, the **bicuspid valve**, and the **aortic valve** (Fig. 3-12).

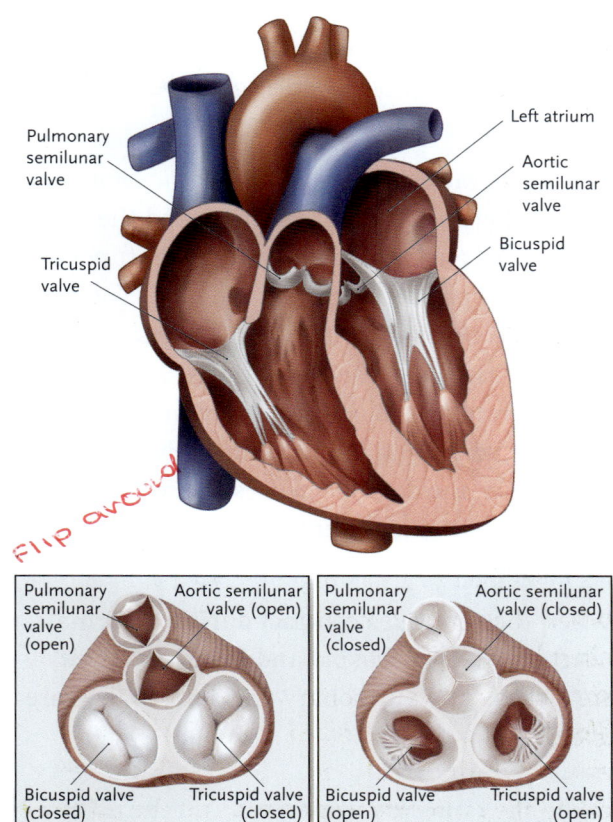

Fig. 3-12. *The valves of the heart work to ensure proper blood flow.*

The tricuspid valve (also called the *right atrioventricular valve*) is between the right atrium and the right ventricle. It is made up of three flaps (or *cusps*). The cusps are connected to special tissues in the ventricular wall that prevent the backward flow of blood when the right ventricle contracts.

The pulmonary valve (also called the *pulmonary semilunar valve*) is between the right ventricle and the pulmonary artery. This valve has three cusps that are shaped like pockets. These pockets fill and close the valve as the pulmonary artery fills and pressure in the pulmonary artery increases. The valve opens again as pressure in the pulmonary artery decreases and pressure in the right ventricle increases.

The bicuspid valve (also called the *mitral valve* or the *left atrioventricular valve*) is between the left atrium and the left ventricle. This valve has two cusps that are connected to special tissues in the ventricular wall. These cusps prevent the backward flow of blood during left ventricular contraction.

The aortic valve (also called the *aortic semilunar valve*) is between the left ventricle and the aorta. This valve consists of three cusps that function like the cusps of the pulmonary valve. The pockets on the cusps fill with blood as pressure in the aorta rises and the valve closes. The closed aortic valve keeps blood from flowing back into the heart, directing blood to the body. As the pressure in the aorta decreases, the ventricular pressure rises due to ventricular systole, and the cusps open.

When the ventricles contract during a normal heart cycle, the tricuspid and bicuspid valves are closed. The pulmonary and aortic valves are open.

Tip

Fast Rates Can Be Dangerous

The coronary arteries branch off from the aorta near the cusps of the aortic valve. When the ventricles relax (diastole), the aortic valve is closed. The coronary arteries receive blood. When the ventricles contract (systole), the aortic valve is open. The cusps of the aortic valve block the coronary arteries. Ventricular diastole is shortened in a fast heart rate. Since this is the stage that allows the coronary arteries to receive blood, the coronary arteries get less blood when the heart rate rises. This can be especially harmful to a heart that is weakened by disease.

8. Describe two circulatory paths: pulmonary and systemic

The term **pulmonary circuit** refers to the circulation of blood between the heart and the lungs (Fig. 3-13).

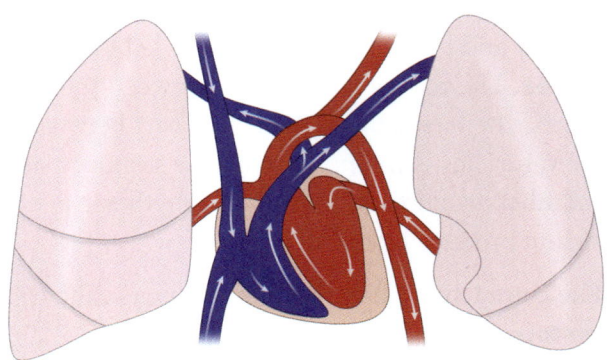

Fig. 3-13. *The pulmonary circuit is the path blood follows from the heart to the lungs and back to the heart.*

The circulation of blood between the heart and the rest of the body is called the **systemic circuit**. This constant, closed circuit maintains homeostasis by delivering substances needed by the cells and removing waste products at **exchange sites** throughout the body. The systemic circuit begins when the left ventricle pumps blood to the aorta. The aorta carries the blood to other major arteries that supply the heart muscle itself, other organs, and the remainder of the body, including the limbs.

The arteries branch into arterioles and then into capillaries or *sinusoids*. Capillaries and sinusoids are the sites where oxygen and carbon dioxide are exchanged, as well as nutrients and waste products. Sinusoids are exchange sites in certain organs, such as the spleen and liver, that do not have capillaries. After leaving the capillaries, blood enters venules and then veins. Veins come together to form the inferior and superior vena cava, which transport the oxygen-depleted blood back to the right atrium of the heart (Fig. 3-14).

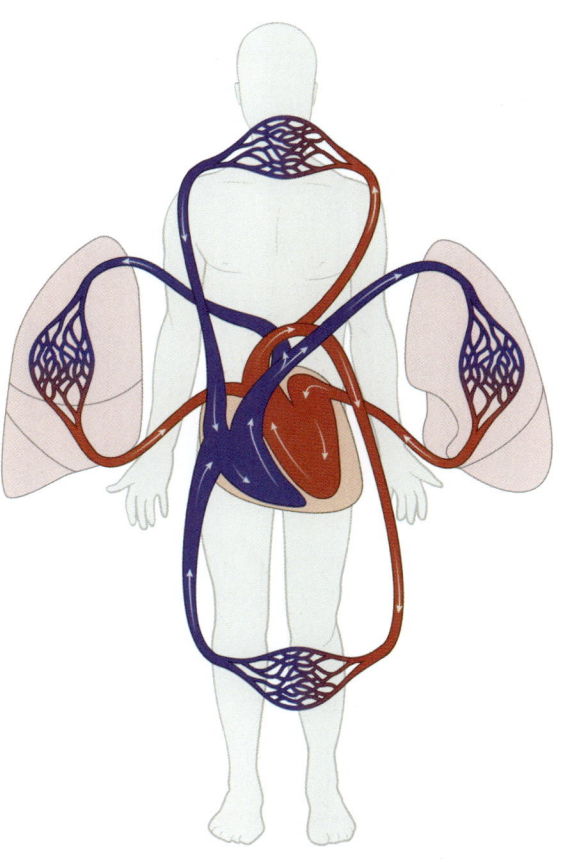

Fig. 3-14. The systemic circuit is the path blood follows as it delivers oxygen and other necessary substances throughout the body and returns to the heart.

9. Discuss the relationship between the cardiovascular system and the respiratory system

The respiratory system and the cardiovascular system work together to provide oxygen to all parts of the body. Anything that goes wrong in one system affects the other.

These examples show the connection between the respiratory and the cardiovascular systems:

- If a patient chokes or suffers an asthma attack, the respiratory tract can become partially or completely blocked. A blockage results in less oxygen being available for exchange. The cardiovascular system may be perfectly healthy, but the blood in the patient's capillaries does not have enough oxygen for the body's cells.

- If a patient has fluid in the lungs as a result of heart failure or pneumonia, the surface of some alveoli will not be able to exchange oxygen and carbon dioxide. Blood flowing to the rest of the body will not have enough oxygen.

- A patient with heavy bleeding from an injury may not have enough blood circulating to take oxygen to the tissues. The respiratory system may be healthy, but the patient does not have enough red blood cells circulating to carry the oxygen throughout the body.

All of these examples result in hypoxia, or inadequate oxygen supply in the tissues. Hypoxia affects the brain. It can cause difficulty staying awake or difficulty responding appropriately. Signs of hypoxia also include **cyanosis**, or blue/gray color in the nail beds and around the mouth. Untreated hypoxia can permanently affect other healthy body systems.

Chapter Review

- *Anatomy* and *physiology* are the studies of the cells, tissues, and organs that make up the systems of the body and the way they work together to keep the body functioning at its best.

- *Homeostasis* is a state of balance and stability within the body. Body systems work together to maintain this state.

- The cardiovascular system circulates blood, gases, and nutrients to all cells and transports waste products away from the cells. A healthy cardiovascular system is essential to life.

- Body systems work together, and changes in one can influence another. The nervous system and the respiratory system play strong roles in the proper functioning of the cardiovascular system.

- The nervous system, as the control center of the body, sends the signals that cause the heart to beat.

- The respiratory system brings oxygen into the body and removes carbon dioxide from the body. The respiratory system works with the heart to oxygenate blood that is pumped throughout the body.

- The heart is made up of different layers of tissues: an outer layer that protects the heart, a thick middle layer containing the specialized tissues that make the heart beat, and a smooth inner layer that keeps blood moving through the chambers. Valves located between chambers and vessels keep blood flowing in the right direction.

- There are four chambers in the heart: two upper chambers, or atria, and two lower chambers, or ventricles. The right side of the heart receives oxygen-depleted blood from the body and circulates it to the lungs for oxygenation. The left side of the heart receives oxygen-rich blood from the lungs and pumps it to the rest of the body, including to the heart muscle itself.

- The respiratory system and the cardiovascular system work very closely together. Changes or problems in one system can have either an immediate or a long-term effect on the other.

4
Common Cardiovascular Diseases and Disorders

Tip

Technicians Do Not Diagnose

EKG technicians do not diagnose or treat illnesses, but they are likely to work with patients who have the diseases or disorders described in this chapter. Knowing the causes, signs, and symptoms of cardiac disorders can help EKG technicians understand their jobs. The technician should contact a supervisor immediately if she is concerned about symptoms a patient has during EKG testing. Detailed information on responding to emergencies is in Chapter 10.

1. Describe coronary artery disease

Coronary artery disease (CAD) occurs when the arteries that supply the heart muscle become narrowed, thickened, and hardened by the buildup of fatty deposits called **plaque**. The plaque damages the inner lining of the vessel and causes hardening and thickening of the vessel wall (Fig. 4-1). The name for this condition is **arteriosclerosis**.

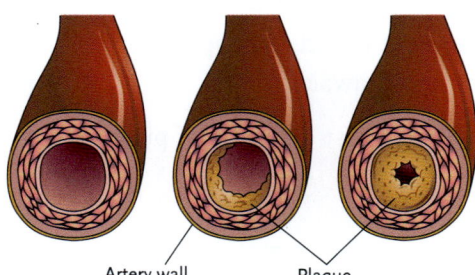

Fig. 4-1. *A buildup of plaque may cause arteries to harden and narrow.*

As CAD progresses, the damaged coronary arteries can cause increased blood pressure and decreased blood flow to the heart muscle. In extreme cases, a total blockage of the artery can result in heart muscle death (heart attack or myocardial infarction, discussed in the next learning objective). Arteriosclerosis can also affect other arteries, including those in the brain and those that supply the arms and legs.

CAD can also cause problems if plaque becomes dislodged from the artery wall or if damage in the artery results in the formation of a **blood clot** (Learning Objective 6). A blood clot or loosened plaque is called a **thrombus** when it forms. It is called an **embolus** when it moves from the original site. An embolus can block the flow of blood to crucial locations in the body, causing serious damage.

2. Describe ischemia and myocardial infarction

When an embolus blocks the coronary artery, the heart muscle does not get enough oxygen, creating a condition called **ischemia**. If ischemia is not treated, it results in cell death. When one or more of the coronary arteries becomes blocked by plaque and cell death results, it is known as myocardial infarction (MI), or heart attack (Fig. 4-2).

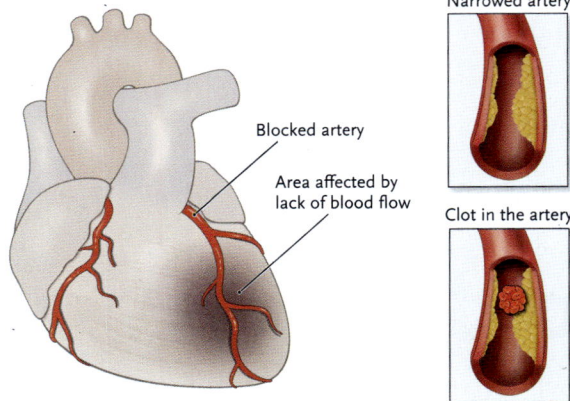

Fig. 4-2. When the heart does not receive enough oxygen it can cause ischemia, chest pain, and, eventually, myocardial infarction.

Ischemia also causes chest pain, called **angina**. Angina is a symptom of arteriosclerosis. Like all the other muscles in the body, the heart muscle needs more oxygen when it is working harder. When the coronary arteries are narrowed, the heart muscle does not get the blood flow it needs. This can cause angina. Because exertion and stress make the heart work harder in order to beat faster, angina usually gets worse with physical effort or stress. Angina that occurs at rest or without stress is called **unstable angina**. Unstable angina may indicate that arteriosclerosis is getting worse and that an MI is more likely.

The area damaged by an MI may be large or small. This depends on the artery involved. This damage can also create other problems in the body. The heart must function properly to keep the body supplied with oxygenated blood. MI can decrease the amount of blood pumped by the heart, called **cardiac output**. Symptoms of low cardiac output include fatigue, changes in level of consciousness, a weak pulse, cold or cyanotic extremities, and low blood pressure. If symptoms are ignored or untreated, a patient may suffer **cardiac arrest**, a total loss of heart function. Cardiac arrest can cause death within minutes.

The signs and symptoms of MI are shown in Figure 4-3 and listed below. Not all patients have these symptoms during an MI.

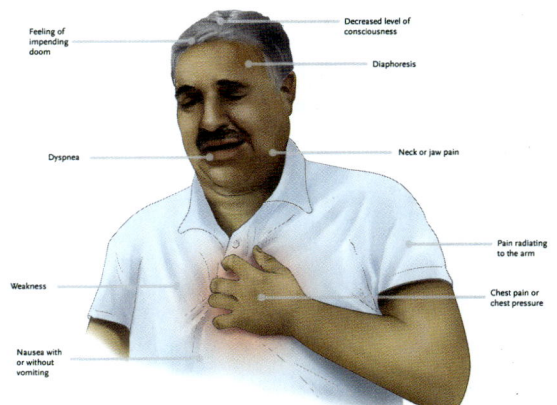

Fig. 4-3. EKG technicians should be familiar with these signs and symptoms of a heart attack.

These signs and symptoms may happen with MI:

- Angina (chest pain) on the right or left side of the chest
- **Diaphoresis** (sweating, especially a large amount)
- Nausea with or without vomiting
- Weakness
- Dyspnea (shortness of breath)
- Neck or jaw pain
- Pain radiating to the arm
- Feeling of impending doom
- Decreased level of consciousness (patient may have difficulty responding to questions or staying awake)
- Cardiac arrest (absence of pulse)

Tip

Differences in MI Symptoms

Signs and symptoms of MI can be very different from person to person. Women may experience MI differently than men. As with men, women may have chest pain or discomfort. Women can also have heart attacks without chest pain or pressure. Women are more likely to have shortness of breath, nausea, lightheadedness, stomach pain, sweating, fatigue, and back, neck, or jaw pain. Some women's symptoms seem more flu-like. Women are also more likely to deny that they are having a heart attack. The provider or nurse should be notified immediately if the EKG technician suspects the patient may be having an MI. An EKG and blood work may be ordered to rule out MI.

3. Describe cardiomyopathy

Changes to the muscular layer of the heart can make it pump less effectively. This is called **cardiomyopathy**. If the heart muscle becomes enlarged, blood begins to back up and causes valve damage (Fig. 4-4). The same can happen if the heart muscle becomes stretched out or thinned. A backup of blood also places increased pressure on the blood vessels.

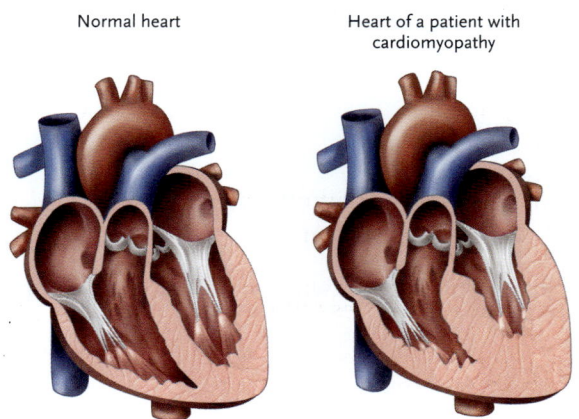

Fig. 4-4. *When the heart is enlarged it does not pump as efficiently as it should.*

Vessel damage and decreased circulation can cause fluid to build up in the lungs and body tissues. **Pulmonary edema** occurs when fluid in the lungs interferes with gas exchange. A patient with pulmonary edema may have shortness of breath, orthopnea, and a cough. Fluid buildup in the body is known as **peripheral edema**. Peripheral edema usually causes swelling in the lower legs, ankles, and feet. In severe cases, swelling can also occur in the abdomen (Fig. 4-5).

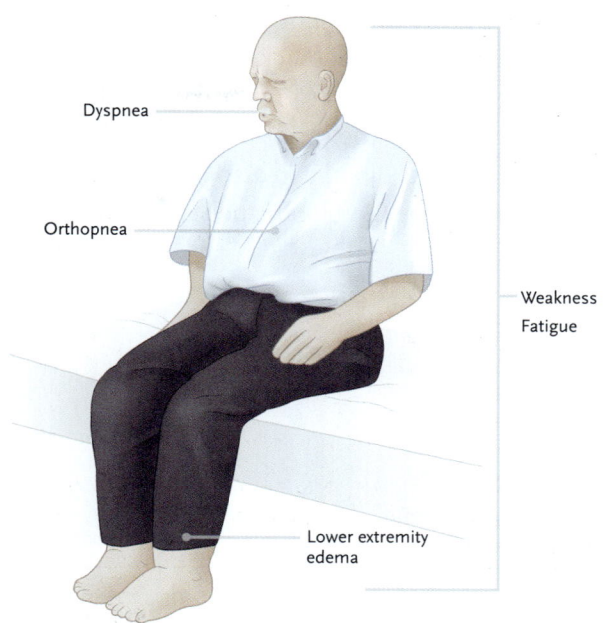

Fig. 4-5. *Signs and symptoms of cardiomyopathy.*

Causes of cardiomyopathy include advanced age, alcoholism, and heredity. There is no cure for cardiomyopathy. Treatment is directed at controlling symptoms with medications that strengthen the heart's action and help the body eliminate excess fluid. If cardiomyopathy is caused by alcoholism, lifestyle changes may slow the disease.

Signs and symptoms of cardiomyopathy include the following:

- Fatigue
- Lower extremity edema (swelling of legs and feet)
- Dyspnea (difficulty breathing)
- Orthopnea (difficulty breathing when lying flat)
- Weakness

4. Describe congestive heart failure

Congestive heart failure occurs when the heart is unable to pump effectively. It can be caused by many different heart diseases, including MI and hypertension (Learning Objective 7). Congestive heart failure can affect the right or left side of the heart. If the dysfunction begins on the right side of the heart, blood backs up in the large veins returning blood from the body to the right atrium, especially the jugular veins on either side of the neck. Blood can also back up in large organs that filter the blood, such as the liver and spleen (Fig. 4-6).

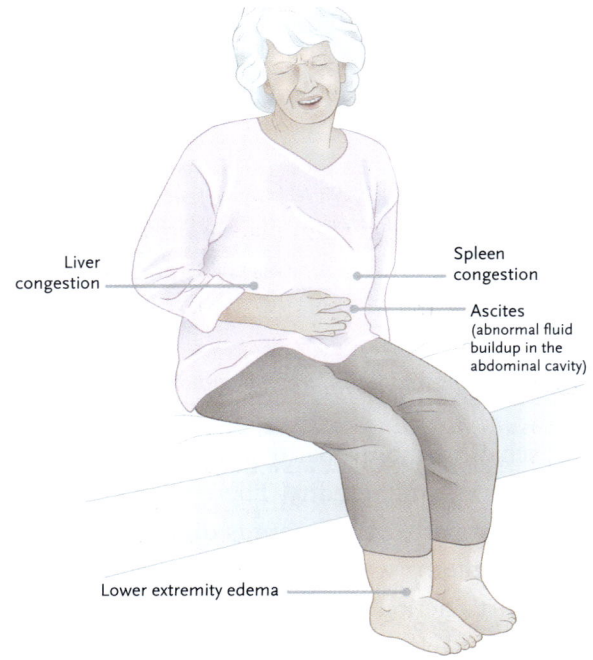

Fig. 4-6. Right-sided congestive heart failure causes blood to back up in the veins returning blood from the body to the heart.

If the dysfunction begins on the left side of the heart, blood will back up into the pulmonary veins and eventually into the lungs, causing fluid buildup (Fig. 4-7). This fluid can leak from the pulmonary capillaries and collect in the alveoli. This results in dyspnea, orthopnea, and a productive cough with frothy **sputum** (mucus coughed up from the lungs). Untreated left-sided congestive heart failure eventually causes right-sided heart failure.

Signs and symptoms of right-sided congestive heart failure include the following:

- Liver congestion
- Spleen congestion

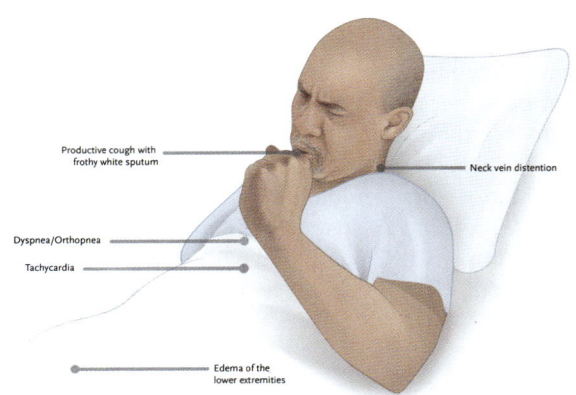

Fig. 4-7. Left-sided congestive heart failure causes blood to back up into the pulmonary veins and lungs.

- **Ascites** (abnormal fluid in the abdominal cavity)
- Lower extremity edema

Signs and symptoms of left-sided congestive heart failure include the following:

- Edema of the lower extremities
- Tachycardia (rapid heart rate)
- Dyspnea
- Orthopnea
- Neck vein distention
- Productive cough with white frothy sputum

5. Describe heart valve disease

The heart valves prevent regurgitation of blood as the heart pumps. **Regurgitation**, also called *backflow,* occurs when blood leaks back into the chamber from which it is being pumped rather than moving further through the heart or into an artery (Fig. 4-8). Heart valves can be damaged by complications of some infections, such as strep throat. Valve function may also be affected by a problem that happened before birth, called a **congenital defect**. Mitral valve prolapse is one example of heart valve disease. In the case of mitral valve prolapse, one or both of the valve flaps does not close properly.

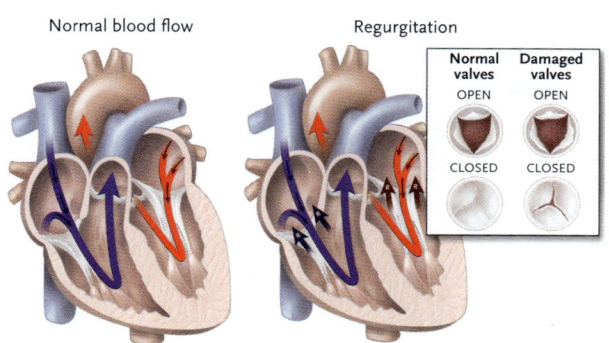

Fig. 4-8. Regurgitation from damaged or impaired valves (marked R in the illustration) creates more work for the heart.

The regurgitation caused by mitral valve prolapse and other heart valve diseases increases the workload of the heart. The backflow of blood also increases the risk of blood clots. As valve disease gets worse the patient may have lower extremity edema, weakness, chest pain, and heart palpitations (Fig. 4-9). Treatment depends on the severity of the disease and can range from medications to surgical valve replacement.

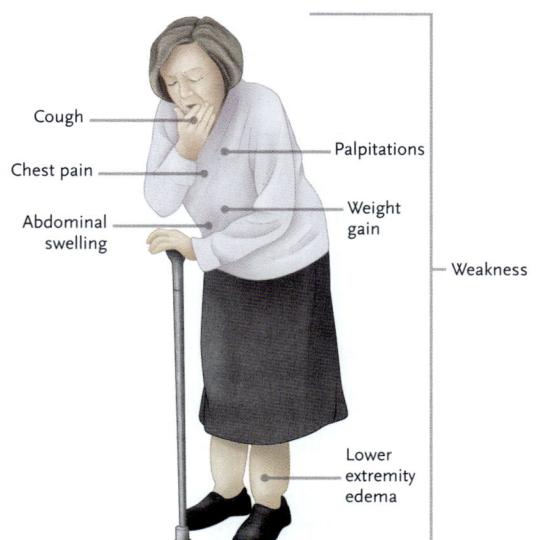

Fig. 4-9. Signs and symptoms may increase as valve disease gets worse.

Signs and symptoms of valve disease include the following:

- Lower extremity edema
- Weakness
- **Palpitations** (a feeling of the heart fluttering or beating in the chest)
- Chest pain
- Abdominal swelling
- Cough
- Weight gain

6. Describe blood clots and possible complications

Blood clots can occur when blood flows through damaged arteries, when plaque breaks loose from the artery wall, or when blood pools in the heart or in the veins of the lower extremities. Some people also have conditions that make their blood more likely to clot. The clot, or thrombus, can **occlude**, or plug up, a vessel where it forms. It can also become an embolus and move to the heart, lungs, or brain before it occludes a vessel. Blood clots begin within the cardiovascular system, but they can have serious effects on other body systems.

When a clot blocks a blood vessel, the tissue supplied by that vessel dies. Damage can vary depending on the location of the clot and the length of time before it is treated. In a condition called **deep vein thrombosis** (**DVT**) a blood clot forms in the veins of the legs or, less commonly, the pelvis or arms. This type of clot may stay where it forms and not travel. In this case it may not cause symptoms or it may only cause symptoms in the immediate area.

Signs and symptoms of deep vein thrombosis include the following:

- Pain and swelling in the affected extremity
- Increased warmth in the affected extremity
- Redness in the affected extremity

The greatest danger of deep vein thrombosis is that a clot may travel to the lungs. Because they interfere with breathing and circulation, clots in the lungs carry a high risk of immediate death.

This condition is called **pulmonary embolism** (**PE**) and is most often caused by clots originally formed in the lower extremities (Fig. 4-10).

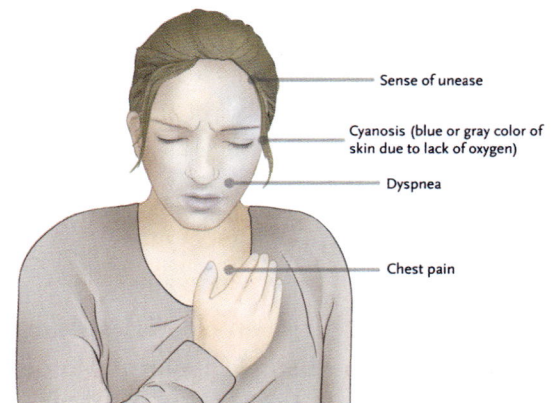

Fig. 4-10. *Pulmonary embolism can cause death. It is important to be aware of the signs and symptoms.*

Signs and symptoms of a pulmonary embolism include the following:

- Dyspnea
- Chest pain
- Sense of unease
- Cyanosis (blue or gray color of skin due to lack of oxygen)

Clots formed in the arteries can also be very dangerous. Clots that block blood flow through the coronary arteries can cause MI. Clots that block the arteries leading to the brain, or that travel to the brain, can cause a **cerebrovascular accident** (**CVA**), also known as a *stroke* (Fig. 4-11).

Signs and symptoms of a cerebrovascular accident include the following:

- **Aphasia** (difficulty speaking)
- Confusion
- **Hemiparesis** (weakness on one side of the body)
- **Hemiplegia** (paralysis of one side of the body)
- Facial droop

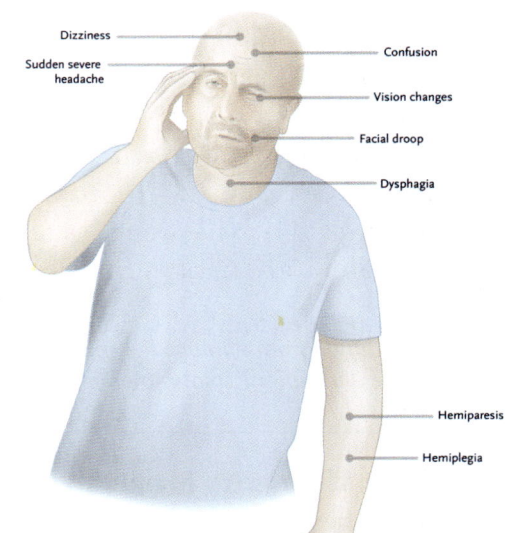

Fig. 4-11. *Recognizing the signs and symptoms of CVA (stroke) and providing prompt treatment can make a significant difference in the patient's recovery.*

- Sudden severe headache
- Dizziness
- Vision changes

Recognizing and treating blood clots quickly can decrease the chance of permanent damage and disability. Treatment is based on the location and size of the clot. Some clots can be surgically removed or dissolved using "clot buster" medications. Treatment may also include long-term blood-thinning medications.

7. Describe hypertension

Hypertension, or high blood pressure, can be a chronic disease on its own or a sign of other diseases of the cardiovascular system. As described in Chapter 2, blood pressure is a measurement of the pressure in the arteries during the contraction and relaxation of the heart. Hypertension is diagnosed when systolic pressure is consistently 130 or higher and/or diastolic pressure 80 or higher.

High blood pressure can occur without symptoms and can continue undetected until it causes a stroke, heart failure, or kidney damage.

The cause of hypertension is often hard to find, but these are known risk factors: smoking, obesity, a diet high in fat or salt, stress, and heredity. Black patients are at a greater risk for inherited hypertension. Annual blood pressure screening is recommended for all patients, especially those in high-risk groups. Treatment consists of medications, monitoring, and lifestyle changes.

Signs and symptoms of hypertension include the following (Fig. 4-12):

- Headache
- Blurred vision
- Dizziness
- Fatigue
- Nausea
- Nosebleed

> **Tip**
>
> **COVID-19 and Heart Disease Risk**
>
> Early in the COVID-19 pandemic doctors reported cardiovascular problems in some patients. Now studies have confirmed that even mild cases of COVID-19 can increase the risk of heart problems and stroke for a year or more after recovery. Risk is especially high for heart attack, heart failure, and stroke. Blood clots and dysrhythmias also happen at higher rates in recovered COVID-19 patients. Patients should be asked about past COVID-19 infection as part of their medical history. It is a risk factor for cardiovascular disease.

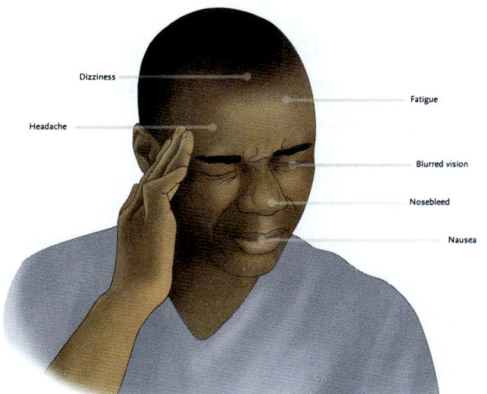

Fig. 4-12. *Hypertension is sometimes called a silent killer because it may not cause symptoms, but in some patients these signs and symptoms may be present.*

Chapter Review

- A number of diseases and conditions can affect the cardiovascular system.

- Diagnosis and treatment are not part of an EKG technician's scope of practice. EKG technicians need to have a basic understanding of these conditions and the signs and symptoms associated with them.

- Some cardiac conditions, like MI or blood clots, can cause immediate and serious damage or even death. Altered mental status, difficulty breathing, chest pain, fainting, abnormal vital signs, and diaphoresis must be reported immediately (see Chapter 10 for more details).

- Some cardiac conditions, including cardiomyopathy, heart valve disease, congestive heart failure, and hypertension can be more or less dangerous, depending on each patient's case. These conditions must be monitored and treated by a healthcare provider to make sure they do not become life-threatening.

- Other body systems can be affected by disorders that begin in the cardiovascular system. For example, stroke affects the nervous system and pulmonary embolism affects the respiratory system.

5 Introduction to EKG Technology and Applications

1. Describe the electrical activity of the heart and how it is recorded by EKG machines

An electrocardiogram shows the electrical activity of the heart. The heart's electrical activity causes the muscle contractions that pump blood. This activity occurs in patterns. These patterns are shown on the EKG.

The heart's electrical activity triggers the muscle contractions that pump blood. *Cardiac conduction is the movement of electrical signals in the heart.* Normal cardiac conduction starts in the upper part of the heart. It moves on a set path through the heart. Conduction is continuous. Changes in its pattern may be a sign of a heart problem.

The electrical activity recorded by the EKG is caused by chemical changes in the heart's cells. **Depolarization** is a change in electrical charge from negative to positive. Each heartbeat begins with one small area of the heart muscle depolarizing. Depolarization then quickly spreads to the next cell and throughout the heart. This causes the heart muscle to contract and pump blood.

Repolarization is a change in electrical charge from positive back to negative. This causes the heart muscle to relax. During each cardiac cycle, the atria and ventricles have depolarization and repolarization phases at opposite times. As this happens, the chambers fill and then pump blood.

EKG machines are connected to patients using **electrodes**. These are pads that conduct electricity. Electrodes are attached to **lead wires** (also sometimes called *EKG cables* or *electrode cables*). The lead wires transmit the heart's electrical signals to the EKG machine. The EKG machine can measure the electrical activity of the heart in several ways. It takes information from different electrodes to create different "views" of the heart. These different views are called **leads**. Each lead provides different information about the heart. The information is based on the electrical activity between two or more electrodes. The EKG records this activity on graph paper that moves though the machine at a fixed rate. The result is called an **EKG tracing**.

> **Tip**
>
> **Electrodes Are Not Leads**
> Many people, even healthcare workers, use the word *leads* to refer to the electrodes used in EKG tests. This can be confusing because in cardiology, the word *leads* has a very specific meaning. Leads are measurements of the heart's electrical activity, and each EKG lead provides information about a different part of the heart. More than one electrode is used to create each measurement. In this book, the word *lead* is only used to describe these views of the heart. The word *electrode* is always used to describe the pads applied to the patient's skin.

The muscle contractions of the heart are the heart's *mechanical activity*. EKGs do not give direct information about the heart's mechanical activity. They only record the heart's electrical activity. They give information about the location, rate, and rhythm of that activity. If information about the mechanical activity of the heart is needed, the doctor may order an **echocardiogram**. The echocardiogram uses sound waves to visualize the heart. Echocardiograms are performed by specially trained technicians.

2. Discuss the portable EKG machine

EKG machines measure small differences in electrical charge, or **voltage**, between electrodes on a patient's body. This creates a record of the heart's electrical activity. The portable EKG machine includes a screen, keyboard, and printer. It is often on a wheeled cart (Fig. 5-1). The machine has a long cable that branches into 10 lead wires (Fig. 5-2). Each wire attaches to an electrode placed on the patient's body. This completes an electrical circuit with the EKG machine. The machine reads and records the electrical activity from the different leads. The leads are created by combinations of signals from two or more lead wires.

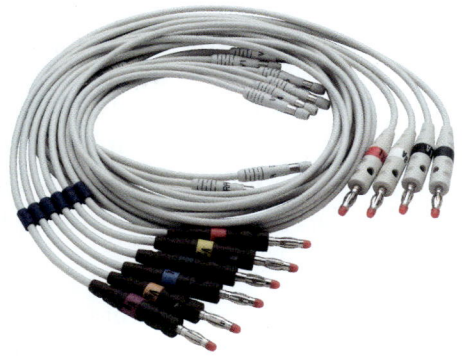

Fig. 5-2. Lead wires connect the EKG machine to the electrodes that are placed on the patient. (WELCH ALLYN™ IS A TRADEMARK OF HILL-ROM SERVICES, INC. © 2022 HILL-ROM SERVICES, INC. REPRINTED WITH PERMISSION - ALL RIGHTS RESERVED;)

Electrodes attach to the lead wires using snaps or clips (Fig. 5-3). They are placed on the patient's chest and limbs in specific locations (Learning Objective 5). Different types of electrodes are used for different EKG tests. Thin, flat electrodes called *resting electrodes* are used for routine screening EKGs. Circular pad electrodes called *monitoring electrodes* are used for continuous monitoring. They may also be used when resting electrodes cannot be attached to the patient due to diaphoresis. Electrodes contain a special gel that conducts electrical signals from the skin to the lead wire. The electrodes should be stored according to the manufacturer's recommendations. This prevents the gel from drying out. Many electrodes have a specific use-by date.

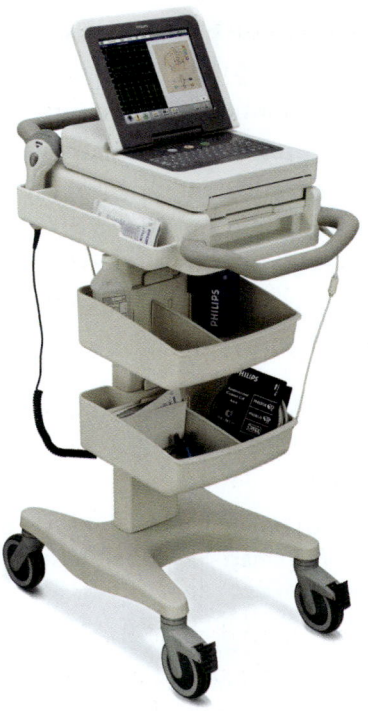

Fig. 5-1. EKG machines are often on wheeled carts. (COURTESY OF ROYAL PHILIPS.)

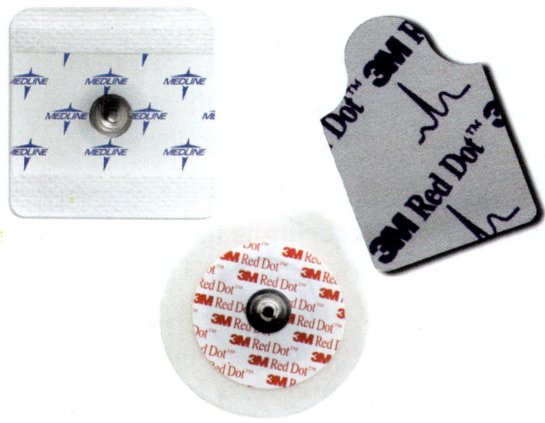

Fig. 5-3. Several different types of electrodes are used in EKG testing. (TOP LEFT: IMAGE COURTESY OF MEDLINE INDUSTRIES, LP. USED WITH PERMISSION. TOP RIGHT: SOURCE REFERENCE: RESTING ELECTRODE. COURTESY OF 3M. © 3M 2012. ALL RIGHTS RESERVED. BOTTOM PHOTO: SOURCE REFERENCE: MONITORING ELECTRODE. COURTESY OF 3M. © 3M 2013. ALL RIGHTS RESERVED.)

3. Describe the types of EKG-based tests and discuss the indications for each

EKG technicians perform several different types of EKG tests. Different tests use different numbers and types of electrodes and leads. A healthcare provider orders a specific type of EKG based on the information she needs.

If the patient's EKG must be monitored for an extended time, either 3 or 5 leads are used. This type of monitoring is often done in emergency care settings. It allows the provider to continuously assess the patient's rate and rhythm (Fig. 5-4).

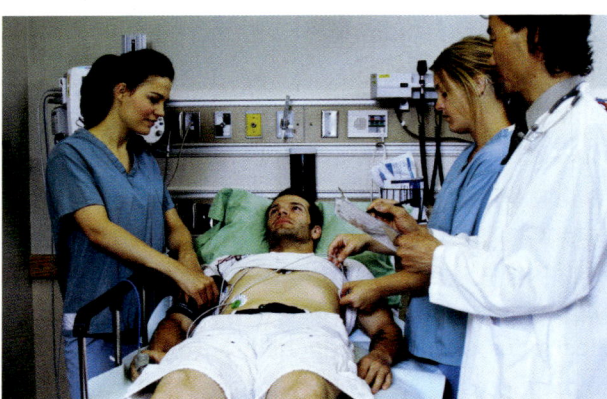

Fig. 5-4. EKG technology allows for constant monitoring of a patient's heart.

Telemetry monitoring is used in large facilities. It monitors a patient's EKG on an ongoing basis (Fig. 5-5). The patient wears a small device with 5 lead wires. The device transmits information to a central monitoring station. Specially trained healthcare workers view the patient's cardiac activity. They alert the nurse or doctor if the patient's heart rate or rhythm changes.

Ambulatory monitoring is used when a patient is not hospitalized and the provider needs information about the heart over a longer period of time. An ambulatory monitor stays with the patient. **Holter monitors** are one common type of ambulatory monitor. These monitors are usually placed on the patient in a medical office and removed after 24–48 hours (Fig. 5-6).

The information stored in the machine is then evaluated by the provider.

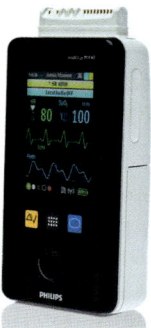

Fig. 5-5. This telemetry pack stays with the patient. It allows the patient to be monitored remotely. (COURTESY OF ROYAL PHILIPS.)

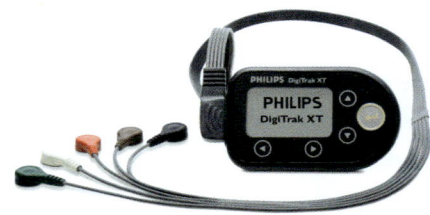

Fig. 5-6. A Holter monitor allows the patient to continue everyday life while being monitored. (COURTESY OF ROYAL PHILIPS.)

Event monitors are another type of ambulatory monitor. They only record the heart's electrical activity when the patient presses a button. Pressing the button indicates that he is having symptoms. Sometimes these monitors are returned to the provider's office for evaluation. Sometimes the information is sent in by telephone or through an internet connection. **Mobile cardiac telemetry** is a type of ambulatory monitoring that automatically alerts a healthcare professional if an irregular heart rate or rhythm is detected.

> **Tip**
>
> **Personal EKGs**
>
> EKG devices for home use are becoming more common. Some smart watches, fitness trackers, and handheld devices can record EKGs, usually in a single lead. Data from these devices syncs to a smartphone. It can also be shared with a provider. Some manufacturers offer monitoring services for a monthly fee.

These devices can detect occasional rhythm problems that may not be found during a routine EKG. They are more convenient than ambulatory monitors. The data they provide is not as complete, though. They cannot detect all dysrhythmias. They cannot detect a heart attack or high blood pressure. Harmless changes in rhythm may cause users unnecessary worry. Users with serious cardiac symptoms may ignore them if the EKG device does not indicate a problem. Personal EKG devices are best used with guidance from a healthcare provider.

The most common EKG test for screening and diagnosis is the **12-lead EKG**. The 12-lead EKG is also used during **stress tests**. These tests monitor how the heart responds to physical activity on a treadmill or stationary bicycle (Fig. 5-7). If the patient cannot exercise for a stress test, the stress can be created by giving the patient medications that speed up the heart.

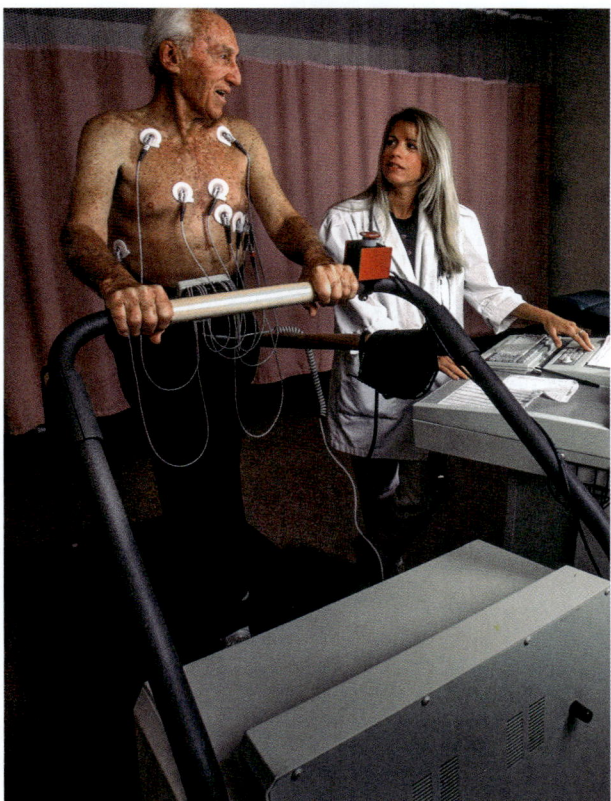

Fig. 5-7. *An exercise stress test uses a treadmill or a stationary bicycle to increase a patient's heart rate while blood pressure and a 12-lead EKG are monitored.*

This Quick Reference chart summarizes the five types of EKGs and the indications for each.

Quick Reference

EKG test type	Purpose
Continuous monitoring	Monitors heart rate and rhythm using a bedside monitor. Produces a longer record of the heart's electrical activity to help identify rhythm problems.
Telemetry monitoring	Allows heart rate to be monitored at a remote station. Produces a longer record of the heart's electrical activity to help identify rhythm problems.
Holter monitoring and other ambulatory monitoring systems	Monitors heart rate and rhythm using a portable machine worn by the patient. Allows provider to check for signs of heart problems over an extended time. Holter monitors are worn for 24–48 hours; other types are worn for as long as a month.
12-lead EKG	Used to assess rate, rhythm, and signs of acute or chronic heart disease when patient is experiencing symptoms, or as a screening tool.
Stress test	Used to assess cardiac symptoms under stress (caused by exercise or medication). Can help track recovery after an MI.

4. Identify EKG leads and lead groups

The 12-lead EKG test is one of the most common uses of EKG technology. A standard 12-lead EKG shows a 2.5-second recording, or tracing, of each of 12 leads. The tracings are arranged in a grid with four rows and three columns. Tracings are recorded in sequence by the EKG machine, switching from one lead to the next every 2.5 seconds (Fig. 5-8).

A 12-lead EKG also includes a fourth row, called a **rhythm strip**, which is a 12-second tracing of lead II. Lead II is the lead most commonly used to examine the patient's heart rate and rhythm. It is also used when a patient's EKG must be continuously monitored. More about the different leads is found in the next part of this learning objective.

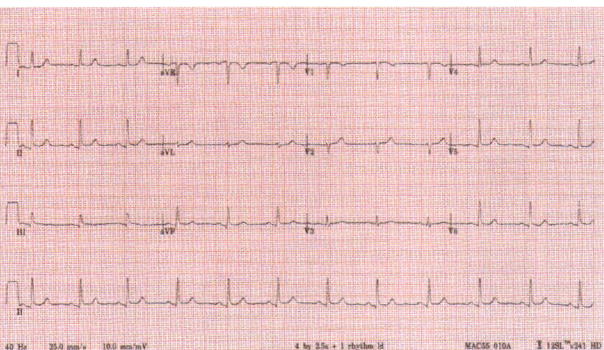

Fig. 5-8. The 12-lead EKG cycles through different leads every 2.5 seconds. The fourth row shows a full 12 seconds of activity in lead II.

All of the leads used in EKG tests have names and are arranged into groups. The groups also have names. Leads I, II, and III are called the **limb leads**. The limb lead electrodes form the points known as **Einthoven's triangle**. Einthoven was the doctor who first recorded the heart's electrical activity in the early 1900s. The original, most basic EKG recordings were from the limb leads. These leads are also called the **bipolar leads**. This means they measure differences in voltage (electrical force) between an electrically positive point and an electrically negative point.

Points with opposite electrical charges are called *poles*. Lead I measures the voltage between the left arm electrode (the positive pole) and right arm electrode (the negative pole). Lead II records the voltage between the left leg electrode (positive) and the right arm electrode (negative). Lead III records the voltage between the left leg electrode (positive) and the left arm electrode (negative) (Fig. 5-9).

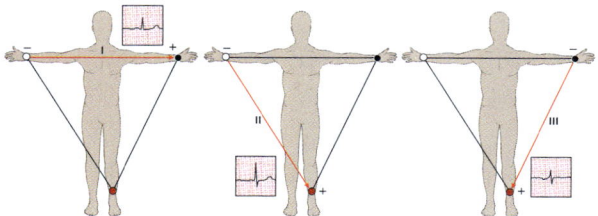

Fig. 5-9. Each of the limb leads has a different appearance on the EKG tracing. Together they form Einthoven's triangle.

Leads aVR, aVL, and aVF are called the **augmented limb leads**. They use the same three electrodes as leads I, II, and III but are **unipolar leads**. Each one focuses on the electrical activity of one positive pole. It measures the flow of electrical current in one direction only. The augmented limb leads measure voltage at a positive pole in comparison to a neutral reference point. *Neutral* means without positive or negative electrical charge. In the augmented limb leads the positive input is recorded at the right arm for aVR, the left arm for aVL, and the left leg for aVF. In each lead the positive input is referenced to a combination of the other two limb leads (Fig. 5-10).

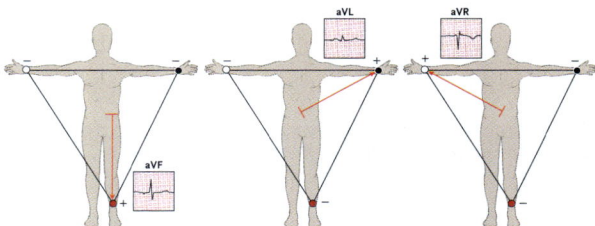

Fig. 5-10. Each augmented limb lead focuses on one particular positive electrode. The use of these leads allows for a much more targeted way to interpret the signals from the heart.

Leads V1, V2, V3, V4, V5, and V6 are known together as the **precordial leads**, or *chest leads*. These leads are also unipolar (Fig. 5-11). The positive input from each of the chest electrodes is measured against a reference point called **Wilson's central terminal**. Wilson's central terminal is the center of Einthoven's triangle. It combines the output of the three limb leads. This allows it to act as a neutral point of reference.

Each lead on the EKG gives information about a specific area of the heart (Fig. 5-12). Leads II, III, and aVF give information about the inferior (or lower) wall of the heart. This is a portion of the left ventricle. Leads V1, V2, V3, and V4 give information about the anteroseptal wall of the heart. The anteroseptal wall is the front part of the wall that divides the right and left sides of the heart. Leads I, aVL, V5, and V6 give information about the left lateral wall of the heart. The left lateral wall of the heart is the wall of the left ventricle.

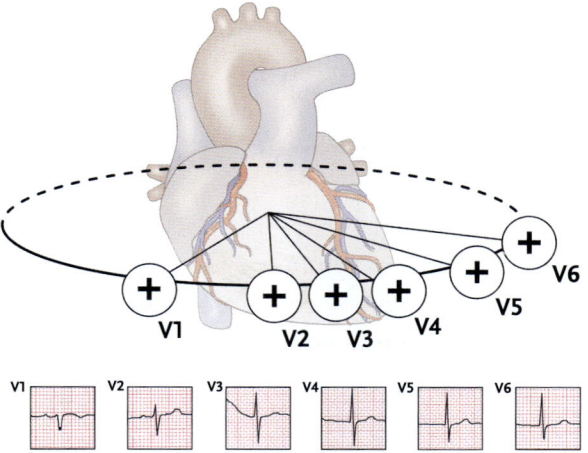

Fig. 5-11. The precordial, or chest, leads are created by electrodes placed in a line across the chest.

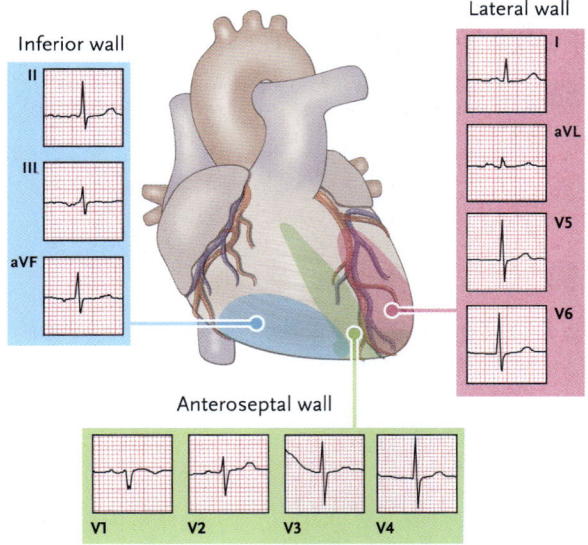

Fig. 5-12. Different leads provide information about the electrical activity in different areas of the heart.

Tip

EKGs and Electrophysiology

A detailed knowledge of an area of medicine called *electrophysiology*, along with more information about physics and chemistry than this book provides, is needed to fully understand how an EKG machine works. The details of electrophysiology are not part of the EKG technician's daily work. The EKG technician's main job is to carefully place electrodes and conduct EKG tests. This creates accurate and easy-to-read tracings. EKG technicians should know the names of leads and lead groups. They should know which leads are bipolar and unipolar. It is also helpful to know the areas of the heart examined by the leads.

5. Describe electrode placement and the use of different leads

EKG tests require different numbers of leads. The following chart shows the number of leads used for different EKG tests:

Quick Reference

Number of leads	Application
3	Continuous monitoring of heart rhythm
5	Continuous monitoring of heart rhythm, telemetry monitoring, ambulatory (e.g., Holter) monitoring
12	Resting 12-lead EKG, stress tests

To record EKG leads, the technician needs to know where to place electrodes on the patient. Incorrect electrode placement creates errors in EKG tracings. Most EKG tests use either 3, 5, or 12 leads with 3, 5, or 10 electrodes. Some leads in a 12-lead EKG share the same electrodes, so only 10 electrodes are needed for that test.

For 3-lead testing, the electrodes are usually placed on the chest and lower torso (Fig. 5-13). The electrodes are called the *right arm*, *left arm*, and *left leg* electrodes, but these electrodes are often placed on the torso. This allows the patient to move more freely. It can also give a more accurate reading. The right arm electrode (RA) is generally placed on the right upper torso, the left arm electrode (LA) on the left upper torso, and the left leg electrode (LL) on the left lower torso.

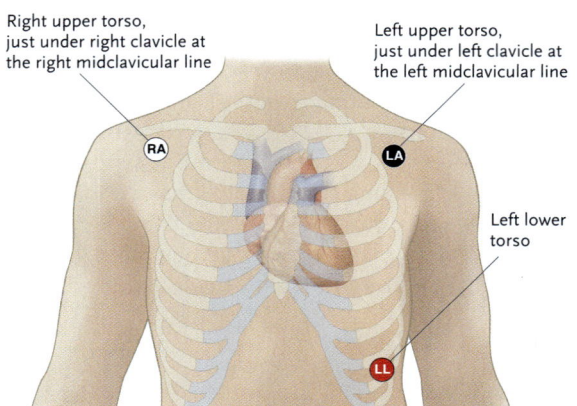

Fig. 5-13. *3-lead applications only use the right arm, left arm, and left leg electrodes.*

Tip

Limb Lead Reversal

One of the most common mistakes in electrocardiography is the reversal of limb leads. This error causes the EKG tracing to be incorrect. EKG technicians should *always* double-check electrode placement. The right arm electrode must be on the patient's right side. The left arm electrode must be on the patient's left side.

In 5-lead testing, the right arm, left arm, and left leg electrodes are placed as in 3-lead testing. The V1 electrode is placed to the right of the sternum at the fourth intercostal space. The right leg electrode (RL) is placed on the right lower torso (Fig. 5-14). This electrode is also sometimes known as the *ground electrode*.

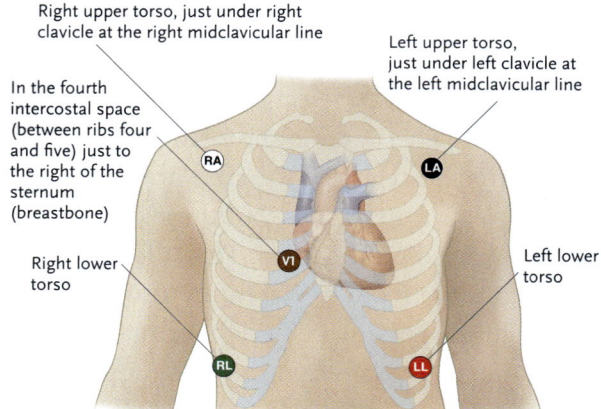

Fig. 5-14. *The 5-lead applications require five electrodes. These are the same electrodes used in 3-lead applications, plus the right leg (ground) electrode and V1 electrode.*

The 12-lead EKG uses 10 electrodes. They are placed in four limb locations and six chest locations. The EKG technician should know the anatomical name and the physical location for each. Correct electrode placement is described in the following chart and shown in Figure 5-15.

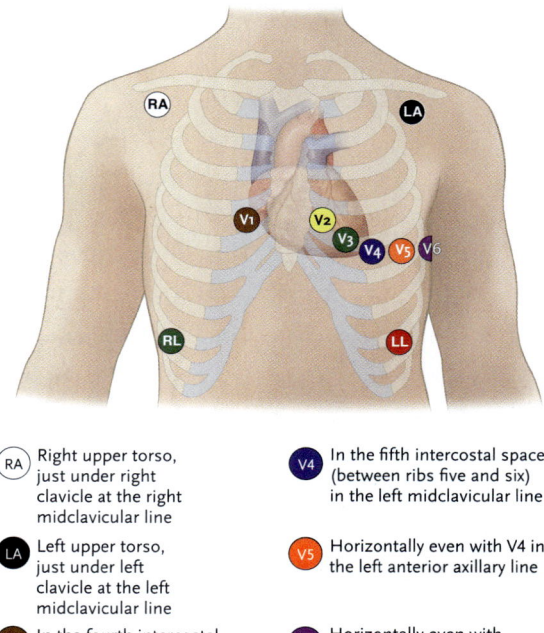

RA	Right upper torso, just under right clavicle at the right midclavicular line	V4	In the fifth intercostal space (between ribs five and six) in the left midclavicular line
LA	Left upper torso, just under left clavicle at the left midclavicular line	V5	Horizontally even with V4 in the left anterior axillary line
V1	In the fourth intercostal space (between ribs four and five) just to the right of the sternum (breastbone)	V6	Horizontally even with V4 and V5 in the left midaxillary line
V2	In the fourth intercostal space (between ribs four and five) just to the left of the sternum (breastbone)	RL	Right lower torso
V3	Between electrodes for V2 and V4	LL	Left lower torso

Fig. 5-15. *There are 10 electrodes required for a 12-lead EKG. Some leads share the same electrodes.*

Quick Reference

Electrode name	Placement
RA	Right arm or right upper torso, just under right clavicle at the right midclavicular line
RL	Right leg or right lower torso
LA	Left arm or left upper torso, just under left clavicle at the left midclavicular line
LL	Left leg or left lower torso

V1	In the fourth intercostal space (between ribs four and five) just to the right of the sternum (breastbone)
V2	In the fourth intercostal space (between ribs four and five) just to the left of the sternum (breastbone)
V3	Between electrodes for V2 and V4
V4	In the fifth intercostal space (between ribs five and six) in the left midclavicular line
V5	Horizontally even with V4 in the left anterior axillary line
V6	Horizontally even with V4 and V5 in the left midaxillary line

In 3-lead and 5-lead EKG applications the limb electrodes are placed on the torso. This leaves the patient free to move more normally. During a resting 12-lead EKG the limb electrodes may be placed on the limbs or on the torso. These variations are shown in Figure 5-16. For stress testing these electrodes are placed on the torso to allow free limb movement.

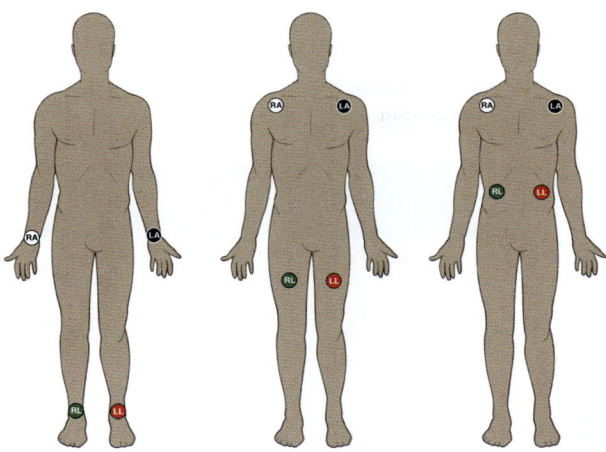

Fig. 5-16. The arm and leg electrodes can be placed either on the torso or on the limbs themselves.

Lead wires are usually color-coded. They are labeled with the name of the proper electrode. The standard colors used for each electrode are shown in this chapter's illustrations and in the chart below.

Quick Reference

Electrode name	Standard color (USA)
RA	White
RL	Green
LA	Black
LL	Red
V1	Brown
V2	Yellow
V3	Green
V4	Blue
V5	Orange
V6	Purple

Changes to electrode placement may be needed for some patients. Chapter 7 describes these situations.

6. Demonstrate proper setup of the EKG machine

The EKG machine must be set up properly before a test. This makes it more likely that the tracing will be accurate and not show interference or distortion, known as **artifact**. (Causes of artifact and ways to correct it are described in detail in Chapter 7.) Most modern machines run an automatic self-test when they are turned on. If the machine fails the self-test, it will display an error message.

Tip

Troubleshooting

EKG technicians should follow facility policy if an EKG machine displays an error message. Some facilities expect EKG technicians to try basic troubleshooting steps described in the user's manual. Some large facilities have a biomedical repair department that can check the machine. If repair is not possible, the EKG technician should try to get another machine to complete the tests ordered. They should notify a supervisor. EKG technicians should never try troubleshooting or repairs that are not authorized.

The EKG machine should be placed close to the patient during testing. This reduces tension on lead wires and electrodes. Some machines are attached to rolling carts. Others have handles so they can be carried. Smaller machines can be placed on a bedside or overbed table. If possible, the machine should be placed to the left of the patient. Electrodes for the precordial leads are placed on the left side of the chest.

EKG technicians should always plug the EKG machine in before starting an EKG. Many machines have a built-in battery, but an older battery may lose its charge and shut off in the middle of the test. If the EKG is done in an area without an electrical outlet, the technician should check the battery indicator to be sure the battery is fully charged.

The lead wires must be plugged into the machine if they are not already attached. The wires can be laid over the machine or beside the patient. The electrodes can be attached to the lead wires before or after they are placed on the patient. Attaching the lead wires to the electrodes before applying them to the patient reduces pressure on the patient's skin.

EKG paper has preprinted grids made up of one-millimeter blocks. The EKG technician can adjust the speed of the paper going through the machine. The default (standard) paper speed is 25 millimeters per second (mm/s). The EKG machine prints the paper speed on each electrocardiogram (Fig. 5-17).

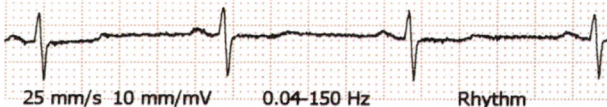

Fig. 5-17. An EKG tracing at the default paper speed of 25 mm/s.

Paper speed can be increased to 50 mm/s if the provider requests it. The faster speed spreads out the tracing. It makes waves easier to see. This can be especially helpful for fast heart rhythms (Fig. 5-18). Instructions for changing the paper speed may vary from one EKG machine to another. They can be found in the manufacturer's manual.

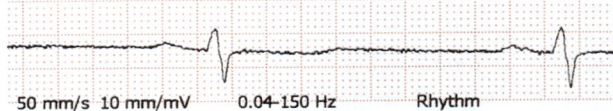

Fig. 5-18. An EKG tracing at the paper speed of 50 mm/s. The tracing is spread out over a wider space, which is especially helpful in viewing fast rhythms.

The **gain control** on an EKG machine can be used to change the sensitivity of the machine. *Gain* is a measurement of how high or low the **stylus** (the part of the machine that makes the marks on the paper) moves. Gain is measured in millimeters per millivolt (mm/mV). Millivolts are a measurement of electricity. The gain setting controls how many millimeters the stylus will move to record each millivolt of electricity. **Standard gain**, or the default gain setting for an EKG machine, is 10 mm/mV. This means that a 1-millivolt electrical signal will produce a mark on the EKG tracing that measures 10 millimeters.

The EKG tracing includes a calibration marker that looks like a vertical rectangle with the bottom line missing (Fig. 5-19). When the machine is operated at default speed and with standard gain, the mark should be 5 millimeters wide by 10 millimeters tall.

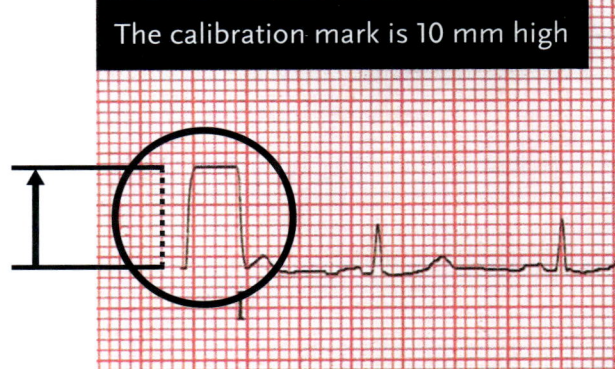

Fig. 5-19. The rectangular calibration mark on an EKG tracing demonstrates the gain control setting on the machine. Standard gain is 10 mm/mV.

Adjusting the gain control changes how the EKG tracing looks (Fig. 5-20). Increasing gain can make the tracing clearer. There may be specific machine settings shown in mm/mV: 5 mm/mV (equal to one half of standard), 10 mm/mV (equal to standard), 20 mm/mV (equal to two times standard), and so on. EKG technicians should use standard gain unless a provider asks for a different setting.

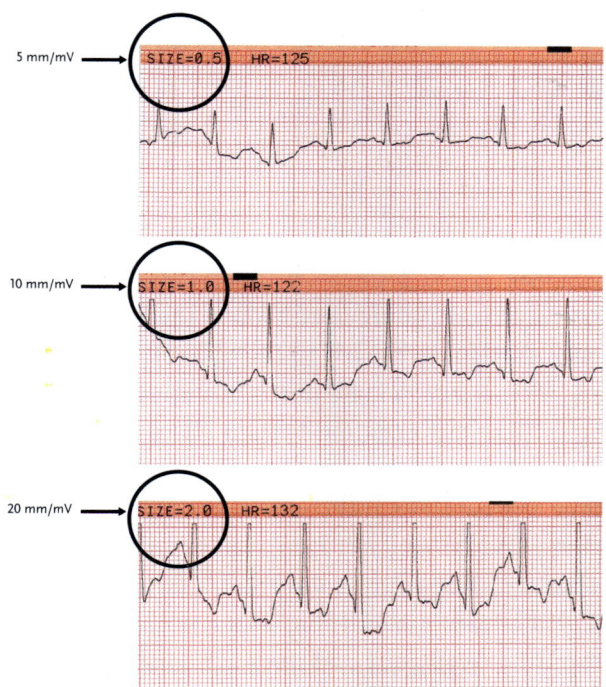

Fig. 5-20. *Higher gain creates a taller tracing. Lower gain creates a shorter tracing. These tracings show gain at 5 mm/mV, 10 mm/mV, and 20 mm/mV.*

Chapter Review

- EKG machines create a visual record of the electrical activity of the heart, called an electrocardiogram.

- Electrodes are placed on a patient's body and attached by lead wires to the EKG machine. Differences between the electrical charges at the electrode sites create different "views" of the heart's activity. These are called *leads*. Each lead records activity in a different location of the heart.

- Each lead has a name and is part of a lead group: the limb leads (bipolar leads), the augmented limb leads, and the precordial (chest) leads.

- Lead II is most commonly used to interpret the patient's heart rate and rhythm.

- EKG technology is used for several types of cardiac testing: routine screening, diagnosis of heart problems, and ongoing monitoring of a patient's heart rate and rhythm.

- EKG technicians need to know how and where to attach electrodes to patients, how to connect the electrodes to the lead wires and the lead wires to the EKG machine, and how to operate the EKG machine.

- Each type of EKG test—the 12-lead EKG, 3- and 5-lead applications (continuous monitoring, telemetry, and ambulatory monitors), and stress tests—has its own set of procedures and its own use in patient care.

6 Basic EKG Procedures

1. Describe patient identification, patient preparation, and response to emergency situations during EKG testing

Before conducting an EKG test, the EKG technician needs to identify and prepare the patient. She must also identify herself by name and by title. Clear communication is key. If the patient does not speak or understand English, the EKG technician must use an interpreter or interpretation service, following facility policy.

> **Tip**
>
> **Understanding Care is a Patient Right**
> Medical interpretation ensures that patients understand the care they receive. It allows them to answer questions from healthcare workers and ask their own questions. Many facilities use a telephone- or computer-based interpretation service. The EKG technician should know the system used in his facility. A patient's friend or family member may help with initial communication, but should not interpret medical information.

Identification is the first step when preparing a patient for EKG testing. Identifying the patient ensures that care is provided to the correct person. Failure to properly identify a patient could link the patient's information to the wrong medical record. It could begin a second, duplicate medical record for the patient. Either situation could keep the provider from finding the results.

Identification must be checked using two identifiers. The patient's full name and date of birth are most commonly used. When the EKG technician introduces herself to the patient, she should ask the patient to state her full name and date of birth. This information is then checked against the provider's order. The technician should not state the patient's information and ask if it is correct. Patients may not hear well or may not understand. They may not want to ask someone to repeat a question and may agree without understanding. A patient's address or room number should not be used as an identifier. These things can change.

A patient may be wearing a wristband for identification. The EKG technician should always make sure that the information in the patient's record matches what the patient says and what is on the wristband. If any information does not match, the technician should report the problem. He should not perform the test until the patient's identity is confirmed. Many facilities now use barcode scanners to identify patients and add information to their medical records. The barcode scanner may not work if the information on the patient's wristband does not match the medical record.

If a facility does not use barcodes, the EKG technician may enter patient information manually into the EKG machine. In most cases, this includes full name, date of birth, gender, race, medical record number, and the name of the provider who ordered the test. Facility policy may require additional information. Medications the patient is taking, symptoms at the time of the test, and special considerations (e.g., medical conditions that require adjustments to electrode placement) may also be entered.

Proper infection control practices are important during testing. Standard Precautions are used in all situations with all patients. A higher level of precautions may be needed in some cases. Chapter 2 provides information on Standard and Transmission-Based Precautions.

The patient's skin should be observed before electrodes are placed. Moisture, dryness, oil, dirt, and body hair can all affect electrode contact. Open sores or scars can prevent placement of the electrodes in the standard positions. Implanted pacemakers or defibrillators also need to be avoided when placing electrodes. Chapter 7 contains more information.

Take Action Now!

The EKG technician must always take precautions to prevent the spread of infection. Gloves should be worn (and changed when needed) if contact with nonintact skin or body fluids is likely. Masks should be worn if a patient has or may have a respiratory illness. An EKG technician should contact her supervisor if she is unsure about what PPE to use.

EKG technicians have an important role in responding to emergency situations that develop during EKG testing. A patient's condition can change at any time. The EKG technician must recognize emergency situations and follow the correct emergency response procedures. They should watch carefully for changes that indicate an emergency may be developing. These situations are discussed in detail in Chapter 10.

2. Demonstrate the performance of the 12-lead EKG test

A 12-lead EKG test is used in many settings. It may be done as a screening procedure during a routine physical. It is also useful as a diagnostic tool for suspected heart problems. The EKG technician should reassure the patient that the test is painless, and that it will give the provider important information about the patient's heart rate and rhythm (Fig. 6-1).

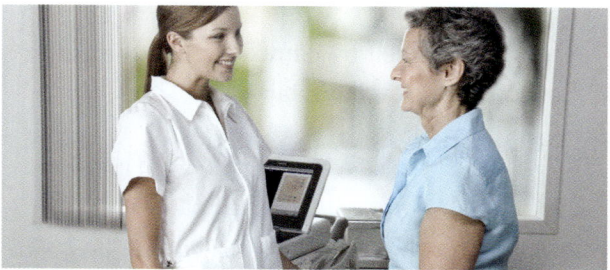

Fig. 6-1. *The EKG technician can help put a patient at ease before conducting a test.* (COURTESY OF ROYAL PHILIPS.)

Tip

Pediatric Patients

Children may be scared of doctors' offices and medical procedures. It is important to reassure pediatric patients that EKG tests do not hurt and only take a few minutes. Children may not understand medical terms. The EKG technician should describe the tests in words they are sure to understand. Electrodes can be called *stickers*. The thorax can be *chest and tummy* or *chest and stomach*, depending on the child's age. Children should also be given a chance to ask any questions they may have before the test is given.

Tip

Patients with Developmental Disabilities

Although needs differ, here are some general guidelines for providing care to patients who have developmental disabilities:

- Adult patients should always be treated as adults.
- Parents or other caregivers may accompany patients with developmental disabilities. They should be allowed to remain in the exam room during the test. They can be an excellent source of information.
- If a patient uses a communication board or sign language, the EKG technician should accommodate these needs.
- Some patients do not like being touched. EKG technicians should explain procedures simply but carefully. They should get the patient's consent before touching the patient.
- If a patient is anxious about the test, the EKG technician should give her time to become more comfortable before starting.

Obtaining a 12-lead EKG

Equipment: EKG machine loaded with paper, lead wires, electrodes, gloves (if needed), patient gown, towel, clippers

1. Identify yourself by name. Identify the patient according to facility policy.

2. Wash your hands.

3. Explain the procedure to the patient. Speak clearly, slowly, and directly. Maintain face-to-face contact whenever possible. For a male patient, explain that chest hair may need to be clipped for proper electrode contact. Reassure the patient that the test is painless and takes only a few minutes.

4. Ask the patient to undress from the waist up and put the gown on with the opening facing forward. Follow facility procedures about asking patients to remove jewelry and about asking a female patient to remove or leave on her bra. The patient should also be asked to remove socks or stockings that would prevent electrodes from being placed on the lower extremities (unless the LL and RL electrodes will be placed on the torso). Provide privacy for the patient to change.

5. After returning to the room, put on gloves if needed.

6. Assist the patient into a supine position (lying flat on his back).

7. Place the EKG machine beside the bed and plug it in to an electrical outlet.

8. Turn the machine on and wait until it completes self-tests.

9. Enter the patient's information into the machine or scan his barcode bracelet. Be sure the machine is showing the right patient information.

10. Prepare the patient's skin, if needed, by drying or removing lotion or by clipping hair that would stop electrodes from sticking. Throughout the procedure, expose only the areas necessary to prepare the skin and run the test.

11. Open the package of electrodes and attach one electrode to each lead wire by snapping or clipping.

12. Attach the electrodes in the correct positions, keeping the patient covered as much as possible. Avoid bony areas, broken skin, scar tissue, and skin over implanted devices.

13. Ask the patient to relax and be as still as possible.

14. When the tracing is clear on the monitor or when the machine shows a green light, print the EKG according to the manufacturer's instructions.

15. Check the EKG for evidence of lethal dysrhythmias or ST segment abnormalities (more information in Chapters 8 and 9). If any are seen, tell the provider immediately.

16. Follow facility policy for processing completed EKGs. EKGs may need to be immediately shown to the provider.

17. Disconnect lead wires, taking care not to pull or tug on the patient's skin (Fig. 6-2). Ask the patient to remove and discard the electrodes. If the patient is not able to do this, remove the electrodes gently and discard them yourself.

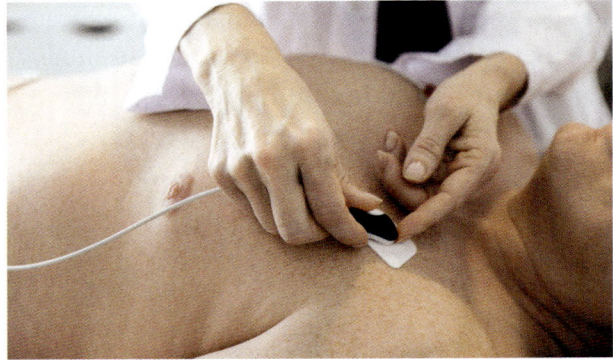

Fig. 6-2. *Be careful to avoid patient discomfort when removing lead wires from electrodes.*

18. Remove and discard your gloves (if used). Wash your hands.

19. Tell the patient where to place the gown and give them privacy for dressing.

20. Upload or file the EKG into the patient's medical record. Document the procedure using facility guidelines.

21. Clean and store the EKG machine and equipment. This may include cleaning the electrode clips and wiping the lead wires with a cleansing agent.

22. Wash your hands.

NOTE: Follow facility policy regarding reuse of electrodes if more than one EKG is conducted on the same patient. Some electrodes perform less effectively once the gel has conducted electrical activity.

Tip

Attaching Electrodes

Electrodes can be attached first to the patient or to the lead wires. If electrodes are attached first to the patient, care is needed when snapping or clipping the lead wires in place. It is important to avoid pulling the patient's skin when attaching clip-style electrodes. It is also important to avoid putting uncomfortable pressure on the patient when attaching snap-style electrodes.

3. Explain patient preparation and monitoring for telemetry

A **telemetry pack** (also called a *telemetry unit*) is used to monitor a patient's heart rate and rhythm. Telemetry technicians monitor signals from multiple patients' telemetry packs at a remote location and notify a nurse or doctor of changes (Fig. 6-3).

Most telemetry units come in a small pouch. The pouch has straps that allow the patient to tie the unit around her neck (Fig. 6-4). Some facilities have patient gowns with a small pocket in the front for a telemetry unit. The patient should be told not to remove the electrodes or wires. The patient must notify the EKG technician or the nurse if the electrodes or wires become loose or fall off. The patient can get out of bed and move around the facility while wearing the telemetry pack.

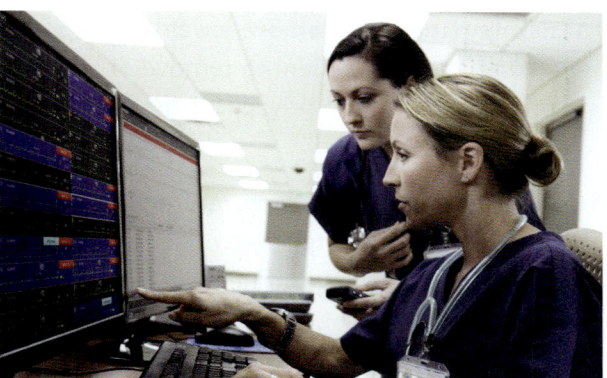

Fig. 6-3. *Specially trained workers monitor several patients at once in telemetry monitoring rooms or stations.* (COURTESY OF ROYAL PHILIPS.)

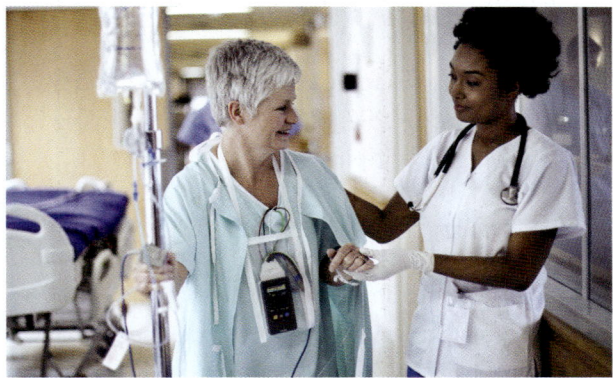

Fig. 6-4. *Telemetry packs can be worn around the neck or in the pocket of a hospital gown. Patients wearing a telemetry pack are free to move around.* (COURTESY OF ROYAL PHILIPS.)

Applying a telemetry pack

Equipment: Telemetry pack with fresh batteries, telemetry pack case, lead wires, electrodes, gloves (if needed), towel, clippers, patient instruction sheet

1. Identify yourself by name. Identify the patient according to facility policy.

2. Wash your hands.

3. Explain the procedure to the patient. Speak clearly, slowly, and directly. Maintain face-to-face contact whenever possible. For a male patient, explain that chest hair may need to be clipped for proper electrode contact.

4. Ask the patient to undress from the waist up and put the gown on with the opening facing forward. Follow facility procedures about asking patients to remove jewelry and about asking a female patient to remove or leave on her bra. Provide privacy for the patient to change.

5. When the patient is ready, return to the care area and place the telemetry pack near the patient. Put on gloves if needed.

6. Prepare the patient's skin, if needed, by drying or removing lotion or by clipping hair that would stop electrodes from sticking. Throughout the procedure, expose only the areas necessary to prepare the skin and apply the electrodes.

7. Open the package of electrodes and attach one electrode to each electrode wire by snapping or clipping.

8. Attach the electrodes in the correct positions, keeping the patient covered as much as possible. Avoid bony areas, broken skin, scar tissue, and skin over implanted devices.

9. Attach the electrode wires to the telemetry pack and turn the unit on.

10. Call the telemetry monitor room to confirm the unit is working properly.

11. Tell the patient to inform you or the nurse if electrodes fall off or the unit is disconnected.

12. Provide privacy for the patient to change into the gown normally worn in the facility. Help the patient to store the telemetry pack in the gown pocket or pouch.

13. Give the patient an instruction sheet and any other information required by facility policy.

14. Remove and discard your gloves (if used). Wash your hands.

15. Document the procedure using facility guidelines.

4. Demonstrate the performance of a stress test

A stress test measures how the heart functions under controlled stress. Stress tests are used to assess heart function and predict future heart problems. They can also be helpful in planning more invasive heart procedures. They may be used as a screening tool for patients 35 years of age and older, especially those with a family history of heart disease. Patients who have had heart surgery usually have a stress test once a year to monitor heart function.

Depending on the patient's condition, cardiac stress can be induced (created) in different ways. Exercise on a treadmill or stationary bicycle is the most common way to raise the heart rate. The provider may inject stimulant medications to raise the heart rate in patients who cannot exercise. Other names for this test include *exercise stress test, exercise tolerance test,* and *treadmill test.* When the stress is created with medications, the test may be called a *pharmacologic stress test.*

A **nuclear stress test** is another type of cardiac stress test. During this test a harmless radioactive substance called a tracer is injected into the patient's bloodstream. Before the stress test is done, the patient is placed in a supine position with her arms over her head. A special camera records the motion of the tracer through the heart. This is repeated after the exercise is complete. This type of test gives the provider more detailed information about possible blockages in coronary arteries.

The patient should receive instructions to prepare for the test. These instructions should include the following:

- Avoid caffeine (coffee, tea, soft drinks, chocolate, certain headache medications) for 24 hours before the exam. Remind the patient that even decaffeinated tea, coffee, and cola products contain some caffeine.
- Follow the provider's instructions about taking any regular medications for 24 hours before the test. Some medications may need to be stopped temporarily.
- Do not eat or drink anything except water for 3 hours before the test. Patients who have diabetes should check with the provider for specific instructions.
- Wear comfortable, loose clothing and rubber-soled shoes or athletic shoes.
- Bring all of your medications on the day of the test.
- The entire procedure will last 2–4 hours.
- A medical professional will be present or nearby for the entire test.

A 12-lead EKG is done before the patient starts exercising and then continuously during the test. The EKG is then repeated at 5, 10, and 15 minutes after the exercise is completed. The patient's vital signs are also monitored every 2.5 minutes during the test.

In order for a stress test to be considered valid, the patient must reach a particular heart rate. The goal is for the patient to reach 85% of a rate called the **age-predicted maximal heart rate**. This rate is calculated by subtracting the patient's age from 220, as shown below:

$$220 - \text{patient's age} = \text{age-predicted maximal heart rate}$$

$$\text{Age-predicted maximal heart rate} \times 0.85 = \text{target heart rate (goal) for stress test}$$

For example, a 54-year-old's maximum heart rate would be calculated in this way:

$$220 - 54 = 166 \text{ beats per minute (BPM), the age-predicted maximal heart rate}$$

The heart rate the patient should achieve during the test is 85% of 166:

$$166 \times 0.85 = 141 \text{ BPM, the target heart rate for the test}$$

This patient must reach a heart rate of 141 BPM for the test to be valid.

Stress testing should only be done by workers trained in CPR. The facility must have oxygen, an automated external defibrillator (AED), and a **crash cart** ready. (A crash cart has supplies needed immediately for a medical emergency.) The test should be stopped immediately if the patient has any of the following:

- Dizziness
- Chest pain
- Shortness of breath
- A sudden increase or decrease in systolic or diastolic blood pressure
- Systolic blood pressure greater than 250 mm Hg
- Diastolic blood pressure greater than 115 mm Hg
- Leg cramps
- Severe fatigue
- Severe diaphoresis
- ST segment changes (described in Chapter 9)
- Worsening or possibly dangerous dysrhythmias (described in Chapter 9)

The test should also be stopped if the patient wants to stop or if the heart rate does not rise above 120 BPM.

The EKG technician continues to monitor the patient after the test is completed until the patient's vital signs return to baseline. The patient should be told to rest and avoid stimulants for the rest of the day.

Conducting an exercise stress test

Equipment: treadmill or stationary bicycle, EKG machine, lead wires, electrodes, gloves (if needed), towel, clippers, sphygmomanometer, pulse oximeter

1. Identify yourself by name. Identify the patient according to facility policy.

2. Wash your hands.

3. Explain the procedure to the patient. Speak clearly, slowly, and directly. Maintain face-to-face contact whenever possible. For a male patient, explain that chest hair may need to be clipped for proper electrode contact. Reassure the patient that the test is painless.

4. Calculate the target heart rate for the stress test. Record it in the patient's chart. The target rate is 85% of the age-related maximal heart rate. (220 − patient's age = age-related maximal heart rate. Multiply this number by 0.85 to calculate the target rate.)

5. Put on gloves if needed.

6. Follow steps 6–15 of the procedure *Obtaining a 12-lead EKG* to get the patient's baseline 12-lead EKG. Place limb electrodes on the torso or near the torso for greater freedom of movement during exercise.

7. Assist the patient to a seated position.

8. Apply the sphygmomanometer cuff and pulse oximetry probe to the patient.

9. Obtain and record baseline measurements for blood pressure, oxygen saturation, heart rate, and respirations. Set monitor to read blood pressure as often as directed (often every two minutes).

10. Tell the provider when the patient is ready to start the test.

11. Repeat the EKG every 2–3 minutes according to facility guidelines.

12. Monitor the patient's EKG, heart rate, blood pressure, respirations, and oxygen saturation readings during the test (Fig. 6-5).

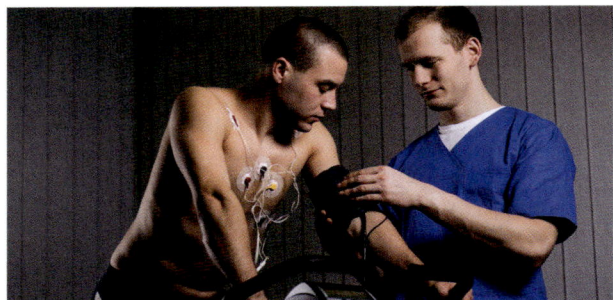

Fig. 6-5. *An EKG technician measures vital signs before, during, and after stress testing.*

13. Assist the provider as requested.

14. Continue to monitor the patient when the stress test is completed. Wait until EKG, heart rate, blood pressure, respirations, and oxygen saturation return to baseline (usually within 15 minutes).

15. Disconnect lead wires, taking care not to pull or tug on the patient's skin. Ask the patient to remove and discard the electrodes. If the patient is not able to do this, remove the electrodes gently and discard them yourself.

16. Remove and discard your gloves (if used). Wash your hands.

17. Give the patient any additional information or directions, following facility policy.

18. Upload or file the EKG and other data into the patient's medical record. Document the procedure using facility guidelines.

19. Clean and store EKG machine and equipment. This may include cleaning the electrode clips and wiping the lead wires with a cleaning agent.

20. Wash your hands.

5. Discuss Holter and other ambulatory monitoring

Holter monitors allow the physician to evaluate cardiac activity over a 24- to 48-hour period. The patient wears a small recording device with lead wires. These are attached to electrodes on the patient's chest. Other types of ambulatory monitors may be worn for longer periods of time.

Most ambulatory monitors use 5 electrodes. The skin may have to be cleaned with soap and water or gently abraded (rubbed) with a piece of gauze. This helps the electrodes adhere (stick) to the skin (Fig. 6-6). The technician should make sure that the monitor batteries are fresh before attaching the electrodes. Some facilities provide extra batteries to patients, along with instructions for changing them if the installed batteries fail.

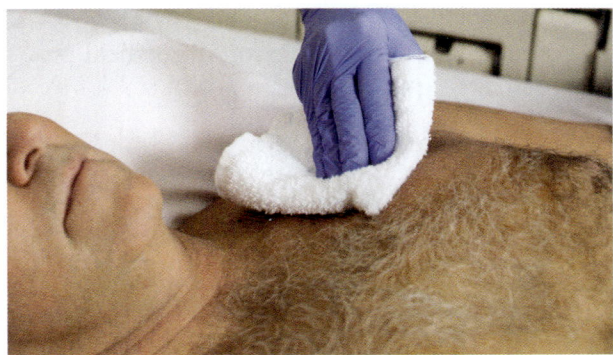

Fig. 6-6. *Gently preparing the skin ensures that electrodes adhere properly.* (SOURCE REFERENCE: CLEANING SKIN OF HAIR. COURTESY OF 3M. © 3M 2015. ALL RIGHTS RESERVED.)

Because patients undergoing ambulatory monitoring continue their everyday activities, electrodes and lead wires may be tugged or strained. This can disrupt the EKG recording or make it harder to read. Some electrodes for ambulatory monitoring have a built-in clip or slot. This allows the technician to create a loop with the lead wire. This is called a **stress loop**. It can reduce tension placed on the electrodes by the patient's movements (Fig. 6-7). A stress loop can also be created by looping the lead wire and then placing tape over the loop.

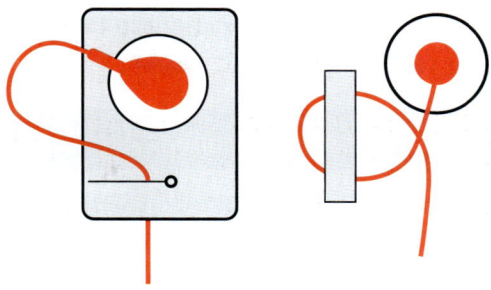

Fig. 6-7. *Stress loops can reduce tugging on the electrodes. This gives a better reading in ambulatory monitoring.*

The technician should give information to the patient about ambulatory monitoring when the monitor is applied (Fig. 6-8). Directions vary for each type of monitoring. The following information should be given to patients for Holter monitoring:

- Call the provider's office if the electrodes become loose or fall off.

- Do not remove the lead wires.

- Do not get the monitor wet. Do not shower or swim with the Holter monitor in place.

- Continue your normal activities.

- Keep an activity and symptom diary. Press the event button on the monitor for any concerning symptom.

- Call 911 for severe chest pain, weakness, or shortness of breath.

- Return all equipment as directed when the test is complete.

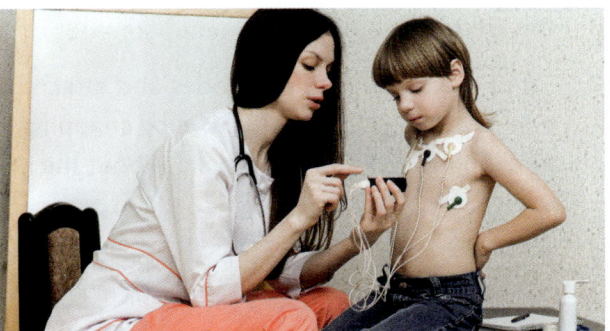

Fig. 6-8. *Patient education is an important part of setting up ambulatory monitoring.*

Most facilities have printed instructions in brochures or booklets for the patient to take home and refer to if needed.

Applying an ambulatory monitor

Equipment: Holter or other ambulatory monitor unit, lead wires, electrodes, gloves (if needed), towel, clippers, patient diary

1. Identify yourself by name. Identify the patient according to facility policy.

2. Wash your hands.

3. Explain the procedure to the patient. Speak clearly, slowly, and directly. Maintain face-to-face contact whenever possible. For a male patient, explain that chest hair may need to be clipped for proper electrode contact. Reassure the patient that the test is painless.

4. Ask the patient to undress from the waist up and put the gown on with the opening facing forward. Follow facility procedures about asking patients to remove jewelry and about asking a female patient to remove or leave on her bra. Provide privacy for the patient to change.

5. After returning to the room, put on gloves if needed.

6. Prepare the patient's skin, if needed, by drying or removing lotion or by clipping hair that would stop electrodes from sticking. Throughout the procedure, expose only the areas necessary to prepare the skin and place the electrodes.

7. Open the package of electrodes and attach one electrode to each lead wire by snapping or clipping. Follow facility policy about the use of stress loops.

8. Attach the electrodes in the correct positions. Avoid bony areas, broken skin, scar tissue, and skin over implanted devices.

9. Remove and discard your gloves (if used). Wash your hands.

10. Give the patient privacy for dressing.

11. Give the patient instructions for the type of monitoring ordered. This includes directions for returning the monitor. Allow the patient to ask any questions he may have. Reinforce instructions.

12. Document the procedure using facility guidelines.

6. Discuss the importance of accurate record-keeping and patient confidentiality

The EKG technician must document EKG tests correctly after they are completed. Most medical facilities use electronic health records (EHRs). The completed EKG must be uploaded into the record so it will be available for all medical providers to view (Fig. 6-9).

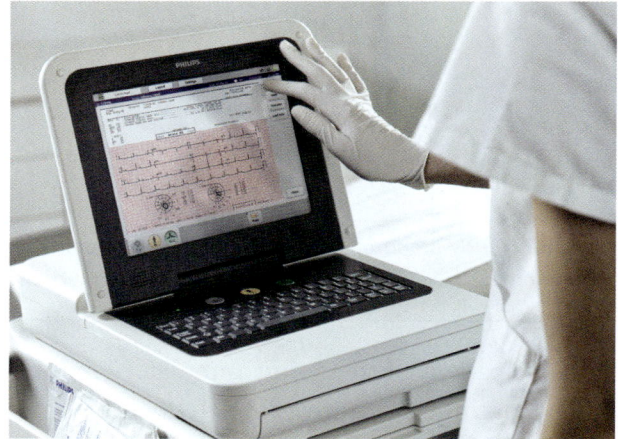

Fig. 6-9. *The EKG technician is responsible for documenting properly after tests are complete.* (COURTESY OF ROYAL PHILIPS.)

Some EKG machines automatically upload EKGs to a patient's EHR. The technician should always check that the EKG is uploaded to the correct patient's chart. In some settings the EKG technician may also be responsible for uploading information created by other healthcare professionals. This information could include the following:

- Discharge (d/c) summaries
- Medications
- Nurses' notes
- A provider's assessment of the patient, sometimes called *systems review*

All care team members must maintain confidentiality when dealing with patients' health information. Protected health information (PHI) must be kept private. PHI includes a patient's name, address, telephone number, social security number, and other identifying information.

Facilities that use EHR assign a username and password to each team member. Computer systems keep a detailed record of who logs in, which records are opened, and what information is entered or changed. It is essential to keep passwords secure and to log out of the system when a task is complete.

Several federal laws address how a patient's medical information can be collected, viewed, and shared. One of these laws is the Health Insurance Portability and Accountability Act (HIPAA). Under HIPAA, healthcare workers can be fined, can lose certification, and can be sentenced to prison for mishandling patients' PHI. This is true even if their actions were not intentional. The Health Information Technology for Economic and Clinical Health (HITECH) Act increased the penalties established by HIPAA and encouraged providers to adopt EHR in place of paper records.

Laws about protected health information apply to all members of the care team. PHI can be shared only with team members involved in the patient's care or with someone who has a legal right to know. PHI should never be discussed over the phone unless the EKG technician is certain she is talking to someone with a legal right to receive the information.

Patients can give others the right to receive their health information by signing a release form. This form must be signed before a patient's records can be shared with any outside person, facility, or organization. Release forms can be several pages long. They may ask the patient about specific situations for information release. For example, they may ask how the patient would prefer her information to be communicated (e.g., by email, fax, text, or voicemail). An EKG technician should always check the patient's release form before sharing PHI with anyone outside the facility. If the technician has any doubts about sharing a patient's PHI, he should contact his supervisor.

Chapter Review

- EKG technicians must always identify patients before conducting tests. They must use proper infection prevention measures during all patient contact. After testing, they must document the results as directed.

- If emergency situations happen during EKG testing, the technician must immediately call for help, following the facility's policies and procedures.

- After completing an EKG test, the technician should follow facility policy for review of results. It is the provider's job to read and interpret the completed EKG.

- All of a patient's medical and personal information, including EKG results, is confidential. It must be protected. Failing to protect confidentiality can result in fines and penalties. This is true even if this is done unintentionally.

7
EKG Adaptations and Troubleshooting

1. Discuss artifact and identify situations that require adaptations during EKG testing

An EKG technician's job is to generate a correct and readable EKG tracing. In some situations, the technician has to make adjustments to improve a tracing. She may also have to adapt how an EKG test is done due to the patient's age or health.

Artifact is any interference with the recording of the EKG tracing. It can be caused by environmental factors, problems with equipment, and patient conditions. Artifact distorts the tracing and may make it impossible for the provider to interpret the rhythm (Fig. 7-1).

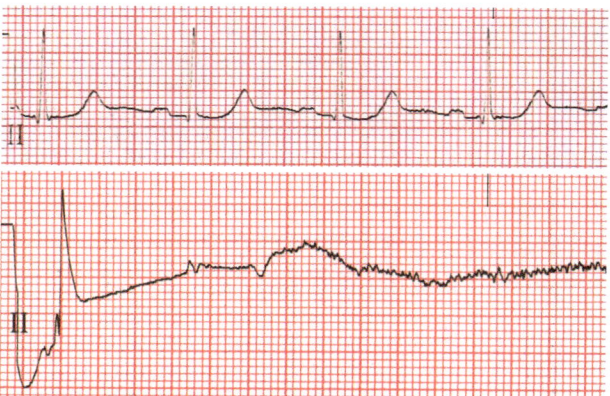

Fig. 7-1. *The first strip shows an artifact-free normal heart rhythm. The second strip shows an EKG tracing disrupted by artifact.*

The EKG technician must be able to recognize types of artifact. Artifact must be reduced or eliminated *before* printing the EKG for the provider. After a tracing has been created and the patient is not connected to the machine, repeating an EKG to fix artifact can delay diagnosis and treatment.

EKG technicians also need to be aware of situations that require changes to the usual EKG test procedures. Physical conditions, such as pregnancy, amputation, or the presence of scar tissue, may require a change in electrode placement or patient positioning. These situations will usually be noted in patient records. EKG technicians should also watch for situations in which changes may be necessary. The following learning objectives describe these situations in detail.

> **Tip**
>
> **Infection Prevention and EKG testing**
>
> EKG technicians must use Standard Precautions at all times with all patients. There are additional testing considerations for some patients under Transmission-Based Precautions. A mask—N95 respirator or other required mask—should be worn when entering the room of a patient under Droplet Precautions. If the patient has to be taken to another area for testing, the EKG technician should ask the patient to put on a mask as well.
>
> Patients under Airborne Precautions may be in a special room called a *negative pressure room*. This type of room keeps pathogens from infecting other areas of the facility. Facilities without negative pressure rooms may put portable air filters in the rooms of patients under Airborne Precautions. EKG technicians should put on N95 respirators *before* entering these rooms and should only open the door to these rooms as necessary.

When doing tests on patients under Contact Precautions, the EKG technician should put on gloves, gown, mask, and eye protection before entering the room. They should follow the correct facility procedures when leaving the room. This usually includes specific instructions for cleaning equipment. All PPE except the mask is usually removed and discarded before exiting. Facilities may use disposable, single-use lead wires in some situations. Methicillin-resistant *Staphylococcus aureus* (MRSA) is a common pathogen that requires Contact Precautions.

The technician should tell a supervisor immediately if she sees signs or symptoms of a communicable illness that is not noted in the patient's record. It is very hard to stop the spread of an illness like MRSA in a hospital or healthcare facility. Early detection is very important to prevent the spread of disease.

2. Demonstrate solutions to different types of EKG artifact

Both patient and environmental factors can interfere with EKG tracings. Newer EKG machines can detect artifact and correct for it. Recognizing and correcting artifact is still an important skill for EKG technicians.

The muscle action involved in any patient movement is recorded on an EKG tracing. This can create two types of artifact: **somatic tremor** and **wandering baseline**.

Somatic tremor artifact makes a fine, choppy distortion on the EKG tracing (Fig. 7-2). This makes the EKG difficult or impossible to read. This interference is usually caused by tremors or shivering. These are ways to reduce somatic tremor artifact:

- Patients who have Parkinson's disease or other conditions that cause tremors can be positioned with their hands under their buttocks. This reduces tremors.
- Placing limb electrodes on the torso, rather than on the limbs, may also help.
- Patients who are shivering should be given a blanket. The room temperature should be adjusted if possible. Pillows can also help make a patient more comfortable and reduce movement.
- Anxious or nervous patients should be reassured that the test is painless.

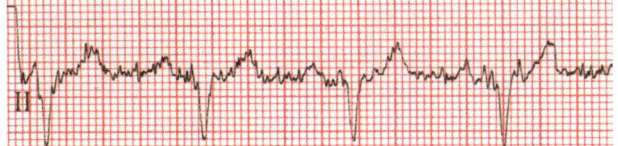

Fig. 7-2. Somatic tremor may occur if a patient is cold or has an illness that causes tremors.

The *baseline* on an EKG is the straight, horizontal line that is supposed to appear between the up-and-down movements that trace electrical activity. (It is also called an *isoelectric line*. It will be described in the next chapter.) In wandering baseline artifact, the normally flat baseline goes up and down across the tracing (Fig. 7-3). It may be hard for the provider to read the EKG. In some cases the tracing goes off the paper.

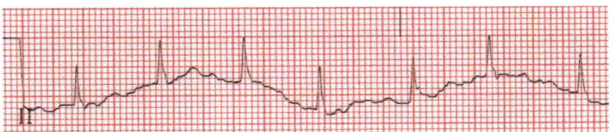

Fig. 7-3. Wandering baseline makes it hard to see the features of the EKG tracing. Sometimes the tracing runs off the paper.

The movement of the muscles used for breathing can cause wandering baseline artifact. The technician should remind patients to breathe as normally as possible and to stay quiet and still during the test. Placing the electrodes for the limb leads on the wrists and ankles can reduce wandering baseline caused by breathing irregularities.

Loose electrodes or poor electrode contact are also common causes of wandering baseline. Sweaty or wet skin, oily or soiled skin, dry skin, and body hair can all interfere with electrode contact. Careful skin preparation is the best way to stop wandering baseline caused by poor electrode contact:

- Sweat or moisture can be removed with a towel, paper towel, or gauze pads.

- Skin oil or other substances like lotion can be removed with soap and water.

- The outer layer of dead skin cells can be removed by gently rubbing, or **abrading**, the skin. This lets the electrode gel come in contact with more conductive tissue. Dry gauze or a special skin-abrading product may be used for this purpose (Fig. 7-4).

- Body hair may need to be removed to increase contact between skin and electrode.

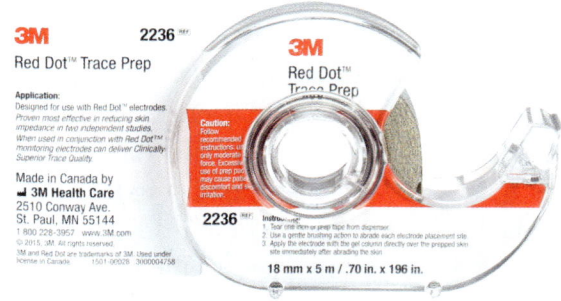

Fig. 7-4. The use of abrading tape can improve skin–electrode contact. (SOURCE REFERENCE: ELECTRODE TRACE PREP. COURTESY OF 3M. © 3M 2016. ALL RIGHTS RESERVED.)

Body hair that prevents electrode contact should only be removed with a razor or electric clippers designed for hair removal in medical settings (Fig. 7-5). Medical clippers are usually powered by rechargeable batteries. They have disposable cutting heads. A standard shaving razor should not be used. It can create microcuts, which increase the chance of infection. The EKG technician can also place paper tape over an electrode to help increase skin contact.

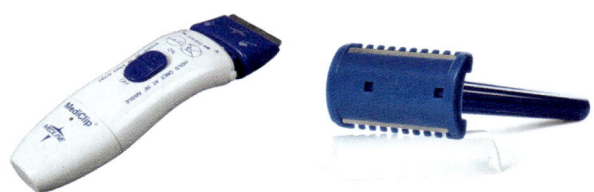

Fig. 7-5. Medical razors or clippers should be used to remove body hair if necessary. Most facilities use electric clippers for this purpose. (IMAGES COURTESY OF MEDLINE INDUSTRIES, LP. USED WITH PERMISSION.)

Other factors can also cause wandering baseline. Electrodes that are expired or dried out may cause wandering baseline. They may prevent the EKG machine from picking up any signals at all. Electrodes should be stored in an airtight container. Any that are dried out or expired should be thrown away. Tension on the lead wires or wires that are not secured well can also cause wandering baseline artifact. The EKG technician should always place the EKG machine so that lead wires are not stretched.

Artifacts called *electrical interference* and *broken recording* can be caused by factors in the care environment. **Electrical interference** is also called *alternating current (AC) interference* or *60-cycle interference*. It can be caused by other appliances or equipment in use in the area near the EKG machine (Fig. 7-6).

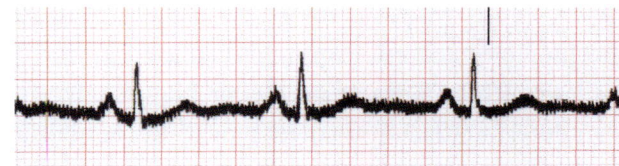

Fig. 7-6. An EKG tracing showing electrical interference is difficult or impossible to read.

The EKG technician needs to look for the source of electrical interference and try to stop it. Electrical interference may be eliminated by

- Turning off other electrical appliances

- Changing the outlet being used to power the EKG machine

- Not plugging the EKG machine into an extension cord

- Making sure the machine is properly grounded. This involves checking that the machine is plugged into a three-prong, grounded outlet.

- Turning off fluorescent lights

EKG machines often have a built-in filter to reduce electrical interference. However, it is still important for EKG technicians to know how to avoid situations that may cause it.

Broken recording, also called *interrupted baseline*, occurs when the EKG machine cannot find a signal. The stylus goes from side to side as the machine searches for a signal (Fig. 7-7). The most common cause of broken recording is frayed or broken lead wires. The EKG technician should check the EKG machine before each use to make sure the lead wires are in good shape. If the lead wires are broken or frayed, he should not use them.

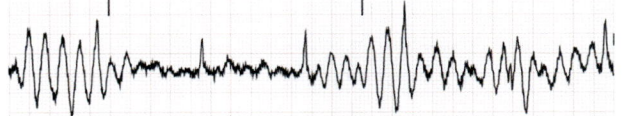

Fig. 7-7. *Broken recording is usually a result of frayed wires.*

Errors in electrode placement can also create EKG tracings that are not accurate. These problems are addressed in Chapter 9, which outlines the different EKG rhythms and how to identify them.

Quick Reference

Type of artifact	Possible cause	Adaptation/solution
Somatic tremor	Patient is cold	Increase room temperature, offer blanket
	Patient is experiencing a seizure	Turn down lights and provide quiet environment; delay EKG until seizure is over
	Patient is experiencing tremor due to Parkinson's disease	Have patient place hands, palms up, under buttocks
	Patient is anxious	Reassure patient and encourage slow breaths
Wandering baseline	Patient's breathing is creating interference due to muscle movement	Encourage slow breaths; do not position limb lead electrodes on torso
	Patient's body hair is preventing skin–electrode contact	Remove body hair using medical clippers or razor
	Natural skin oils or grooming products are interfering with skin–electrode contact	Remove with soap and water and thoroughly dry skin
	Electrode gel is dried out	Discard dry electrodes; store electrodes in airtight containers
	Lead wires are tight or stretched	Place machine close to patient and avoid movement of wires during recording
	Patient is very thin	Place electrodes away from bony areas
Electrical (AC or 60-cycle) interference	There is electrical equipment in the area or being used by patient	Move electrical equipment or turn off if possible
	Unknown source	Turn off fluorescent lights and other nonmedical equipment in the room
		Do not use machine with extension cord
		Be sure machine is properly grounded
		Move machine to another location in the room or to a different outlet
Broken recording	There are frayed or broken lead wires	Check for frayed or broken lead wires and replace
		Clean and store lead wires carefully to prevent wear

3. Demonstrate adaptations to electrode placement and patient positioning

Adaptations, or adjustments to the EKG procedure, may be needed for some patients. For most resting EKGs, the patient is in the supine position with standard electrode placement. Electrode placement is different for pediatric patients. Positioning and electrode placement are changed for certain conditions as well. Any time electrodes are placed in alternate locations, the EKG technician must document the changes. Changes should also be written directly on the EKG tracing. This makes sure the provider is aware of the adaptations. This is important because adaptations can change how the EKG looks.

> **Tip**
>
> **Documenting Adaptations**
> Any adaptation made during an EKG should be documented. Any change from the usual facility procedure, including electrodes placed in nonstandard locations or a patient positioned differently, should be noted in the patient's record. This makes sure the provider has all the important facts when she interprets the EKG tracing.

EKG technicians may need to use alternate electrode placement in these situations:

Dextrocardia: **Dextrocardia** is a rare heart condition. It causes the heart to point to the right side of the chest rather than the left side. The chest electrodes must be placed over the heart on the right side of the chest. Otherwise, the EKG will not be accurate (Fig. 7-8). The patient usually knows about this condition or it is noted in the patient's chart.

Limb amputation/injury: Limb electrode placement must be changed for patients with limb amputations. The electrodes may be placed on the torso, as close as possible to the amputated limb. They may also be placed on the limb itself but closer to the torso (Fig. 7-9). The electrodes should not be placed over scar tissue. The electrode for the unaffected limb should be placed in a mirror image position. The EKG technician should also use this adaptation for a patient who has an injured extremity with open skin, a cast, or a thick bandage. All other electrodes are placed in the standard locations.

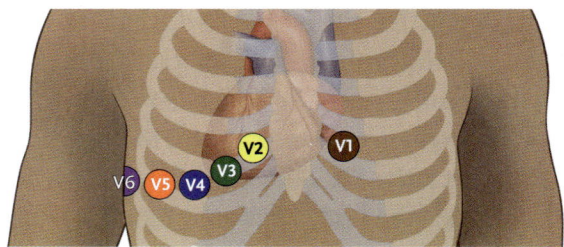

Fig. 7-8. Right-sided placement of the chest electrodes is a mirror image of left-sided placement.

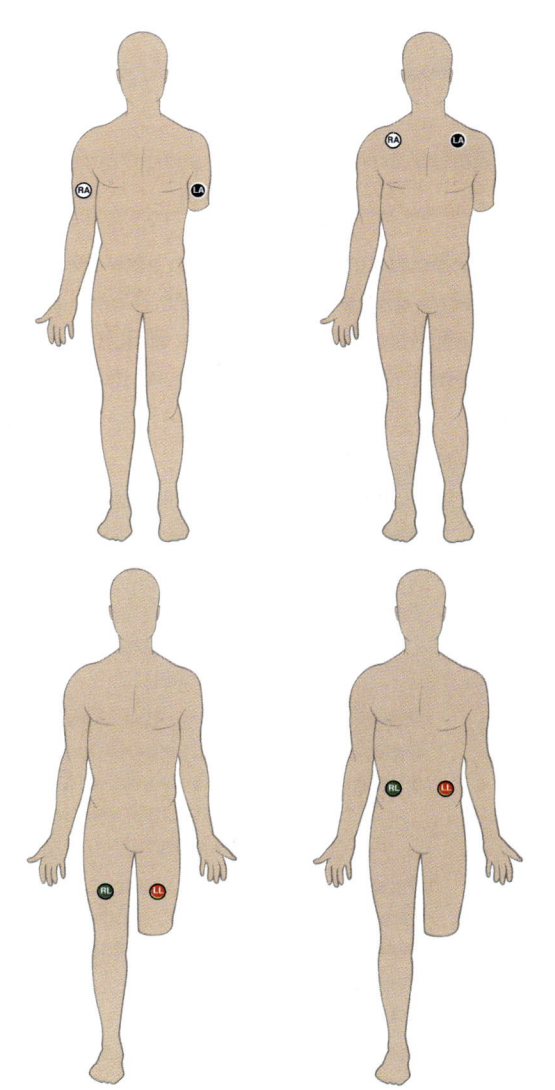

Fig. 7-9. In the case of a patient with an amputation, the electrodes may be moved closer to the torso or may be placed on the torso rather than on the limbs. The limb electrodes on the unaffected side should mirror the electrodes on the affected side.

Scar tissue or injury on the chest wall: The EKG technician should not place electrodes on scar tissue from a mastectomy or other chest wall surgery. Scar tissue can be fragile and may be injured when the electrode is removed. Instead, electrodes should be placed as close as possible to the standard locations (Fig. 7-10).

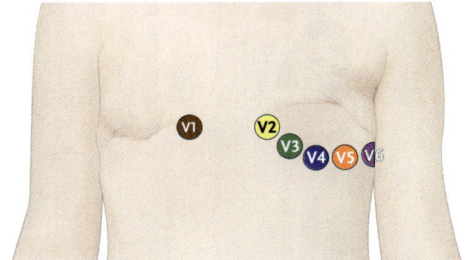

Fig. 7-10. *Electrodes can be placed around mastectomy scars and other scar tissue from chest surgery.*

Medical implants: Electrodes should not be placed over implanted medical equipment, such as a pacemaker, or over breast implants. Instead, the EKG technician should place the electrodes to the side of the implant. They should be as close as possible to the standard positions.

Large breasts: If a patient has large breasts, the breast tissue should be moved away from the electrode site as much as possible. This allows placement of the electrodes on the chest wall. The technician should explain the process to the patient and confirm the patient's consent. The patient can lift her own breast tissue or the technician can move the breast using the back of her hand. The electrodes should be placed close to standard positions. They should not be placed on top of breast tissue.

Pediatric patients: Electrode placement is different for some pediatric patients (Fig. 7-11). Children under 2 require a right-sided EKG (the same electrode placement used for dextrocardia). For children from 2–12, the standard 12-lead electrode placement is used for all electrodes except for V4. The V4 electrode is moved to the right side of the chest at the fifth intercostal space at the midclavicular line. This placement is called V4R.

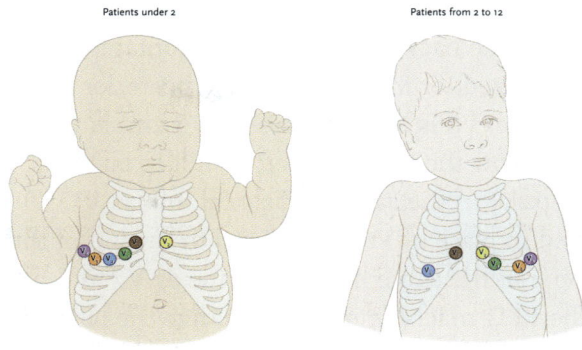

Fig. 7-11. *Pediatric patients have electrodes applied differently than adult patients.*

These adjustments are needed because the right ventricle extends past the right side of the sternum in small children. The EKG technician should label the EKG tracing to note this change. The technician should check with the provider if she does not know which electrode placement to use for a child. Small children may be calmer in a parent's or guardian's arms during an EKG.

Posterior EKG

Sometimes a doctor will ask to have an EKG done using posterior leads. This can help diagnose a type of heart attack called an *inferior wall myocardial infarction*. The EKG technician uses the lead wires commonly used for V4, V5, and V6 and places the electrodes on the patient's back. These locations are called V7, V8, and V9 (Fig. 7-12). The patient is seated while the electrodes are placed on her back. She is then put in the supine position, as usual, for the EKG test itself.

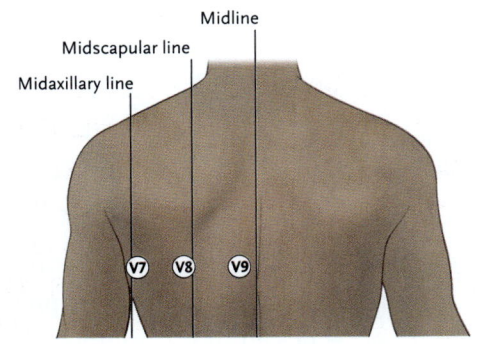

Fig. 7-12. *In a posterior EKG, V7 takes the place of V4, V8 takes the place of V5, and V9 takes the place of V6.*

V7 is used in place of V4. It is located on the left side of the back in the same horizontal line normally used for V4–V6, along the posterior axillary line. V8 is used in place of V5 and is placed just below the tip of the left shoulder blade (scapula) in the same horizontal line as V7. V9 is used in place of V6. It is placed to the left of the spine in the same horizontal line as V7 and V8. The EKG machine may not change the labels on the EKG tracing for a posterior EKG. It is very important for the EKG technician to label the EKG as a posterior EKG (Fig. 7-13).

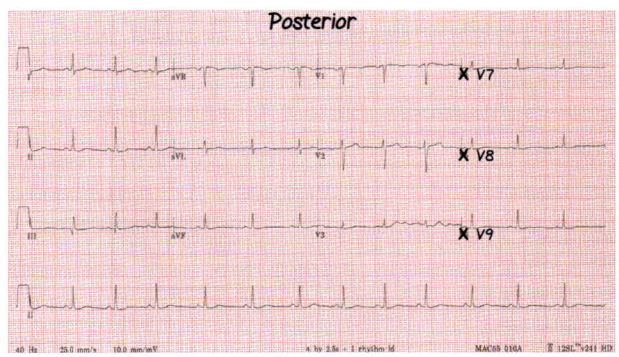

Fig. 7-13. The tracing from a posterior EKG must be clearly marked. Leads V4, V5, and V6 should be crossed out and replaced with V7, V8, and V9 and POSTERIOR written at the top.

Tip

Electrode Placement Adaptations

It is not possible to describe every situation that would change EKG electrode placement. In general, limb electrodes should mirror each other. If the left arm electrode is placed on the left upper arm, the right arm electrode should be placed on the right upper arm. Sometimes it is not possible to reach standard electrode sites. A cast, an injury, or scar tissue may be located where an electrode is usually placed. Electrodes should be placed as close to the standard sites as possible. In the very unusual case that a patient's chest is not accessible, electrodes may be placed on the back. If an EKG technician is unsure about where to place electrodes, he should ask the provider who ordered the test.

Alternate patient positions are also sometimes needed. A patient who is over 6 months pregnant should not be placed in the supine position for an EKG. Lying down in the supine position could cause the fetus to compress the patient's vena cava. This reduces blood return to the heart. The patient could become weak and possibly faint. A pregnant patient should lie down and be tilted slightly (at a 15-degree angle) to the left (Fig. 7-14). A rolled-up blanket or pillow can help make the patient more comfortable.

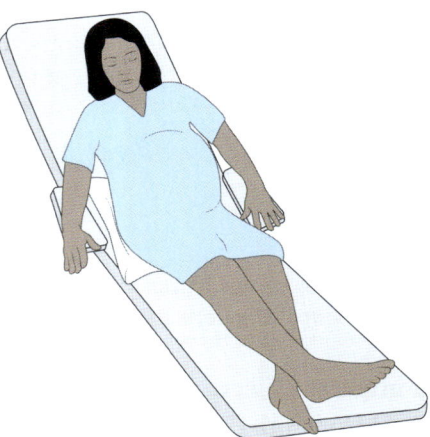

Fig. 7-14. The EKG technician should assist pregnant patients into a modified position, lying down and tilted to the left side.

A patient with respiratory or heart problems may not be comfortable in a supine position for the EKG. If a patient has orthopnea, they should be placed in a semi-Fowler's position (45-degree angle). This will help them breathe during the test (Figure 2-27 in Chapter 2).

Quick Reference

Situation	Placement suggestion
Dextrocardia	Place electrodes and lead wires on right side of chest in same locations as normally used on the left side of the chest.
Limb amputation	Place the electrode on the remaining part of the limb or on the torso near the missing extremity. Place the corresponding electrode on the opposite side in the same location.
Injured extremity	Place the electrode on the closest intact area of the limb or on the torso near the injured extremity. Place the corresponding electrode on the opposite side in the same location.

Mastectomy, implanted pacemaker, or chest wall surgery	Do not place the electrodes on the surgical scar. Place on intact skin as close as possible to regular position.
Breast implants	Place electrodes in regular positions or as close as possible to regular positions. Do not place on skin over implant.
Posterior EKG	Move V4, V5, and V6 electrodes to posterior positions on the left side of the patient's back (V7, V8, and V9).
Large breasts	Use the back of the hand or ask the patient to lift the breast up so the electrode can be placed on the chest wall. Do not place the electrode on top of the breast.
Pediatric patients	Under 2 years old: Place electrodes and lead wires on right side of the chest in same locations as normally used on the left side of the chest. Over 2 years old: Place electrodes in usual locations for 12-lead EKG except V4. Place V4 on right side of chest at fifth intercostal space, midclavicular line. An infant or child can be placed in the arms of parent/guardian to calm him during the EKG.
Pregnancy (past the 6th month)	Place electrodes in regular positions or as close as possible to regular positions. Patient needs to be placed slightly tilted to left side to avoid pressure on the vessels returning blood to the heart.
Orthopnea	Elevate head of exam table or bed to semi-Fowler's position (45-degree angle).

4. Identify sources of information for EKG machine troubleshooting and maintenance

EKG machines should have a user's manual that includes information on safety, operation, setup, cleaning, troubleshooting, and maintenance. Many companies offer free downloads of their manuals online. Some also offer a telephone or internet chat helpline. Some facilities store manuals in an office or work area and others make them available online. Not following the manufacturer's instructions could cause patient injury or damage to the machine.

The EKG technician is usually responsible for basic troubleshooting of EKG machines. This includes checking the battery, checking the paper supply, and making sure supplies have not expired. She may also do basic troubleshooting based on information in the user's manual. If this does not resolve a problem, the machine should be taken out of service until it is fixed. Facilities usually have a backup EKG machine available. If the facility does not have backup equipment, patient appointments may need to be rescheduled.

Most medical facilities have policies and procedures for reporting problems with equipment and for taking equipment out of service. The EKG technician may need to place an *Out of Service* or *Defective* tag on the equipment and/or take it to a different area for service or repair. EKG machines should only be serviced and repaired by approved workers. Proper use, storage, and maintenance reduce the need for repairs.

Chapter Review

- *Artifact* is any interference or distortion that appears in an EKG tracing. Tracings with artifact may be impossible for a provider to read.

- EKG technicians should recognize several types of artifact: somatic tremor, wandering baseline, electrical (also called AC or 60-cycle) interference, and broken recording (also called interrupted baseline). Recognizing and correcting artifact helps create a readable EKG tracing.

- Patient conditions or age may also require changes or adaptations. Patients who have amputated limbs, injuries, or scars affecting the standard electrode placement sites, implanted medical devices, or a condition called *dextrocardia* need alternate placement of some electrodes. Pediatric patients also require alternate electrode placement. Different locations are used for children under 2 and for children between 2–12.

- A provider may order a posterior EKG if she suspects a certain type of heart attack. The electrodes/lead wires usually used for V4, V5, and V6 are placed on the patient's back in positions called V7, V8, and V9. These changes must be noted on the patient's EKG tracing.

- Patients who are more than 6 months pregnant and patients who have trouble breathing when lying down flat should not be placed in the supine position for EKG testing.

- Manufacturers' instructions and facility procedures should always be followed when troubleshooting an EKG machine.

8
The Cardiac Conduction System and EKG Tracings

1. Explain the difference between the mechanical and electrical activity of the heart

Both healthy mechanical function and healthy electrical function are needed for the heart to work properly. The mechanical function of the heart has to do with the heart muscle, heart valves, blood supply, and blood vessels. The electrical function has to do with special tissue in the heart that controls the mechanical function. This tissue begins, or *initiates*, electrical impulses. It then *conducts*, or carries, these electrical impulses through the heart. These impulses are the "spark" that triggers the mechanical actions of the heart muscle.

Cardiac output is the amount of blood, measured in liters, that the heart pumps each minute. It is determined by how much blood is pumped with each heartbeat (stroke volume) and how many times the heart beats each minute (heart rate). Cardiac output must be high enough to carry oxygen and nutrients to all parts of the body.

Both mechanical and electrical problems can affect cardiac output. For example, if electrical impulses are firing very rapidly, the heart's chambers do not have time to fill completely. Cardiac output goes down because there is less blood in the chambers to pump. In this example, an electrical problem in the heart (very rapid impulses) is creating a mechanical problem (not enough blood being pumped out).

The chart below gives examples of how different problems (the medical term is *abnormalities*) can affect how the heart works. Abnormalities in the electrical system of the heart are described in more detail in the next chapter.

Quick Reference

Component	Abnormality	Effect
Mechanical	Severe blood loss	Heart muscle, vessels, and electrical system intact but there is not enough blood to pump
Mechanical	Myocardial infarction (heart attack)	Part of heart muscle dies or is injured so heart cannot pump effectively
Electrical	Absent or extremely slow heart rate	Slow or no electrical impulses fired to prompt heart muscle contraction, which causes lower cardiac output
Electrical	Abnormally rapid rhythms	Rapidly firing electrical impulses do not allow the ventricles time to fill, which causes lower cardiac output

Three things are needed for the heart to pump enough blood to the body. The heart's electrical system must be working properly. The heart muscle and valves must be healthy. There must be enough blood and an intact (complete) vascular system.

2. Explain the electrical conduction system of the heart

The electrical impulses that control the heart's pumping action are arranged in a pathway called the **cardiac conduction system**. This system starts in the upper part of the right atrium. It continues through the heart to the walls of the ventricles (Fig. 8-1). The timing of the electrical impulses makes sure that contractions happen in an organized way. Each part of the cardiac conduction system conducts electrical impulses at its own particular rate, called an **intrinsic rate**. These different rates, specific to each area, ensure that the blood moves through the heart in the correct pattern.

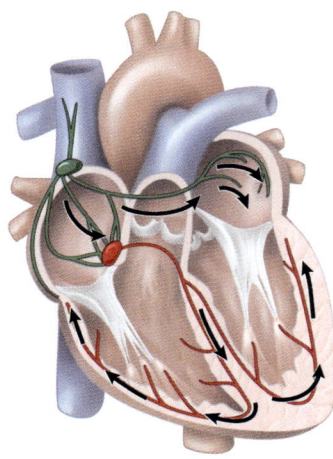

Fig. 8-1. The arrows show the direction of the electrical impulses in the heart.

The **sinoatrial node**, also called the *SA node* or *sinus node*, is in the upper part of the right atrium. It is the main, or primary, **pacemaker** of the heart. This means it sets the timing of the heart's contractions. The sympathetic and parasympathetic nervous systems are both involved in controlling the heart rate. Heart rate can change based on a person's situation and surroundings. The normal firing rate—the intrinsic rate—for the SA node is 60–100 beats per minute (BPM). Sympathetic stimulation (for example, a response to fear or anxiety) can increase the rate to as high as 180 BPM.

From the SA node, the electrical impulse moves to the **atrioventricular node**, also called the *AV node*. The AV node is at the bottom of the right atrium, behind the tricuspid valve. As the impulse enters the AV node it is slowed down by a tenth of a second. Without this delay the atria and ventricles would contract at the same time. Instead, this delay allows the atria to empty and the ventricles to fill before they contract. The intrinsic rate of the AV node is 40–60 BPM.

The electrical impulse then moves through an area known as the **atrioventricular (AV) junction** to the **bundle of His**, or *AV bundle*. The bundle of His is located in the upper part of the wall between the left and right ventricles. This wall is called the interventricular septum. The intrinsic rate of the bundle of His can range from less than 20 BPM to 40–60 BPM.

The bundle of His divides into the right and left **bundle branches**. These branches carry the electrical impulse to the walls of the ventricles. The bundle branches divide into smaller and smaller branches and then form the **Purkinje fibers**. The Purkinje fibers have an intrinsic rate of 20–40 BPM (Fig. 8-2).

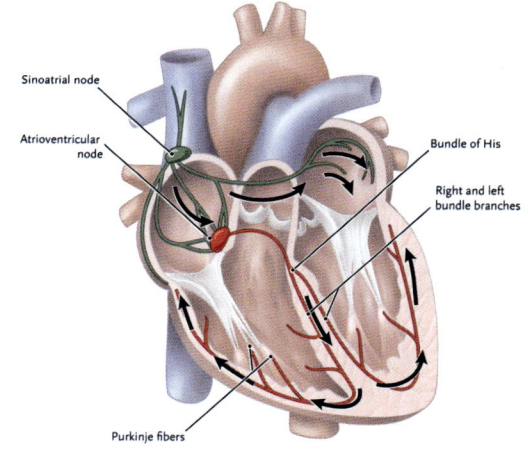

Fig. 8-2. When the heart is healthy, electrical impulses are conducted through these areas and in this pattern. They cause the heart muscles to contract in a regular rhythm and pump blood.

Although the SA node is the primary pacemaker of the heart, other areas of the conduction system can initiate an impulse if the SA node fails. These other areas may also initiate impulses in response to a problem in the heart. For example, lack of oxygen may cause an area to become **irritable**. This means it is more likely to initiate an impulse at the wrong time.

Quick Reference			
Structure	**Location**	**Function**	**Intrinsic rate**
Sinoatrial (SA) node	Upper right atrial wall	Primary pacemaker	60–100 BPM
Atrioventricular (AV) node	Bottom of right atrium behind tricuspid valve	Delays impulse from SA node and relays to bundle of His	40–60 BPM
Bundle of His (AV bundle)	Upper interventricular septum	Relays impulse to right and left bundle branches	40–60 BPM*
Right and left bundle branches	Interventricular septum	Relay impulses to Purkinje fibers	40–60 BPM*
Purkinje fibers	Ventricular myocardium	Relay impulses to ventricular myocardium	20–40 BPM

*Some sources list the intrinsic rates of the bundle of His and bundle branches as low as 20–40 BPM.

3. Understand the features of an EKG tracing

Chapter 5 describes how an EKG machine works. Before learning about the different parts of an EKG tracing, it is important to review this material. The electrical activity of the heart creates changes to the cardiac cells that cause them to contract and relax. These changes are called depolarization and repolarization. During depolarization the cells become more positively charged and they contract. During repolarization they become more negatively charged and they relax, or return to a resting state.

An EKG machine records the voltage, or difference in electrical charge, created by depolarization and repolarization. Graph paper moves through the machine at a controlled speed, creating the EKG tracing (Fig. 8-3). Trained providers read, or interpret, these tracings. Because the electrical activity of the heart prompts the mechanical activity of the heart, EKG tracings make it possible to see problems with a patient's cardiac function.

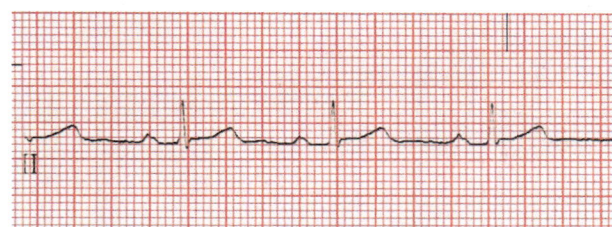

Fig. 8-3. This is an example of a clear, accurate EKG tracing.

Interpreting an EKG tracing (also called an *EKG strip*) is beyond the scope of practice for an EKG technician. The EKG technician's job is to generate a good tracing. To do this, EKG technicians need to know what a tracing should look like and what each part of the tracing shows.

EKG features are shown in Figure 8-4 and described in the Quick Reference chart that follows. The **isoelectric line**, also called the *baseline*, is the straight line between the upward and downward movements on the EKG strip. Those upward and downward movements are called **waves**. A *deflection*, or movement, upward from the isoelectric line is a positive wave. A deflection downward is a negative wave. The area between two waves, where the EKG goes back to the baseline, is called a **segment**. A wave and a segment taken together form an **interval**. Several waves considered together are called a **complex**. The term **morphology** is used to describe the shape and direction of waves, complexes, and segments on an EKG tracing.

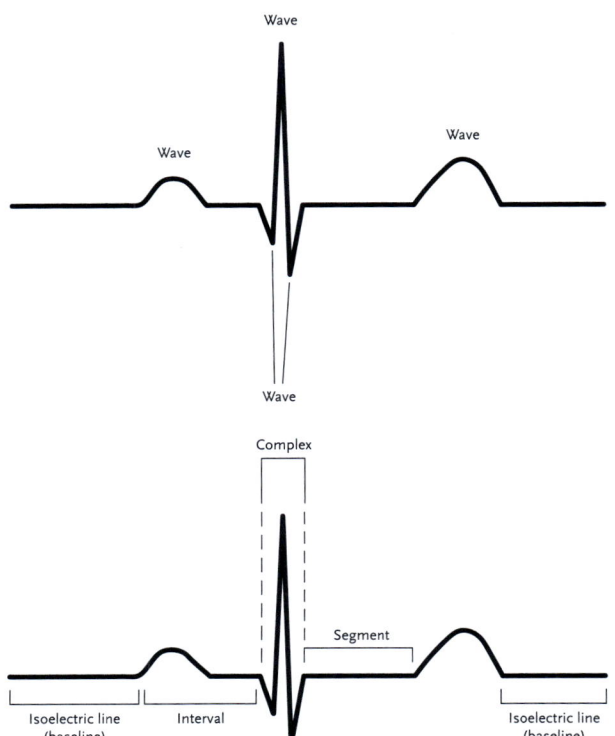

Fig. 8-4. *The isoelectric line, waves, segments, intervals, and complexes are the essential features of the EKG.*

Quick Reference	
Feature	**Definition**
Isoelectric line (baseline)	Flat portion of EKG tracing
Wave	Deflection or movement away from the isoelectric line • Positive is upward • Negative is downward
Segment	Isoelectric area between two waves
Interval	Wave plus a segment
Complex	Several waves that are measured together

When the heart is functioning normally, the EKG shows a pattern called **normal sinus rhythm** (NSR). Chapter 9 contains more detail on NSR and other rhythms. This chapter describes the basic features of an EKG tracing using NSR, showing how each part of the tracing matches up to the mechanical action of a healthy heart.

Normal sinus rhythm on an EKG can look different from person to person. It also looks different in different leads on the same person. However, it will include some version of each of the features described in this learning objective. The basic features of a normal EKG complex in lead II—the view commonly used for routine monitoring—are shown in Figure 8-5. Each part of the tracing is given a letter name that is used to label and describe waves, intervals, and complexes in EKG analysis. These letters do not stand for words or have meaning. They are just labels to refer to the features of the EKG.

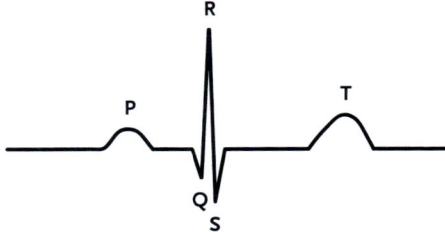

Fig. 8-5. *This image represents a normal sinus rhythm EKG. Each wave is named by a letter. P, Q, R, S, and T waves are the waves most commonly seen.*

Tip

U Waves

Not all EKG waves appear in every EKG tracing. Some waves only appear in certain conditions. Some blend in with other waves and are hard to see. One wave only visible on some EKGs is the U wave. The normal U wave is a small, rounded wave that comes after the T wave and is shorter than the T wave (Fig. 8-6). If the U wave is large it may indicate that the patient has a low potassium level. If the U wave is negative or inverted (goes down from the isoelectric line), it can be a sign of heart disease or an MI. As always, if an EKG technician has a concern about something that appears on a patient's EKG, she should bring it to the provider's attention.

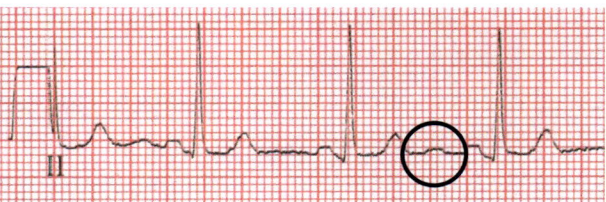

Fig. 8-6. *The U wave does not always appear, but when it does appear it falls after the T wave.*

When the heart is working properly, there is a correlation between the electrical and mechanical actions of the heart. In other words, each electrical change matches up with a mechanical action (as shown in the Quick Reference chart below). The **P wave** is the first positive deflection, or upward movement, in the complex. It represents atrial depolarization. The mechanical activity related to the P wave is contraction of the atria.

The **QRS complex** is made up of three waves:

- The Q wave is the first negative deflection, or downward movement, after the P wave (though it is not always seen in all leads)
- The R wave is the next positive deflection
- The S wave is the next negative deflection

The QRS complex represents ventricular depolarization. The related mechanical action is the contraction of the ventricles. The **T wave** comes after the QRS complex. It shows ventricular repolarization. When this happens, the ventricles relax.

Quick Reference

EKG feature	Electrical activity	Mechanical activity
P wave	Atrial depolarization	Contraction of the atria
QRS complex	Ventricular depolarization	Contraction of the ventricles
T wave	Ventricular repolarization	Relaxation of the ventricles

Tip

Important EKG Changes

The appearance of different waves and complexes gives providers important information. Because the P wave is related to the contraction of the atria, for example, changes in the P wave could be due to a problem like atrial enlargement. Abnormal QRS complexes could indicate a problem with the ventricles. This is one reason EKG technicians need to know the normal appearance of these features. Changes may be signs of serious problems.

4. Identify important intervals and segments on the EKG tracing and list normal measurements

Several intervals and segments are important to observe and measure when reading an EKG. These include the **PR interval**, **QRS interval** (the time associated with the QRS complex), **R-R interval**, and **ST segment** (Fig. 8-7). The graph paper used for EKGs allows a provider or other trained person to measure the amount of time associated with each feature. The measurement of an interval starts from the point where the wave first leaves the baseline. It continues to the point where the next wave leaves the baseline. The measurement of a segment starts from the point where a wave ends (returns to the baseline). It stops where the next wave begins (leaves the baseline). The next learning objective has more detail on how these measurements are made.

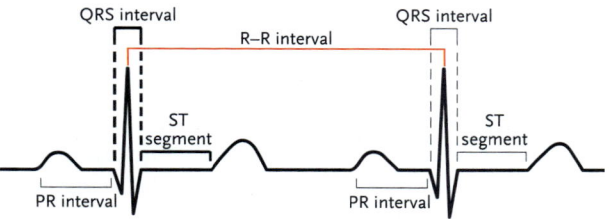

Fig. 8-7. The PR interval, QRS interval, R-R interval, and ST segment are some of the most important features to recognize and measure in an EKG tracing.

Quick Reference

Interval or Segment	Definition	Normal
PR interval	From the beginning of the P wave to the beginning of the QRS complex; this may be the Q wave or the R wave, as Q does not always appear	0.12–0.20 s

QRS interval	Combination of the Q, R, and S waves; measured from where the Q or R wave first leaves the baseline to where the S wave returns to baseline	Less than 0.12 s
R-R interval	Distance between the peak of the R wave of one complex and the peak of the R wave of the next complex	Should be regular
ST segment	From the end of QRS, where the S wave returns to the baseline, to the beginning of the T wave	Should stay at baseline, not deviating above or below

Take Action Now!

EKG technicians should also be familiar with the QT interval. It starts at the beginning of the Q wave and ends when the T wave returns to the baseline. This interval represents the complete cycle of depolarization and repolarization of the ventricles. The normal range for the QT interval differs based on the gender of the patient and the patient's heart rate. It is usually between 0.36 and 0.44 seconds long.

A QT interval that is too long or too short can be a sign of cardiac problems. Analysis of the QT interval is beyond the scope of practice for an EKG technician, but EKG technicians should know that it is an important measurement. QT intervals that are unusually long or unusually short should be reported to a provider.

5. Demonstrate the measurement of time on the EKG tracing using small and large blocks

The electrical and mechanical actions of the heart must happen with correct timing. This helps maintain healthy heart function. EKG graph paper can be used to measure the timing of each EKG feature. The paper is divided into small blocks measuring 1 millimeter (mm)

high and 1 mm wide. Each small block on the horizontal axis (the line going from left to right) represents 0.04 seconds. There is a darker line every fifth block, both vertically and horizontally. These darker lines form larger blocks (Fig. 8-8). Each large block measures 5 mm high and 5 mm wide. A large block on the horizontal axis represents 0.20 seconds (5 × 0.04). Many EKGs also mark 1-, 3-, and 6-second intervals along the top of the paper.

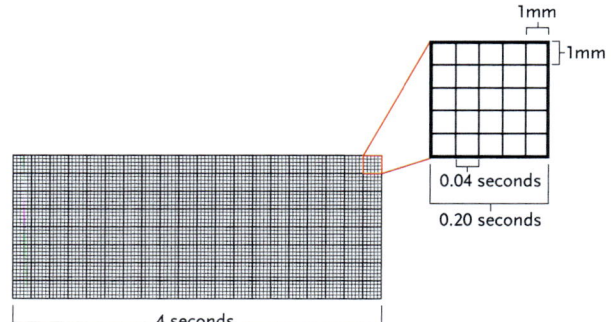

Fig. 8-8. *EKG graph paper is printed with small blocks and large blocks. Measuring the features on an EKG tracing can measure the time involved in the heart's actions.*

6. List the 6 steps used to analyze an EKG tracing

EKG analysis and any related diagnosis is the job of a provider. EKG technicians are responsible for generating a good tracing. They should also know how to recognize potentially dangerous rhythms and take the right action. Because of these responsibilities it is important for EKG technicians to understand the basics of EKG analysis.

EKG tracings show a series of complexes that must be measured and analyzed to determine a heart rhythm. *Heart rhythm* and *heart rate* may sound like the same thing, but they are not. The **heart rhythm** is the overall pattern of the heartbeat. The **heart rate** is the speed at which the heart is beating.

Five pieces of information are needed to analyze a heart rhythm. These are shown in steps 1–5 below. The sixth step is the naming, or identification, of the type of rhythm seen on the tracing. At least six seconds' worth of cardiac activity, or 30 large blocks on an EKG tracing, is needed to accurately analyze a heart rhythm.

Quick Reference

Steps to Analyze Heart Rhythm
1. Determine heart rate in beats per minute (BPM).
2. Check the rhythm for regularity (a clear pattern or lack of pattern).
3. Note presence or absence of identical P wave before each QRS interval.
4. Measure length of PR interval.
5. Measure length of QRS interval.
6. Identify the rhythm.

These steps are always used to analyze and identify heart rhythms. The next several learning objectives describe how to gather the information needed for steps 1 through 5. Chapter 9 addresses the final step: how to identify different heart rhythms using this information.

7. Discuss the first step in analyzing heart rhythms: three methods to determine heart rate from the EKG tracing

The first step in analyzing heart rhythms is to determine the heart rate. There are three methods that can be used. The quickest method is called the **6-second method**. The technician counts the number of complete QRS complexes in a 6-second section (Fig. 8-9). That number is then multiplied by 10 to get an approximate number of beats per minute. This is the only method that can be used on rhythms that are irregular (Fig. 8-10).

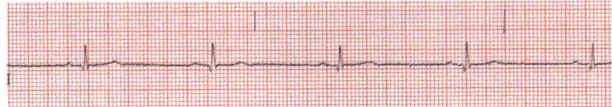

Fig. 8-9. Illustration of a regular 6-second strip. Because 5 QRS complexes are visible, the heart rate is 50 BPM.

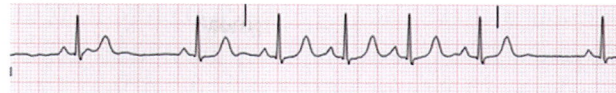

Fig. 8-10. Illustration of an irregular 6-second strip. Because 7 QRS complexes are visible, the heart rate is 70 BPM.

The second method for determining heart rate is called the **large block method**. To use the large block method, the EKG technician finds two consecutive R waves (R waves that are next to each other) and counts the number of large blocks between them. This number corresponds to a particular heart rate, as shown in the chart below.

Quick Reference

Number of large blocks	Corresponding heart rate (BPM)
1	300
2	150
3	100
4	75
5	60
6	50

Figure 8-11 shows an EKG strip with each large block marked to show the heart rate associated with a second R wave at that location. In this strip the second R wave appears with almost 4 large blocks between it and the first R wave. This means the heart rate is close to 75 BPM.

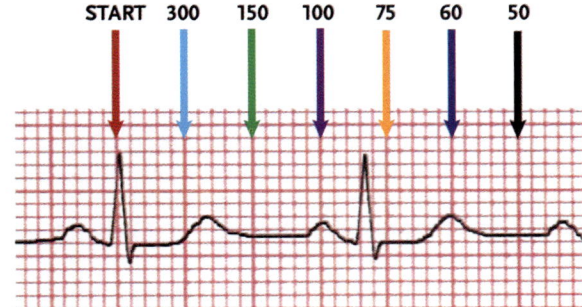

Fig. 8-11. The large block method considers the number of large boxes between R waves.

The chart shown here simplifies the large block method, but this method can also be used without a chart. Each large block represents 0.20 seconds. This means that there are 300 large blocks in a 1-minute EKG strip (60 ÷ 0.20 = 300). The heart rates on the chart are found by dividing the number of large blocks between R waves into 300. Since there are 300 large blocks in a 1-minute section of the EKG, this shows the number of R waves in 1 minute of activity. The method is also called the *300 method*.

The third method for determining heart rate is the **small block method**. This method uses the 1500 small blocks in a one-minute EKG strip to calculate heart rate. It is also called the *1500 method*. The first step in this method is to count the small blocks between any two consecutive R waves. The example in Figure 8-12 shows 13 small blocks between R waves. The second step is to divide 1500 by this number, rounding up or down as needed. Using the numbers shown in Figure 8-12, 1500 ÷ 13 = 115.38. This can be rounded down to 115 BPM.

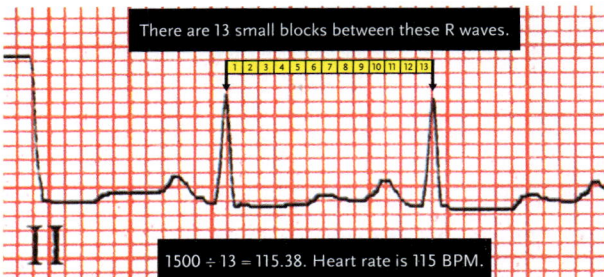

Fig. 8-12. The small block method considers the number of small boxes between R waves.

Tip

Ventricular and Atrial Rates

The methods described in this learning objective are used to calculate the heart's *ventricular rate*. This is the number of times the ventricles contract each minute. All of these methods look at QRS complexes or the distance between R waves because these features represent electrical activity in the ventricles. In most cases, finding the ventricular rate is all that is needed. For some rhythms, though, it might be necessary to find both the ventricular rate and the *atrial rate*. This is the number of times the atria are contracting each minute. Any time there is not a QRS complex following every P wave, the atrial and ventricular rates will be different. Measuring atrial rate involves counting the number of P waves in a 6-second strip and then multiplying by 10. Chapter 9 describes the cardiac rhythms, including which ones have different atrial and ventricular rates.

8. Discuss the second step in analyzing heart rhythms: how to examine an EKG tracing for regularity

The second step in analyzing heart rhythms is to examine the strip for regularity. QRS complexes are categorized as **regular**, **irregular**, or **regularly irregular**. In a regular heart rhythm, QRS complexes occur in a pattern that looks the same each time. The pattern repeats with consistent timing (Fig. 8-13). In an irregular heart rhythm, the QRS complexes may look alike or different from each other. They do not repeat with consistent timing (Fig. 8-14). In a regularly irregular rhythm the QRS complexes may or may not look alike, but they appear in a clear, repeating pattern (Fig. 8-15).

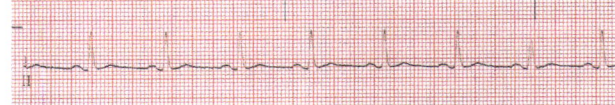

Fig. 8-13. EKG strip showing a regular heart rhythm.

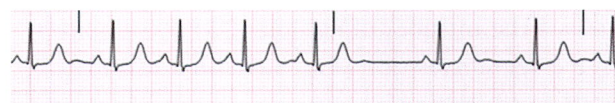

Fig. 8-14. EKG strip showing an irregular heart rhythm.

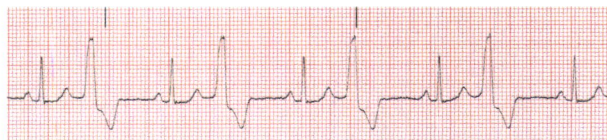

Fig. 8-15. EKG strip showing a regularly irregular heart rhythm.

Tip

Irregularities

The different categories used to describe the regularity of heart rhythms can be confusing. The key is to see if there is a clear pattern to the rhythm. A regular rhythm has a clear and repeating pattern with consistent timing. A regularly irregular rhythm also has a clear and repeating pattern, but that pattern includes abnormal elements. An irregular rhythm may also be called *irregularly irregular* since there is no pattern to the irregularity.

An abnormal heartbeat may come either too early or too late. It is important to know how to tell the difference. This can be done using either paper scraps and pen or pencil or by using a tool called **calipers**. Calipers have two adjustable arms and fine points at the end of each arm (Fig. 8-16). They can be used to measure EKG features.

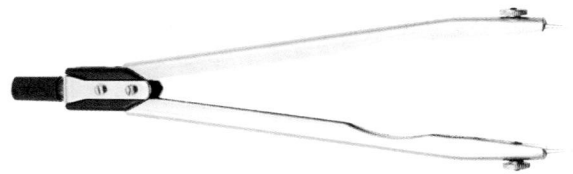

Fig. 8-16. *Calipers have adjustable arms for measuring different EKG intervals and complexes.*

The illustrations in Figure 8-17 show how to check for early or late beats using calipers. First, the distance between the two R waves of a normal beat is measured. Then, the left point of the caliper is placed at the peak of the last R wave before the abnormal beat. If the abnormal beat comes before the right point of the caliper, the beat is early. If it comes after the right point of the caliper, it is late.

This can also be checked by making marks on the edge of a piece of scrap paper, showing the R-R interval of a normal beat. The first mark on the scrap paper is lined up with the last R wave before the abnormal beat. If the abnormal beat comes before the second mark on the scrap paper, the beat is early. If it comes after the second mark on the scrap paper, the beat is late (Fig. 8-18).

Measurement between two normal R waves (a normal R-R interval)

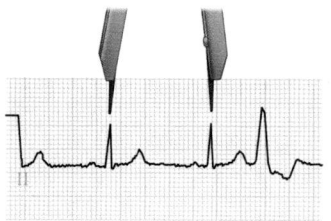

An early beat

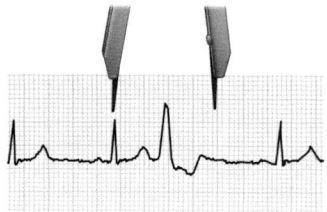

Measurement between two normal R waves (a normal R-R interval)

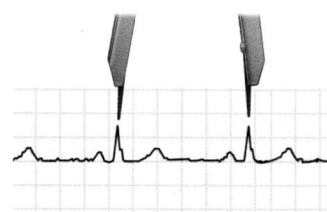

A late beat

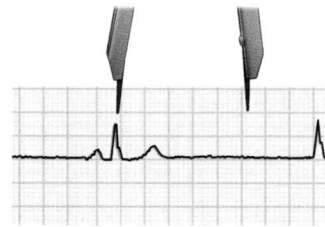

Fig. 8-17. *Calipers can be used to see if an abnormal beat is early or late.*

A normal R-R interval

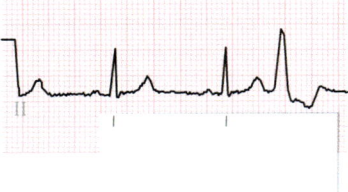

An early beat

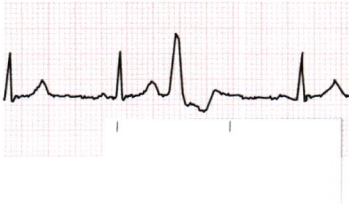

A normal R-R interval

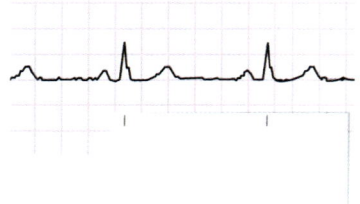

A late beat

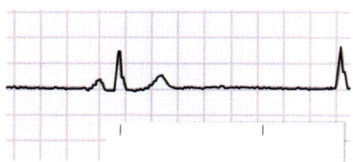

Fig. 8-18. A piece of scrap paper and a pencil can also be used to check for early or late beats.

9. Discuss the third step in analyzing heart rhythms: examining the P wave on an EKG tracing

The third step in analyzing the heart rhythm involves looking closely at the P waves. The P wave is the first positive deflection, or upward movement, from the baseline. An EKG showing a normal heart rhythm has a rounded P wave before every QRS complex. In some abnormal heart rhythms the P wave is missing. It may also be shaped differently (not rounded) or may not be associated with the QRS complex (Fig. 8-19). The EKG technician must observe whether the P wave appears and note its size and shape.

Normal P wave

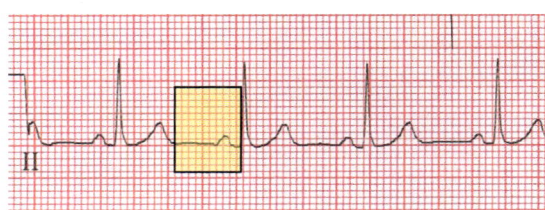

Absent P wave

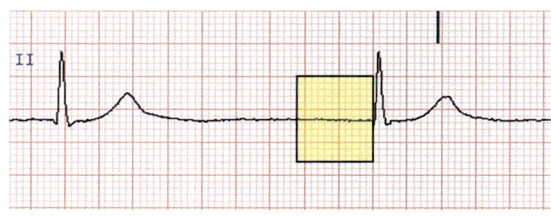

Abnormal P waves

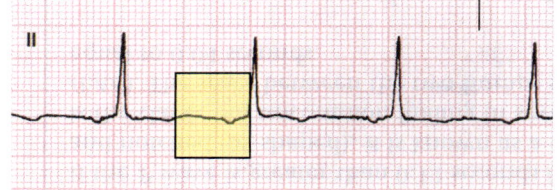

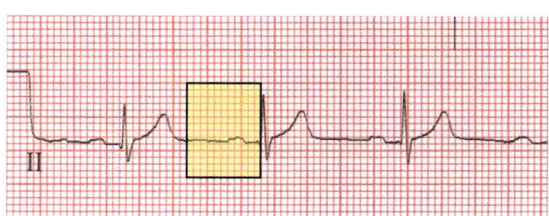

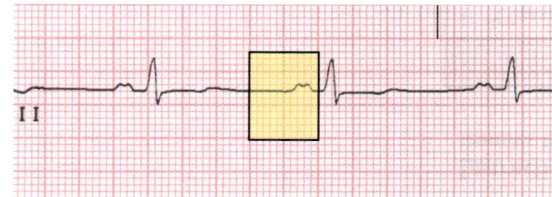

Fig. 8-19. The P wave should appear before the QRS complex. In some rhythms it does not appear or has an unusual appearance.

10. Discuss the fourth step in analyzing heart rhythms: measuring the PR interval on an EKG tracing

The fourth step in analyzing heart rhythms is to measure the PR interval. Measurement of the PR interval starts at the beginning of the P wave—where it leaves the baseline—to the beginning of the QRS complex. (The QRS complex begins where it first leaves the baseline.) This measurement can be made using calipers or scrap paper. After measuring the length of the PR interval, its duration (length of time) can be determined. Either the left caliper point or the first mark on the paper should be lined up with a dark line on the EKG graph paper. This makes it easier to count the number of small boxes between points. To find the duration of the PR interval, this number is multiplied by 0.04 (Figs. 8-20 and 8-21). The normal range for the PR interval is 0.12–0.20 seconds.

Find and measure the PR interval

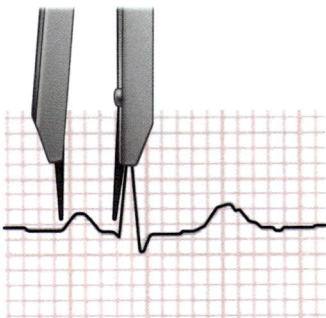

This interval is four small blocks long, which means its duration is 0.16 seconds (4 x 0.04 = 0.16)

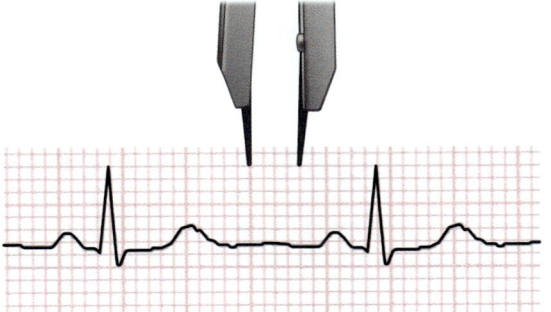

Fig. 8-20. *Determining the length of the PR interval using calipers.*

Mark the length of the PR interval on a piece of paper

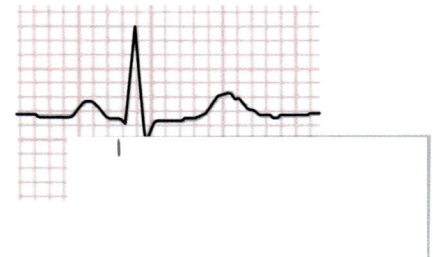

This interval is four small blocks long, which means its duration is 0.16 seconds (4 x 0.04 = 0.16)

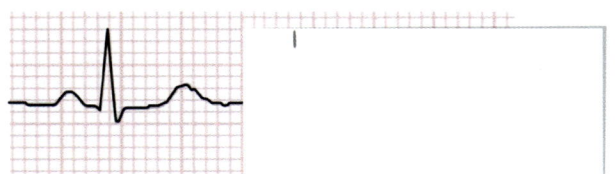

Fig. 8-21. *Determining the length of the PR interval using paper.*

Since P waves and QRS complexes look different from person to person, finding these measurement points takes practice. Measuring several PR intervals on the same strip is a good way to check that measurements are correct. Many abnormal heart rhythms have no measurable PR intervals. If a PR interval is not measurable, that fact should be documented as part of the rhythm analysis. These rhythms are discussed in the next chapter.

PRACTICE

Measure the PR interval in the following complexes.

1. 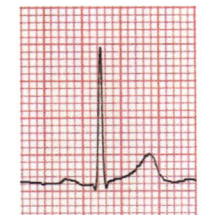 PR interval: _____ seconds

2. 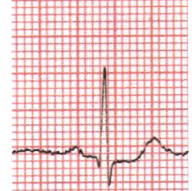 PR interval: _____ seconds

3. 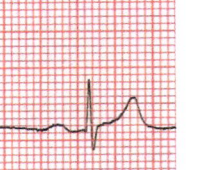 PR interval: _____ seconds

4. 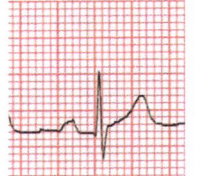 PR interval: _____ seconds

5. 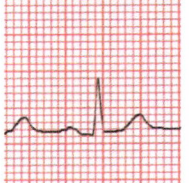 PR interval: _____ seconds

6. 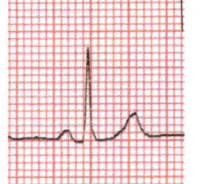 PR interval: _____ seconds

7. 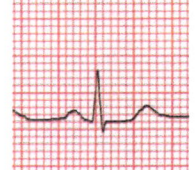 PR interval: _____ seconds

8. 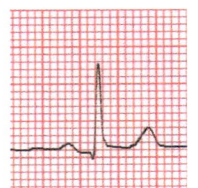 PR interval: _____ seconds

9. 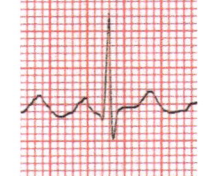 PR interval: _____ seconds

10. 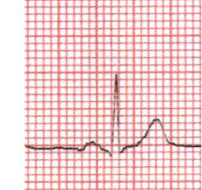 PR interval: _____ seconds

11. Discuss the fifth step in analyzing heart rhythms: measuring the QRS complex on an EKG tracing

The fifth step in heart rhythm analysis is measuring the duration of the QRS complex. This measurement is taken from the point where the first wave of the complex leaves the isoelectric line to the point where the last wave begins to level, or flatten out (Fig. 8-22). The name *QRS complex* can be misleading. QRS complexes do not always have all of these waves. The QRS complex can look very different from one tracing or rhythm to another. Mastering measurement takes a lot of practice. The methods shown for measuring PR interval—calipers and paper—can also be used to measure QRS complexes. The normal value for the duration of the QRS complex is less than 0.12 seconds (<0.12 s). Values between 0.10 s and 0.12 s may be considered slightly prolonged, but not abnormal.

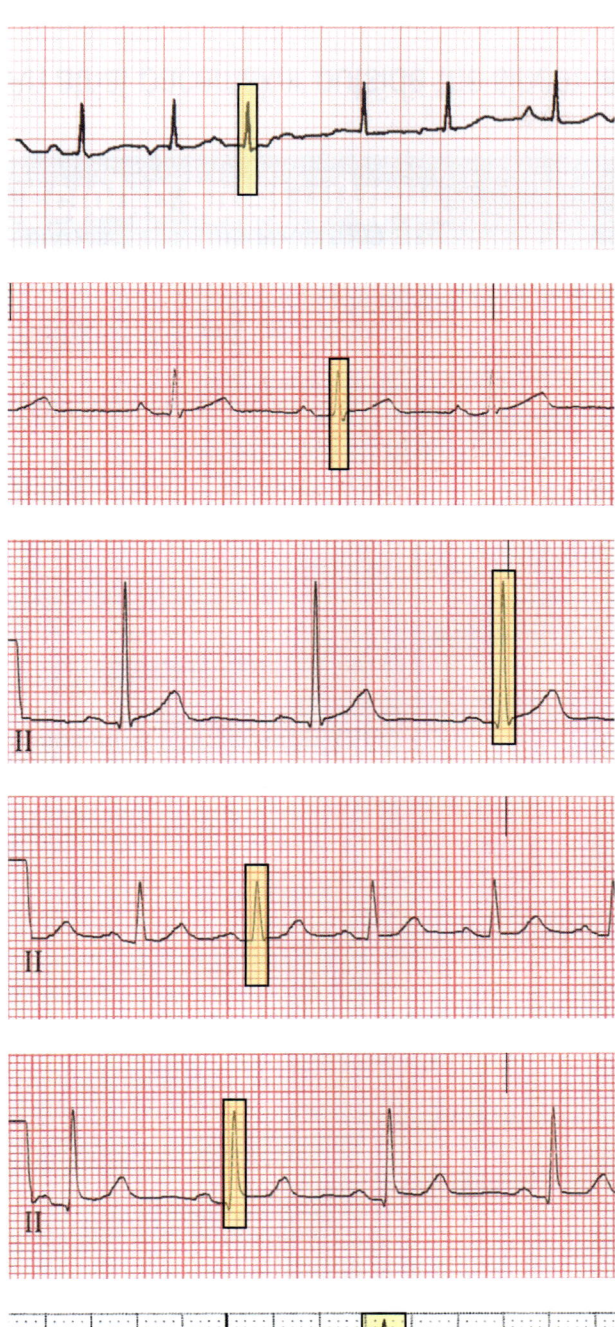

Fig. 8-22. *Different QRS complexes.*

PRACTICE

Measure the duration of the QRS complex in the following complexes:

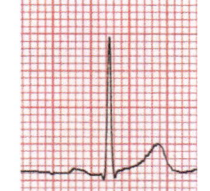
1. QRS duration: _____ seconds

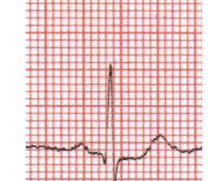
2. QRS duration: _____ seconds

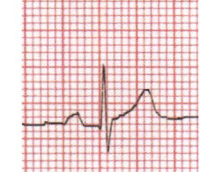
3. QRS duration: _____ seconds

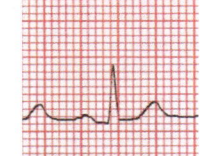
4. QRS duration: _____ seconds

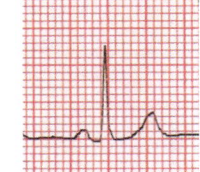
5. QRS duration: _____ seconds

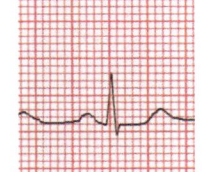
6. QRS duration: _____ seconds

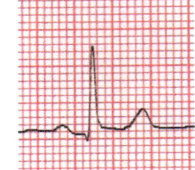
7. QRS duration: _____ seconds

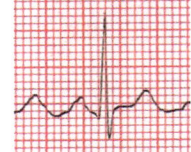
8. QRS duration: _____ seconds

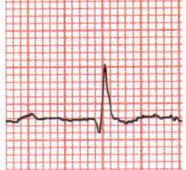
9. QRS duration: _____ seconds

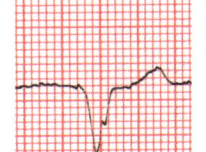
10. QRS duration: _____ seconds

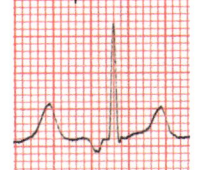
11. QRS duration: _____ seconds

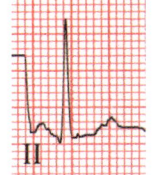
12. QRS duration: _____ seconds

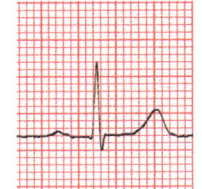
13. QRS duration: _____ seconds

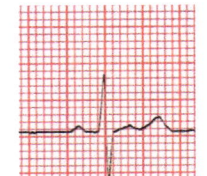
14. QRS duration: _____ seconds

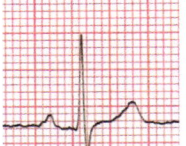
15. QRS duration: _____ seconds

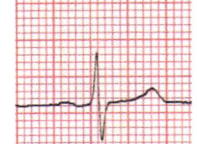
16. QRS duration: _____ seconds

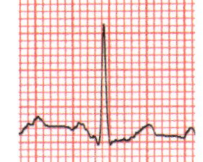
17. QRS duration: _____ seconds

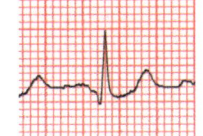
18. QRS duration: _____ seconds

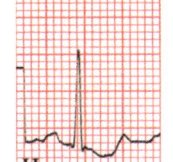
19. QRS duration: _____ seconds

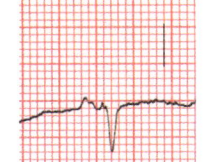
20. QRS duration: _____ seconds

12. Discuss the importance of following each step when analyzing an EKG tracing

Once these 5 steps are complete, all of the information needed for the sixth and final step—identifying the heart rhythm—has been gathered. Chapter 9 provides in-depth information on this step. It is important for a technician to follow each of these steps for every EKG she analyzes. Practicing these steps on different EKG tracings will help the technician master them.

PRACTICE

Complete the first 5 steps of EKG analysis using the strips shown below.

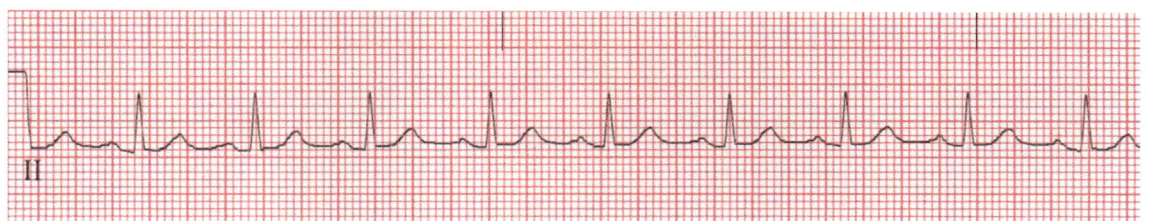

1. Heart rate _____   Regular? _____
   P wave _____   PR interval _____
   QRS duration _____

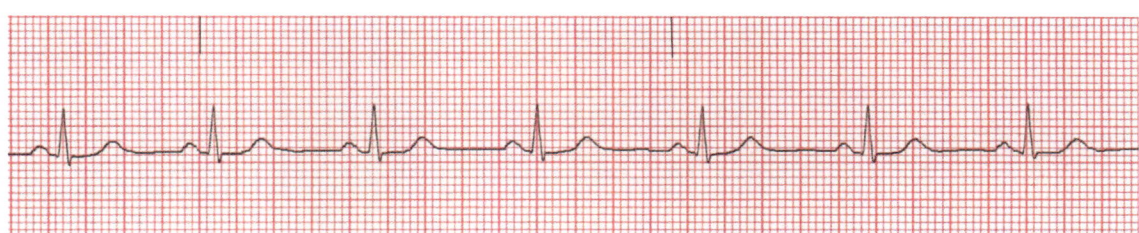

2. Heart rate _____   Regular? _____
   P wave _____   PR interval _____
   QRS duration _____

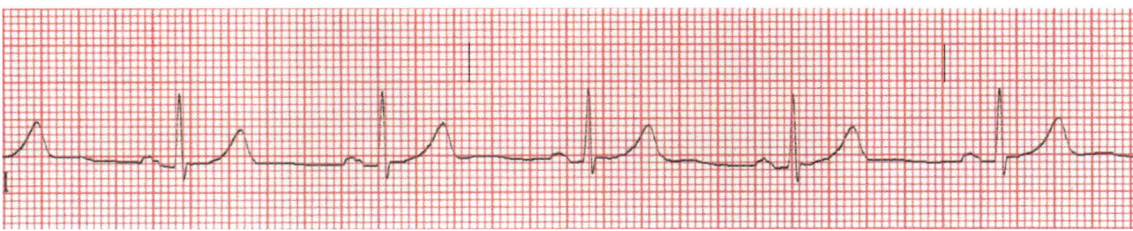

3. Heart rate _____   Regular? _____
   P wave _____   PR interval _____
   QRS duration _____

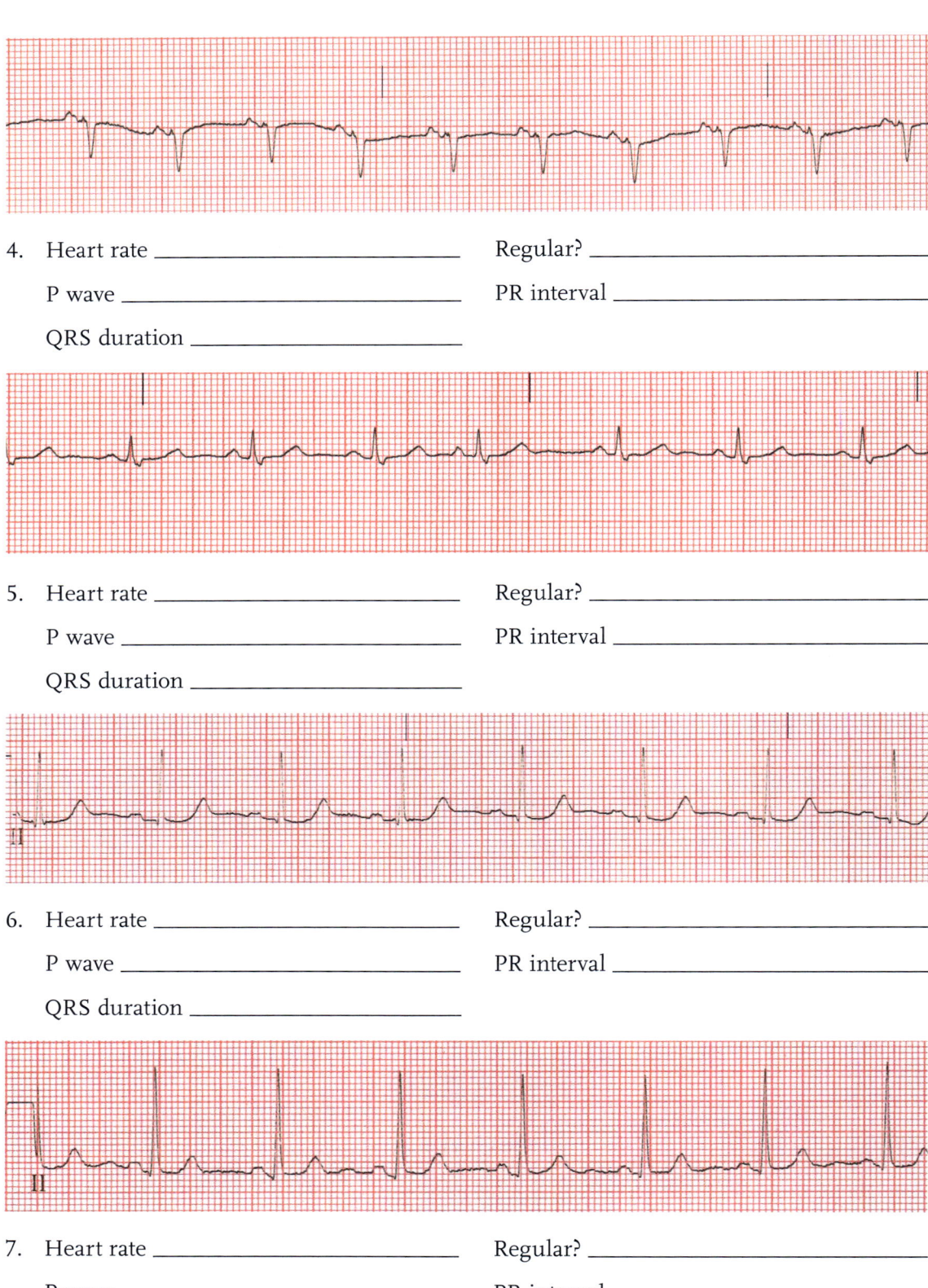

4. Heart rate _____ Regular? _____
   P wave _____ PR interval _____
   QRS duration _____

5. Heart rate _____ Regular? _____
   P wave _____ PR interval _____
   QRS duration _____

6. Heart rate _____ Regular? _____
   P wave _____ PR interval _____
   QRS duration _____

7. Heart rate _____ Regular? _____
   P wave _____ PR interval _____
   QRS duration _____

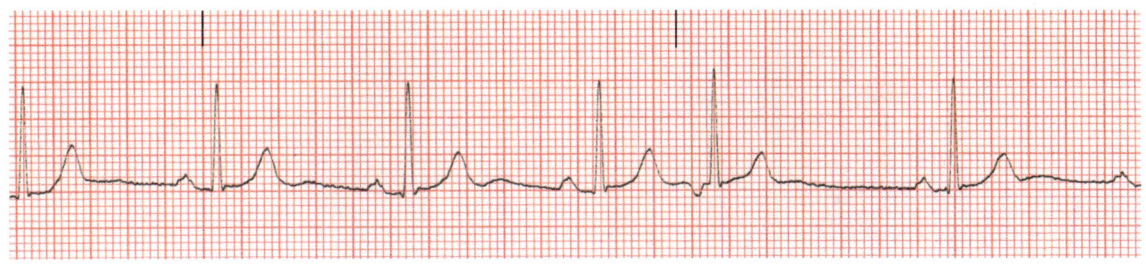

8. Heart rate _____ Regular? _____

   P wave _____ PR interval _____

   QRS duration _____

Chapter Review

- Electrical changes in the heart match up with specific mechanical actions, such as the contraction or relaxation of a particular part of the heart.

- EKG machines measure electrical changes in the heart. They produce EKG tracings (or strips). Reading EKGs gives a provider information about the mechanical actions of a patient's heart.

- EKG strips make it possible for a provider to analyze different features and their timing. These can show if the patient has normal cardiac function.

- The 6 steps used in analyzing an EKG are
  1. Determine the heart rate in beats per minute (BPM).
  2. Check the rhythm for regularity.
  3. Note the presence or absence of identical P waves before each QRS interval.
  4. Measure the duration of the PR interval.
  5. Measure the duration of the QRS complex.
  6. Identify the rhythm.

- EKG interpretation and diagnosis are the responsibilities of a provider. Understanding heart rhythms helps an EKG technician generate high-quality tracings and recognize emergency situations.

9 Overview of Rhythm Interpretation

This chapter contains many illustrations of different heart rhythms. Most of these illustrations include a section of EKG tracing that are as wide as the page. Each one is marked to show the most important feature of the rhythm. A 6-second EKG tracing is needed to identify most heart rhythms. Most of these illustrations are at least 30 large boxes wide. Gray boxes below the tracings give information about the rhythm in general. Measurements for that specific strip are in parentheses. For regular rhythms, the small box method was used to calculate the heart rate. For irregular rhythms, the 6-second method was used. Because these are all real tracings, they look different from one another. The ink from the EKG stylus may be darker or lighter, or the paper different colors. Whenever possible the strips are shown at actual size.

1. Explain how EKG rhythms are named and discuss the importance of recognizing cardiac rhythms

The SA node is the heart's primary pacemaker. It sends electrical impulses through the heart, which causes depolarization in an organized pattern. The SA node is at the top of the cardiac conduction system, followed by the AV node, bundle of His, bundle branches, and Purkinje fibers (shown in Figure 8-2). Another way to think about the conduction system is to arrange the parts of the system from higher to lower (Fig. 9-1).

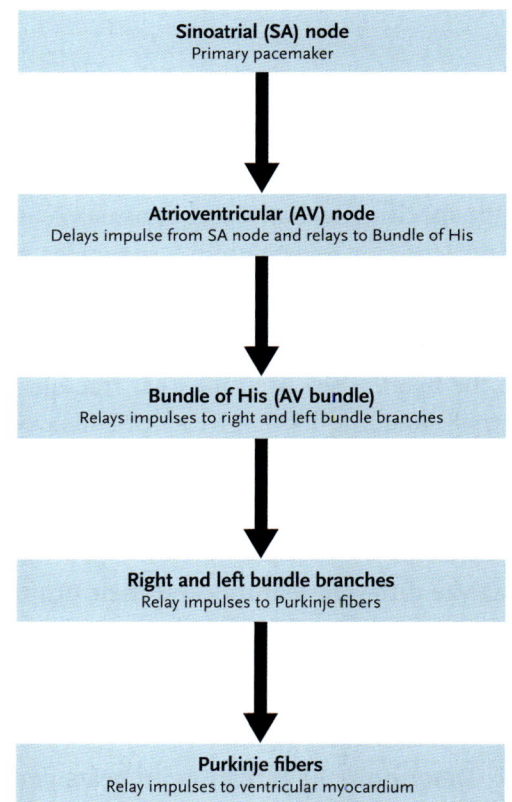

Fig. 9-1. Electrical impulses follow this path downward through the heart.

Heart rhythm is affected by problems in the cardiac conduction system. If the SA node does not generate an impulse, another part of the electrical system can generate it. This causes a late heartbeat called an **escape beat**. An escape beat may be an isolated beat or it may occur regularly. An **escape rhythm** is created when an area other than the SA node acts as the primary pacemaker of the heart.

Abnormal rhythms can also develop when parts of the cardiac conduction system become irritable. Hypoxia, MI, or other medical problems can cause this. The irritable area can generate an impulse even when the SA node is working normally. This is called an **ectopic focus** or *ectopic pacemaker*. Isolated early beats caused by ectopic foci (plural of *focus*) are very common. They are not necessarily caused by a disorder. Problems are more likely when there are several ectopic beats in a row.

Dysrhythmia (commonly called *arrhythmia*) means *difficult or abnormal rhythm*. It includes rhythms that are too fast or too slow or that begin in an area of the heart other than the SA node. Cardiac rhythms can start in five different areas of the heart's conduction system. Each rhythm is named for the area where it begins. A rhythm that starts in the sinoatrial node is called a **sinus rhythm**. Rhythms beginning in the atria, the AV junction, and the ventricles are called **atrial**, **junctional**, and **ventricular rhythms**, respectively. **Heart blocks**, also known as *AV blocks*, are caused by problems in the conduction of electrical impulses between the atria and ventricles.

Tip

Checking for Errors

Before generating an EKG tracing it is important to be sure that electrodes are properly attached and to eliminate as much artifact as possible. Reversal of limb leads, for example, can create tracings that could be mistaken for a dangerous rhythm. The most common limb lead reversal is the incorrect placement of the right and left arm electrodes. This error causes a negative deflection of QRS complexes in lead I and positive deflection of QRS complexes in lead aVR.

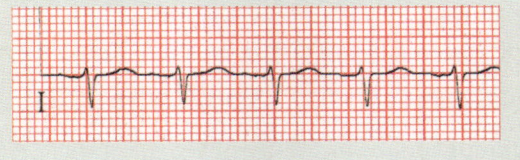

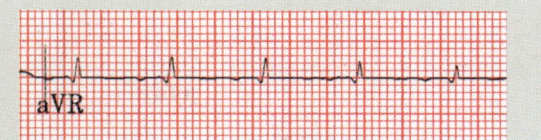

Any limb lead reversal can cause incorrect EKG interpretation and may lead to an incorrect diagnosis. The best time to catch errors is before the tracing is created. If a tracing is unclear or does not seem to match the patient's condition, the technician should double-check electrodes and lead wires. Once a clear and correct tracing is made, analysis can begin.

Quick Reference

Step	Normal characteristics
1. Determine rate.	60–100 beats per minute (BPM)
2. Examine rhythm for regularity.	Regular R-R intervals
3. Note P wave.	One before each QRS complex; all identical
4. Measure PR interval.	0.12–0.20 seconds
5. Measure QRS interval.	<0.12 seconds

The rest of this chapter shows how to complete the sixth and final step in EKG analysis: identifying or naming the rhythm. Some tracings may have more than one name. Tracings may show an **underlying rhythm**, which is the basic rhythm of the patient's heart. They may also show some abnormal heartbeats. These are often called *irregular complexes*. Both the underlying rhythm and the irregular complexes must always be named. For example, a patient's EKG may show an underlying rhythm of sinus bradycardia but also show a type of irregular complex called a premature ventricular contraction. Both should be noted in step 6 of rhythm analysis.

Tip

The Human Touch Matters

Most EKG machines analyze tracings automatically. Even so, EKG technicians should not simply assume that the EKG machine will give an accurate interpretation. If something looks abnormal it must be reported, even if the EKG machine does not indicate a problem.

Quick Reference	
This word	Means the rhythm/complex
Sinus	begins in the sinus node
Atrial	begins in the atria
Junctional	begins in the area of the AV junction
Ventricular	begins in the ventricles
Supraventricular	begins somewhere above the ventricles
Bradycardia	is slow
Tachycardia	is fast
Premature	comes earlier than expected
Escape	comes later than expected
Multifocal	originates from multiple locations in the heart
Paroxysmal	comes and goes in bursts
Uniform	stays the same
Monomorphic	has a key feature (e.g., the QRS complex) that stays the same every time
Polymorphic	has a key feature that changes from beat to beat

EKG technicians must be able to recognize common cardiac rhythms. They must know when an EKG tracing indicates a problem that needs immediate medical attention. Diagnosing a patient is the provider's job, but when EKG technicians understand what a tracing can mean for a patient's health, they can work more effectively. Each learning objective describing a category of rhythms is followed by a learning objective describing possible causes, treatments, and other considerations related to those rhythms.

The best way for EKG technicians to learn to identify normal and abnormal EKG rhythms is through practice. The discussion about each category of rhythm ends with practice EKG strips illustrating the rhythms. Handout 9-1 is a template that can be used to make a reference sheet for rhythm identification. It can be used along with the exercises in this chapter.

2. Identify sinus rhythms

Rhythms that originate in the sinus (SA) node are called *sinus rhythms*. Normal sinus rhythm shows these characteristics: a heart rate between 60 and 100 BPM; a regular rhythm; an identical, positive P wave before each QRS complex; a PR interval between 0.12 and 0.20 seconds; and a QRS interval of less than 0.12 seconds (Fig. 9-2).

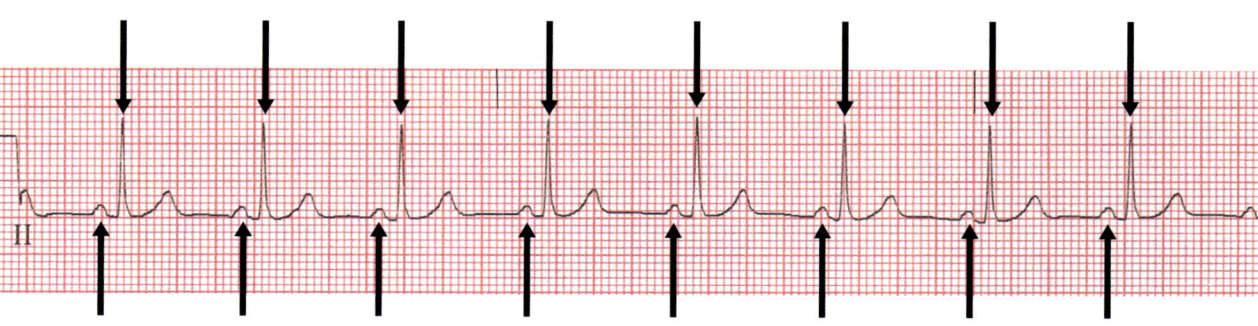

Name of rhythm: Normal sinus rhythm
Rate: 60–100 BPM (70 BPM)
Rhythm pattern: Regular
P wave characteristics: Upright and uniform
PR interval: 0.12–0.20 seconds (0.12 s)
QRS duration: <0.12 seconds (0.08 s)
Unique identifier: All complexes, intervals, rate, and rhythm normal

Fig. 9-2. *EKG tracing showing normal sinus rhythm.*

Sinus rhythms can also be too fast, too slow, or irregular. In **sinus tachycardia** the heart rate is fast, with a rate over 100 beats per minute, but all other characteristics are normal (Fig. 9-3).

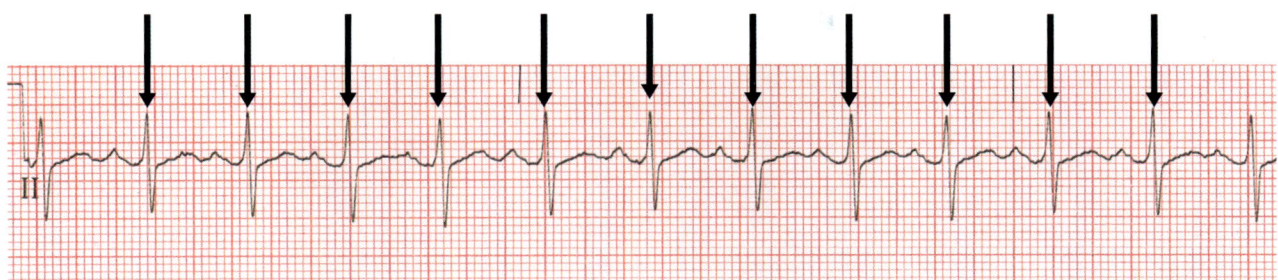

Rhythm is regular, but rate is faster than normal

Name of rhythm: Sinus tachycardia
Rate: 100–160 BPM (107 BPM)
Rhythm pattern: Regular
P wave characteristics: Upright and uniform

PR interval: 0.12–0.20 seconds (0.20 s)
QRS duration: <0.12 seconds (0.08 s)
Unique identifier: All features normal with fast rate

Fig. 9-3. *EKG tracing showing sinus tachycardia.*

In **sinus bradycardia** the heart rate is slow and all other characteristics are normal (Fig. 9-4). Any sinus rhythm with a rate less than 60 BPM is considered bradycardia.

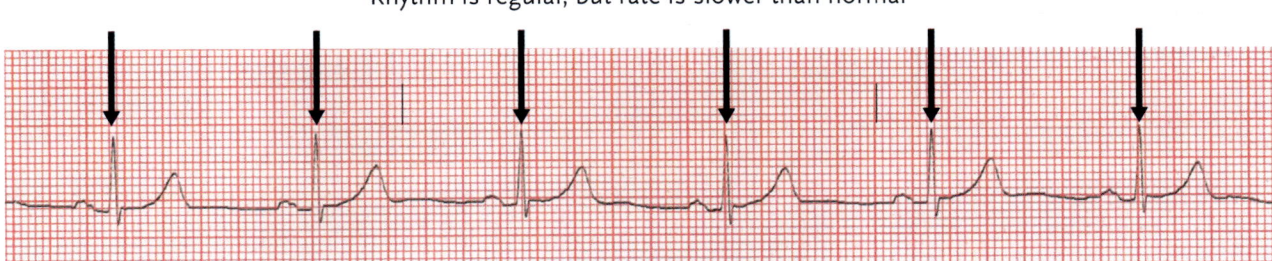

Rhythm is regular, but rate is slower than normal

Name of rhythm: Sinus bradycardia
Rate: <60 BPM (55 BPM)
Rhythm pattern: Regular
P wave characteristics: Upright and uniform

PR interval: 0.12–0.20 seconds (0.16 s)
QRS duration: <0.12 seconds (0.08 s)
Unique identifier: All features normal with slow rate

Fig. 9-4. *EKG tracing showing sinus bradycardia.*

Sinus arrhythmia is a sinus rhythm in which all characteristics are normal except for the R-R intervals (distance between R waves). In sinus arrhythmia the R-R intervals are irregular, meaning that the rhythm does not repeat with consistent timing—an abnormal result for the second step, checking the rhythm for regularity (Fig. 9-5). The irregularity of the rhythm usually varies with the patient's breathing. The rate increases with inhalation and decreases with exhalation.

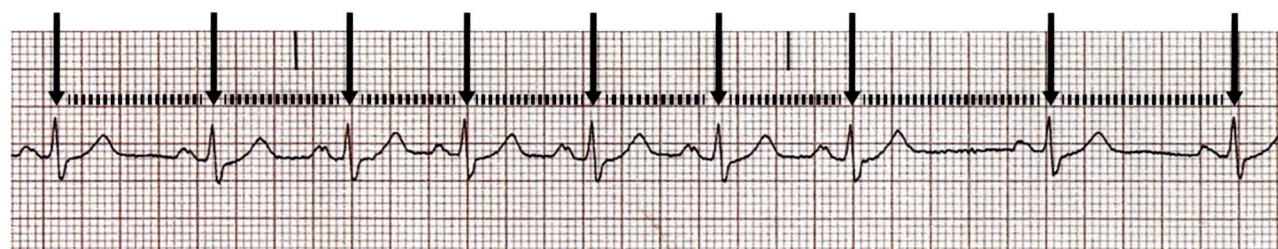

Name of rhythm: Sinus arrhythmia

Rate: 60–100 BPM (70 BPM)

Rhythm pattern: Irregular

P wave characteristics: Upright and uniform

PR interval: 0.12–0.20 seconds (0.16 s)

QRS duration: <0.12 seconds (0.10 s)

Unique identifier: All complexes normal but rate changes with respiration

Fig. 9-5. *EKG tracing showing sinus arrhythmia.*

Sinus arrest or *sinus pause* occurs when the SA node does not initiate an impulse at the right time. This creates pauses in the heart's electrical activity (Fig. 9-6). The complexes that do occur are normal, but the rhythm pattern examined in step 2 is irregular. When analyzing this rhythm it is helpful to note the length of the pause.

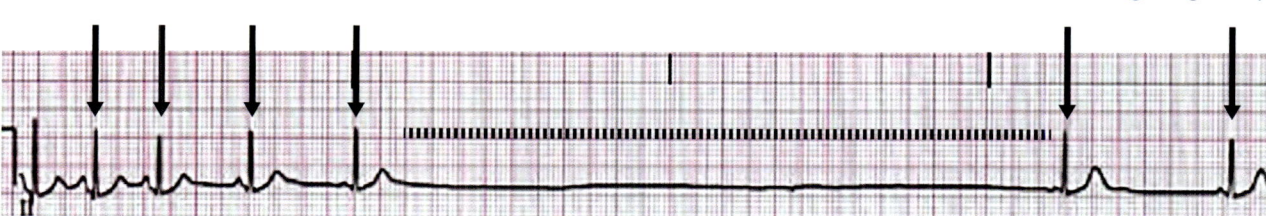

Name of rhythm: Sinus arrest

Rate: Varies due to length and frequency of pause (50 BPM)

Rhythm pattern: Irregular

P wave characteristics: Upright and uniform

PR interval: 0.12–0.20 seconds (0.12 s)

QRS duration: <0.12 seconds (0.08 s)

Unique identifier: Normal complexes alternating with arrest periods

Fig. 9-6. *EKG tracing showing sinus arrest.*

3. Discuss what sinus rhythms mean for the patient

A healthy heart has a normal sinus rhythm. The heart rate can vary due to activity, stress, or medical conditions. The normal range also varies by age (as shown in Chapter 2). Many of these variations are not dangerous for the patient. They may be described as *not of clinical concern*. Sinus bradycardia, for example, may be the normal rhythm for a well-conditioned athlete. Sinus node firing can also be slowed by stimulation of the vagus nerve, which is part of the parasympathetic nervous system. This happens when a person strains to have a bowel movement, for example, or splashes cold water on her face. These changes are not of clinical concern.

It is important to know whether the patient with bradycardia is **symptomatic**, or experiencing cardiac symptoms. Sinus bradycardia can decrease cardiac output, causing symptoms such as dizziness, weakness, or syncope (fainting). It can also cause chest pain, shortness of breath, clammy skin, low blood pressure, or changes in mental status.

Sinus tachycardia may be a side effect of medication, a response to stress, or the heart's response to the body's need for additional oxygen. Fever, exercise, fear, and low blood volume are also possible causes of sinus tachycardia. This rhythm can be harmful to a patient with a history of coronary artery disease. The treatment depends on the cause of the tachycardia. The patient may need medication to control a fever or intravenous fluids to increase blood volume. Sometimes having the patient rest can decrease the heart rate.

Sinus arrhythmia happens naturally in some children and adults. It does not usually need to be treated unless the heart rate slows enough to cause problems with circulation or cardiac output. Medication may be used to treat a patient with sinus arrhythmia that causes symptoms (*symptomatic* sinus arrhythmia).

Sinus arrest may be caused by SA node damage, medications, or increased vagal tone. *Vagal tone* is controlled by the vagus nerve, a part of the parasympathetic nervous system. When the vagus nerve is stimulated by pain, the sight of blood, or straining to have a bowel movement, the heart rate may slow dramatically. This can cause syncope. The decision to treat these conditions is based on how often the arrest happens. Some patients may be **asymptomatic** (having no symptoms). Other patients may be treated successfully with medication.

PRACTICE

Analyze the sinus rhythm strips below using the 6 steps.

1. Heart rate _____   Regular? _____
   P wave _____   PR interval _____
   QRS duration _____   Rhythm name _____

2. Heart rate _____   Regular? _____
   P wave _____   PR interval _____
   QRS duration _____   Rhythm name _____

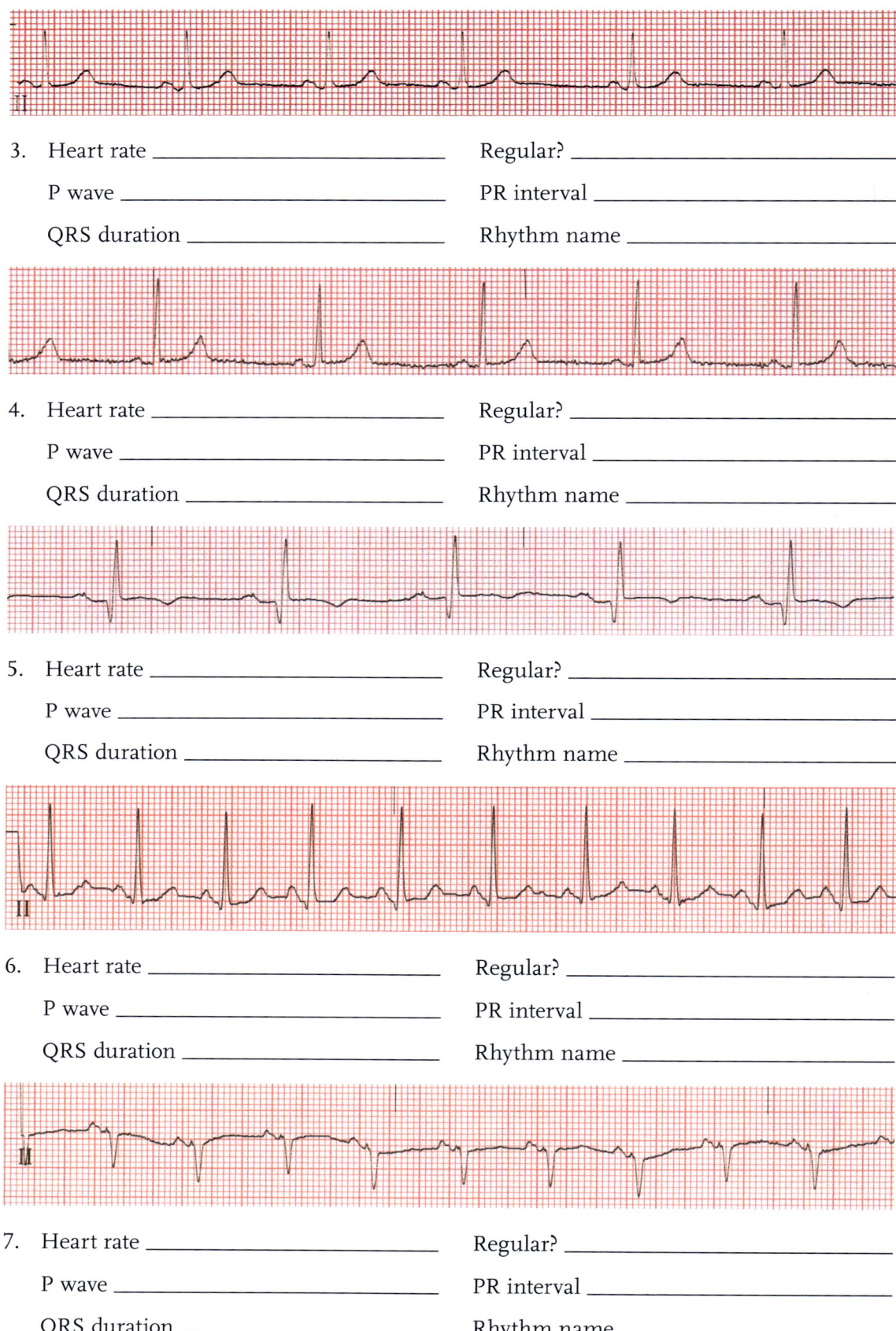

3. Heart rate _____ Regular? _____

   P wave _____ PR interval _____

   QRS duration _____ Rhythm name _____

4. Heart rate _____ Regular? _____

   P wave _____ PR interval _____

   QRS duration _____ Rhythm name _____

5. Heart rate _____ Regular? _____

   P wave _____ PR interval _____

   QRS duration _____ Rhythm name _____

6. Heart rate _____ Regular? _____

   P wave _____ PR interval _____

   QRS duration _____ Rhythm name _____

7. Heart rate _____ Regular? _____

   P wave _____ PR interval _____

   QRS duration _____ Rhythm name _____

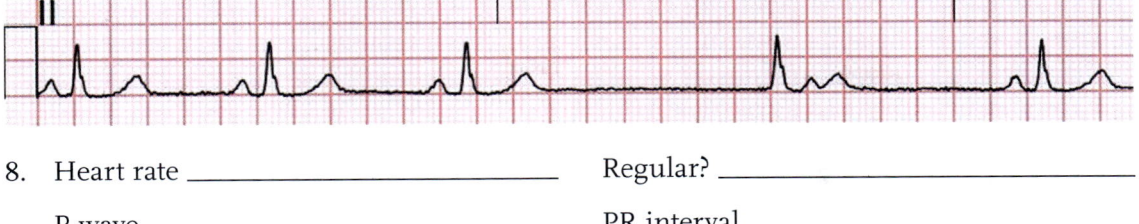

8. Heart rate _____ Regular? _____

   P wave _____ PR interval _____

   QRS duration _____ Rhythm name _____

4. Identify atrial rhythms

Atrial rhythms are caused by an electrical impulse that starts in the atria, but not in the SA node. The P wave on an EKG shows atrial depolarization, which prompts the contraction of the atria. In atrial rhythms, the electrical impulse travels to the AV node on a different path than usual. This means the P waves for these rhythms are different from normal sinus rhythm P waves. P waves in an atrial rhythm may be flattened, pointed, notched, or biphasic (having a positive and a negative deflection). They may be hidden. A hidden P wave cannot be seen because it is lost in the T wave of the complex before it (Fig. 9-7).

a)

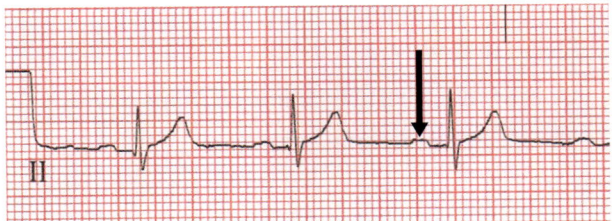

b)

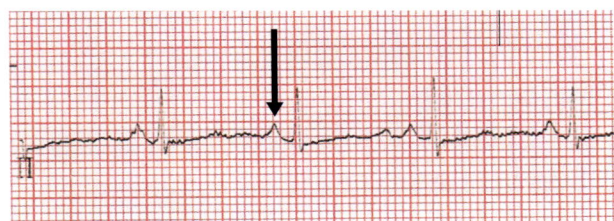

c)

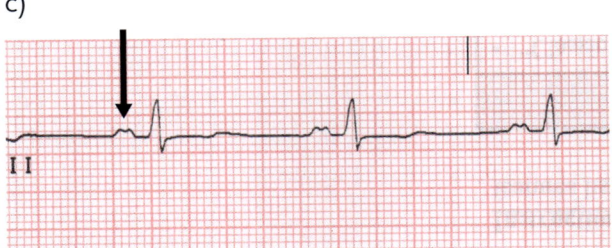

d)

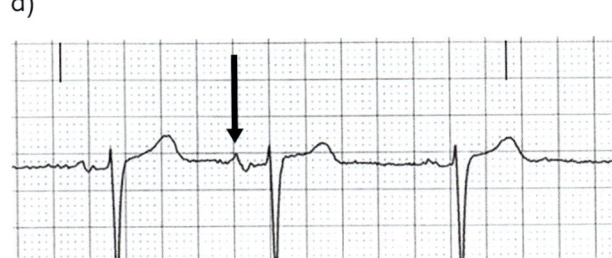

e)

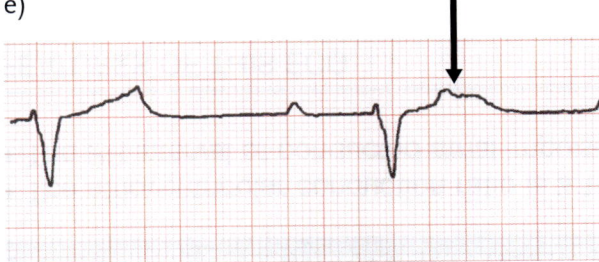

Fig. 9-7. *Illustrations of P wave variations for atrial rhythms: a) flattened; b) pointed; c) notched; d) biphasic; e) hidden in the T wave of the previous complex.*

Premature atrial complexes (**PACs**) begin in the atria and have an underlying sinus rhythm (Fig. 9-8). The underlying rhythm is often normal, but there are obvious early (premature) beats. The QRS complex and the T wave in a premature atrial complex are normal, but the P wave is not normal. The P wave in these early beats may be taller and more pointed than the P wave of the normal sinus complexes in the underlying rhythm. The PR interval may be shortened.

When analyzing a strip that contains PACs, the underlying rhythm should be named. Underlying rhythms can include NSR and sinus bradycardia, among others. The rate of the tracing is based on the rate of the underlying rhythm.

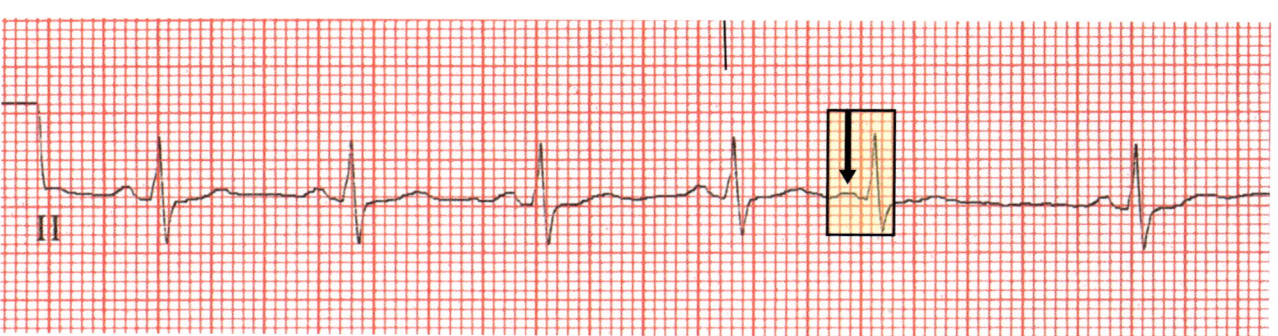

Name of rhythm: PAC with underlying sinus rhythm

Rate: 60–100 BPM (83 BPM)

Rhythm pattern: Irregular

P wave characteristics: Abnormal for premature beats (possibly taller or pointed; flattened in this example)

PR interval: <0.20 seconds (0.16 s)

QRS duration: <0.12 seconds (0.08 s)

Unique identifier: Normal except for obvious early beats which may feature abnormal P waves and shortened PR intervals

Fig. 9-8. *Illustration of PAC with underlying normal sinus rhythm.*

Wandering atrial pacemaker, also called *multiformed atrial rhythm*, occurs when impulses begin in several different areas. These areas may include various locations in the atria, the AV node, and the SA node. P waves vary in shape, size, and direction from beat to beat. The rhythm is irregular. The PR interval varies and the QRS is normal (Fig. 9-9).

P waves look different in every beat; rhythm is irregular

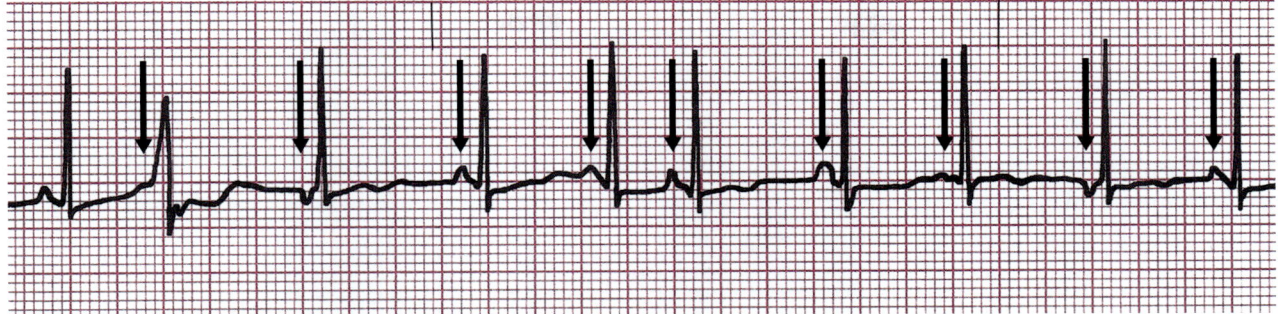

Name of rhythm: Wandering atrial pacemaker (WAP)

Rate: 60–100 BPM (90 BPM)

Rhythm pattern: Irregular

P wave characteristics: Changing configurations

PR interval: Varies

QRS duration: <0.12 seconds (0.06 s)

Unique identifier: Changing P wave—at least three variations in one lead

Fig. 9-9. *Illustration of wandering atrial pacemaker rhythm.*

Atrial tachycardia is a fast rate caused by irritability in the atria (Fig. 9-10). In this rhythm the P wave may be partly or completely hidden in the T wave of the beat that comes before it. Because of this, the PR interval cannot be measured. The rhythm is regular and has a normal QRS complex. It has a rate of 100–250 beats per minute.

PR interval is not measurable but QRS complexes are normal and regular

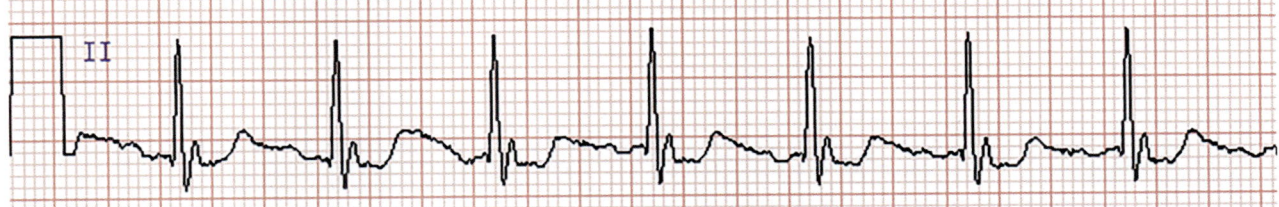

Name of rhythm: Atrial tachycardia

Rate: 100–250 BPM (100 BPM)

Rhythm pattern: Regular

P wave characteristics: May be hidden in previous T wave

PR interval: Not measurable

QRS duration: <0.12 s (0.08 s)

Unique identifier: Fast rate; P wave partly or completely hidden in T wave of previous beat

Fig. 9-10. *Illustration of atrial tachycardia.*

Multifocal atrial tachycardia (MAT) is a rhythm similar to wandering atrial pacemaker. Impulses begin in different areas. In MAT, the ventricular rate is greater than 100 beats per minute (Fig. 9-11).

Variations in P waves due to different areas initiating the electrical impulse

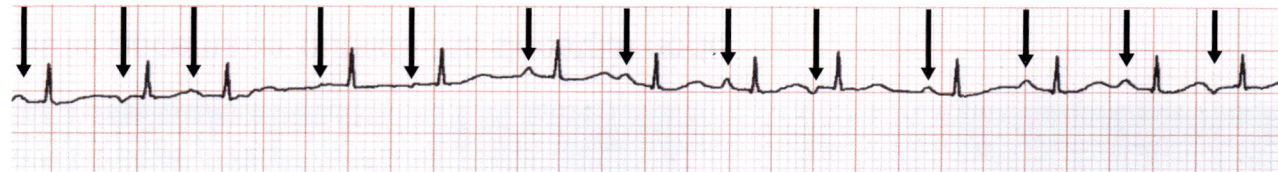

Name of rhythm: Multifocal atrial tachycardia (MAT)

Rate: 100–150 BPM (130 BPM)

Rhythm pattern: Irregular

P wave characteristics: Changing configurations

PR interval: Varies

QRS duration: <0.12 s (0.04 s)

Unique identifier: Changing P wave—may be upright, rounded, inverted, biphasic, hidden in QRS; normal QRS duration

Fig. 9-11. Illustration of multifocal atrial tachycardia.

Another form of tachycardia that can begin in the atria, but may also begin in other locations, is called **supraventricular tachycardia** (Fig. 9-12). It originates above the ventricles but its exact origin is hard to find. The P wave is usually difficult or impossible to see. The PR interval is impossible to measure. The rate is very fast: 150–250 BPM. The QRS complex is normal. This rhythm is also called *narrow complex tachycardia*.

P wave is usually difficult or impossible to see

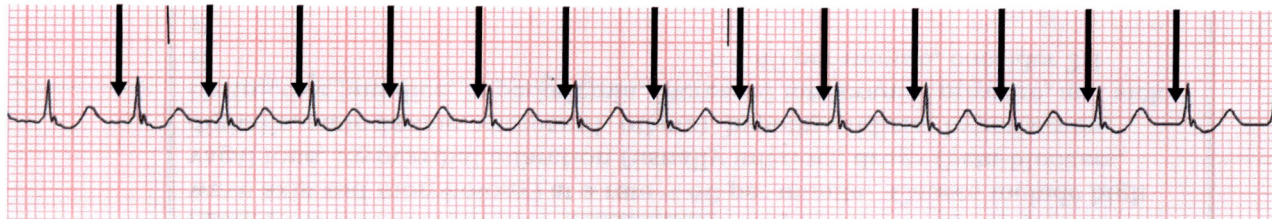

Name of rhythm: Supraventricular tachycardia

Rate: 150–250 BPM (150 BPM)

Rhythm pattern: Regular

P wave characteristics: Difficult or impossible to see

PR interval: Not measurable

QRS duration: <0.12 s (0.08 s)

Unique identifier: Very fast rate; hard to discern P waves; narrow QRS

Fig. 9-12. Illustration of supraventricular (narrow complex) tachychardia.

Tip

Supraventricular Tachycardia

The term *supraventricular tachycardia* may be used to refer to a specific dysrhythmia. It may also be used as a general category of abnormal rhythms. All tachycardias that begin in the SA node, the atria, or the AV junction can be considered supraventricular tachycardias. The prefix *supra* means *above*, and all of these areas are above the ventricles. Because the P waves in these rhythms (if they are visible at all) can be impossible to analyze, the provider may give the patient medication to slow the heart rate. The P waves can then be seen more clearly. This makes it easier for the provider to find the origin of the rhythm. Treatment is based on the origin of the rhythm.

Atrial fibrillation (often called *AFib*) is a very common dysrhythmia. It is especially common in older patients. In this rhythm, multiple irritable sites are firing, or creating impulses in the atria. Atrial fibrillation makes the baseline of the EKG wavy and irregular. There are no clear (or *discernible*) P waves. The QRS complex looks normal and has a normal duration, but the R-R interval is irregular.

The wavy baseline in atrial fibrillation shows the irritable sites firing in the atria. The wavy line is made up of tiny P waves. The contraction of the ventricles that follows the P wave is called *ventricular response*. The QRS complex on an EKG shows ventricular response. The faster the ventricular response in an AFib rhythm, the more QRS complexes there are on the EKG. This makes the rhythm more dangerous for the patient.

The AV node slows down ventricular response. It protects the ventricles by not allowing all of the P waves through. If the heart rate is 100 beats per minute or faster, the rhythm is referred to as *uncontrolled* atrial fibrillation, or atrial fibrillation with **rapid ventricular response** (RVR) (Fig. 9-13a). If the ventricular rate is slower than 100 beats per minute, the rhythm is referred to as *controlled* (Fig. 9-13b).

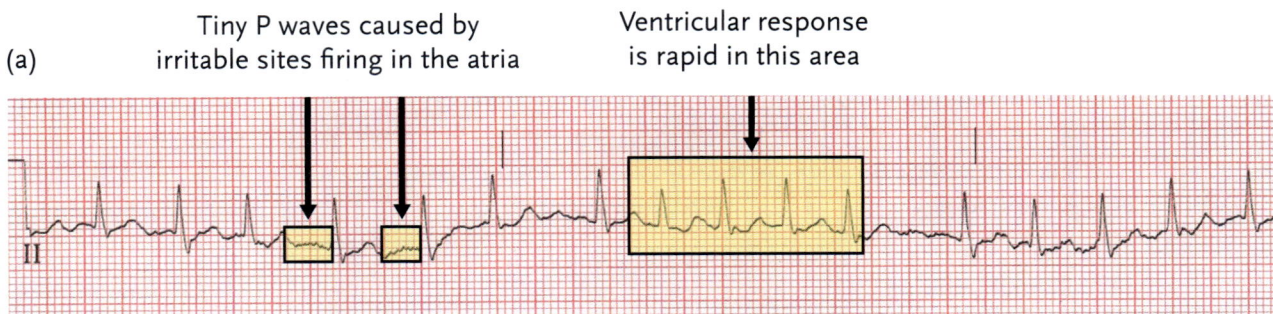

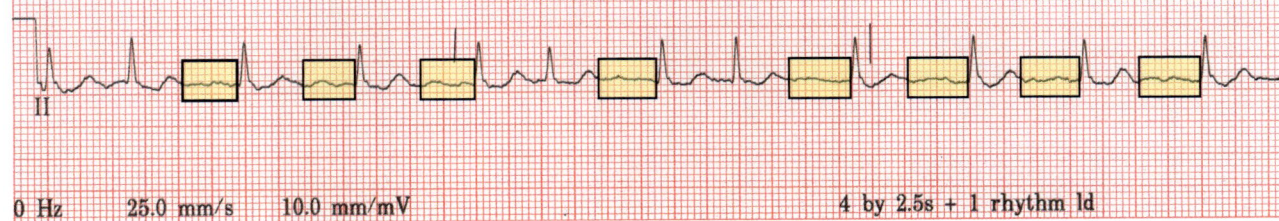

Name of rhythm: Atrial fibrillation, (a) uncontrolled and (b) controlled

Rate: (a) ≥100 BPM for uncontrolled (130 BPM); (b) 60–99 BPM for controlled (80 BPM)

Rhythm pattern: Irregular

P wave characteristics: Not visible

PR interval: Not measurable

QRS duration: <0.12 s (0.08 s in both examples)

Unique identifier: No identifiable P waves; irregular but normal QRS

Fig. 9-13. *Illustration of (a) uncontrolled and (b) controlled atrial fibrillation.*

Atrial flutter happens when an irritable site in the atria fires at a very rapid rate (Fig. 9-14). The AV node does not usually conduct impulses at a rate faster than 180 impulses per minute, so it blocks many of these impulses. The EKG tracing shows more P waves—renamed *F* or *flutter*

waves in this rhythm—than QRS complexes. **F waves** are also called *sawtooth* or *picket fence* waves.

The relationship between F waves and QRS complexes varies. It is expressed as a ratio, or a relationship between the numbers. If two F waves appear for each QRS complex, the rhythm has 2:1 (*two-to-one*) conduction. If three appear, it is 3:1 conduction, and so on. The PR interval is not measurable in atrial flutter because of the distorted P waves. The QRS complex is usually normal. If the ventricular rate is 100 beats per minute or higher, the rhythm is called *uncontrolled* atrial flutter. If the ventricular rate is less than 100 beats per minute, the rhythm is called *controlled* atrial flutter.

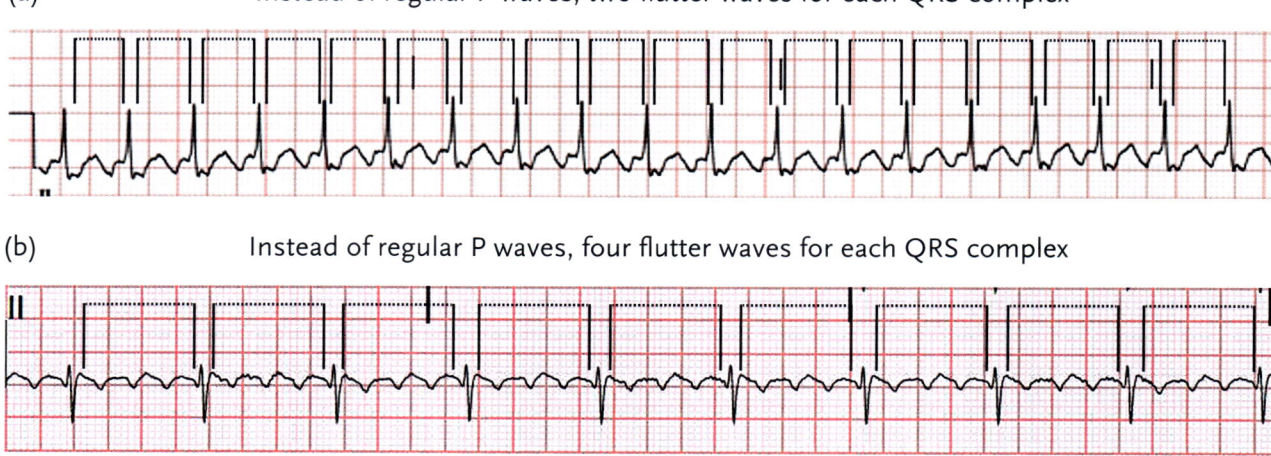

Name of rhythm: Atrial flutter with (a) 2:1 conduction and (b) 4:1 conduction	**P wave characteristics:** Sawtooth, more than one
Atrial rate: 250–300 BPM [(a) 272 BPM; (b) 300 BPM]	**PR interval:** Not measurable
	QRS duration: <0.12 s (0.08 s in both strips)
Ventricular rate: Varies depending on ratio of conducted beats [(a) 136 BPM; (b) 75 BPM]	**Unique identifier:** Sawtooth P waves; more than one P wave for each QRS; P waves may be hidden in QRS or T wave
Rhythm pattern: P-P regular, R-R regular	

Fig. 9-14. *Illustrations of atrial flutter with (a) 2:1 conduction and (b) 4:1 conduction.*

Tip

Atrial Rhythms and Ventricular Rates

The atrial rate in atrial flutter is usually around 300 BPM. The AV node cannot conduct this fast. Not all of the impulses in the atria are sent along to the ventricles. The ventricular rate is 150 if every other impulse is blocked. It is 100 if two out of every three impulses are blocked. This means the tracing will show more P waves (or distorted P waves) than QRS complexes. Any time there is not a QRS complex for every P wave, the atrial and ventricular rates are different. The atrial rate is higher in these rhythms than the ventricular rate. The ventricular rate is the rate at which the heart actually beats.

5. Discuss what atrial rhythms mean for the patient

Premature atrial complexes are common. They are not usually treated if the patient is asymptomatic. If treatment is needed, it is often directed at finding and correcting the underlying cause. Causes may include electrolyte imbalances, stimulant medication side effects, anxiety, and heart disease. The underlying rhythm should also be identified. If it is abnormal, it may also require treatment.

Wandering atrial pacemaker may occur naturally. It can also be caused by dangerous levels of a drug called *digitalis*. This situation is called *digitalis toxicity*. Digitalis slows and strengthens the contraction of the heart to increase cardiac output. If digitalis toxicity may be causing a wandering atrial pacemaker rhythm, a blood test is done to check the level of digitalis in the blood. The drug is stopped until the level returns to a normal range.

Multifocal atrial tachycardia is treated based on the underlying cause and the patient's condition. A provider makes this assessment. Medications may be used to correct the rhythm. A provider may also direct the patient to perform **vagal maneuvers**. These are actions taken to stimulate the vagal nerve and slow the heart rate. One common vagal maneuver is called a *Valsalva maneuver*. The patient takes a deep breath and bears down as though he is having a bowel movement. An EKG technician should only direct a patient to do a vagal maneuver if ordered by a provider. The patient's heart must be monitored during the maneuver.

Treatment for atrial tachycardia involves finding and correcting the underlying cause. Causes may include imbalances in electrolytes that occur naturally in the body, digitalis toxicity, infection, stimulant medication side effects, anxiety, and heart disease. This rhythm may be treated with medications. Atrial tachycardia may also require a treatment called *synchronized cardioversion*. In this treatment, a low-level electrical shock is used to return the heart to a regular rhythm.

Atrial fibrillation may be a **transient rhythm**, meaning it comes and goes. It may also be a **sustained rhythm**, meaning it is always happening. Treatment is based on the patient's symptoms and the rate of ventricular response. Ventricular rates of 100 beats per minute or higher are particularly dangerous. This rapid rate stops the heart from pumping efficiently.

Blood can pool within the atria. It can clot there, putting the patient at risk of stroke. This risk may be reduced by treating the patient with blood thinners.

A patient with AFib may also need an artificial pacemaker or a procedure called *catheter ablation*. Catheter ablation stops abnormal electrical signals from moving through the heart. AFib can be caused by heart disease, pulmonary (lung) disease, diabetes, alcohol abuse, or medication side effects. It is also commonly caused by aging. The provider's decision about treatment is based on the patient's medical history and how much the atrial fibrillation is affecting the patient's health.

Atrial flutter can also be a transient or sustained rhythm. Treatment is based on the patient's symptoms and the correction of underlying causes. Causes may include heart disease, pulmonary disease, MI, pulmonary embolism, or digitalis toxicity. Treatment includes medications and/or synchronized cardioversion.

> **Tip**
>
> **AFib Is Common and Serious**
>
> Atrial fibrillation is the most commonly treated cardiac dysrhythmia. The risk for developing AFib goes up with age, and it is more common in women than in men. It is also more common in people of European ancestry.
>
> AFib does not always cause serious symptoms, but it can be very dangerous. People with AFib have twice the risk of death from cardiac problems and five times the risk of stroke. Not all patients understand these risks. Providers can help explain how patients can reduce the danger.
>
> Patients who use smart watches or other personal EKG devices may be alerted to AFib rhythms. If an EKG technician thinks she sees atrial fibrillation on a patient's EKG, she should be sure to alert the provider. Only the provider can make a diagnosis and discuss treatment with the patient.
>
> Treatments may include blood thinners to prevent pooled blood from clotting, which increases stroke risk. Medications that control heart rate or regulate heart rhythm may also be prescribed.

PRACTICE

Analyze the atrial rhythm strips below using the 6 steps. Some rhythms may have both an atrial rate and a ventricular rate. Note both rates when appropriate (mark A for *atrial* and V for *ventricular*).

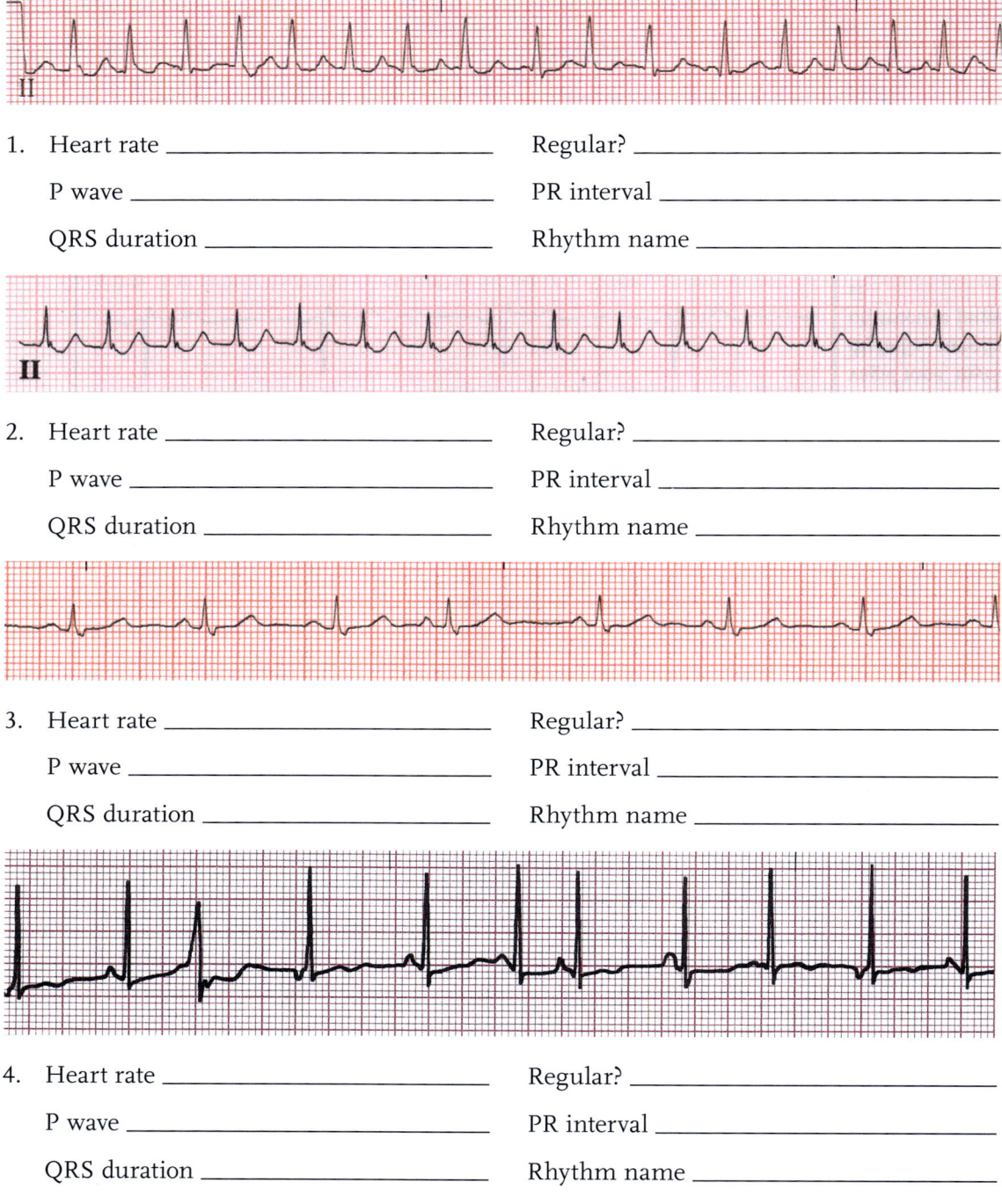

1. Heart rate _____   Regular? _____
   P wave _____   PR interval _____
   QRS duration _____   Rhythm name _____

2. Heart rate _____   Regular? _____
   P wave _____   PR interval _____
   QRS duration _____   Rhythm name _____

3. Heart rate _____   Regular? _____
   P wave _____   PR interval _____
   QRS duration _____   Rhythm name _____

4. Heart rate _____   Regular? _____
   P wave _____   PR interval _____
   QRS duration _____   Rhythm name _____

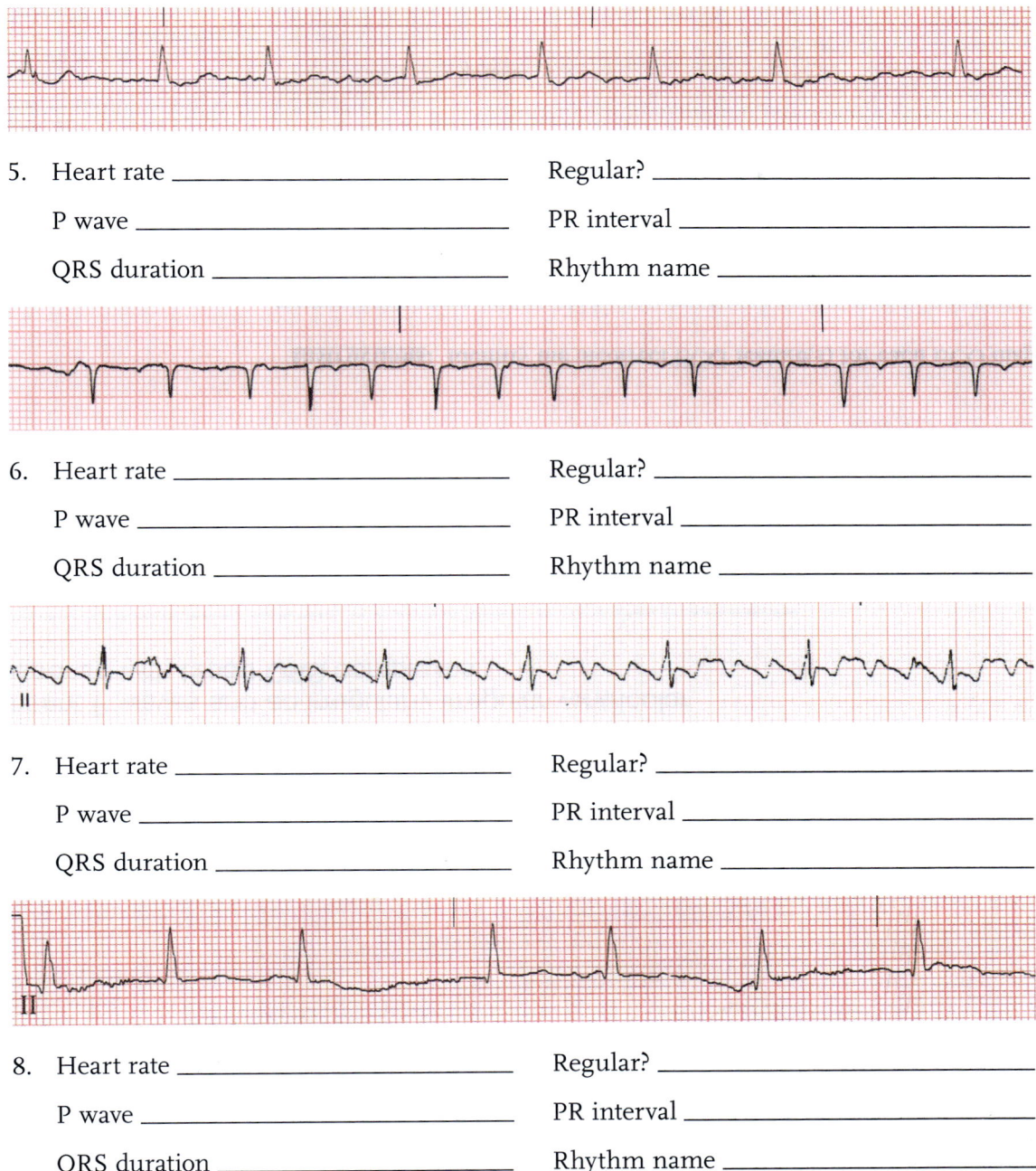

5. Heart rate _____ Regular? _____

   P wave _____ PR interval _____

   QRS duration _____ Rhythm name _____

6. Heart rate _____ Regular? _____

   P wave _____ PR interval _____

   QRS duration _____ Rhythm name _____

7. Heart rate _____ Regular? _____

   P wave _____ PR interval _____

   QRS duration _____ Rhythm name _____

8. Heart rate _____ Regular? _____

   P wave _____ PR interval _____

   QRS duration _____ Rhythm name _____

ADVANCED PRACTICE

Analyze the strips on the following pages using the 6 steps. This set of strips includes both sinus and atrial rhythms. Some rhythms may have both an atrial rate and a ventricular rate. Note both rates when appropriate (mark A for *atrial* and V for *ventricular*).

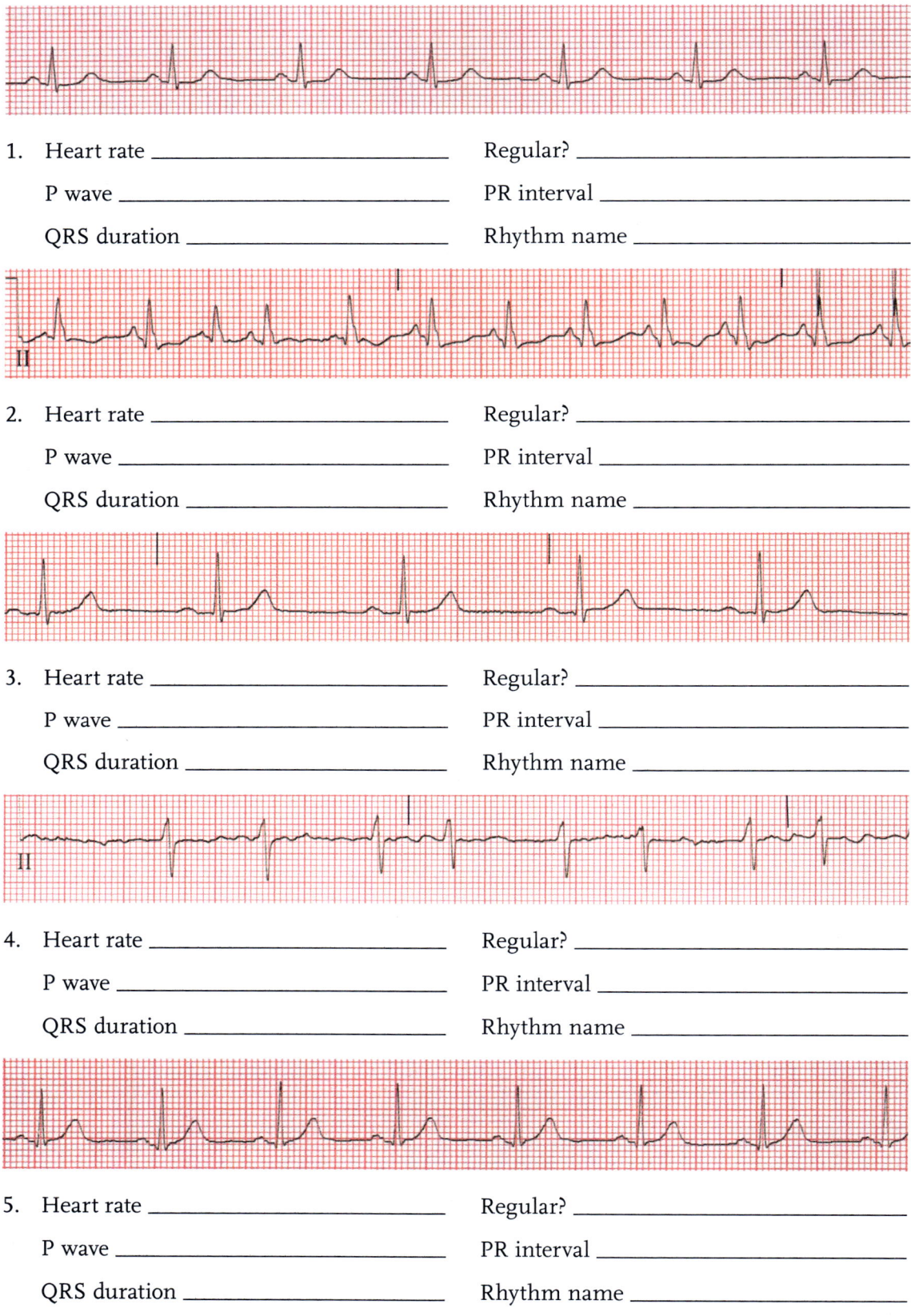

1. Heart rate _____ Regular? _____
   P wave _____ PR interval _____
   QRS duration _____ Rhythm name _____

2. Heart rate _____ Regular? _____
   P wave _____ PR interval _____
   QRS duration _____ Rhythm name _____

3. Heart rate _____ Regular? _____
   P wave _____ PR interval _____
   QRS duration _____ Rhythm name _____

4. Heart rate _____ Regular? _____
   P wave _____ PR interval _____
   QRS duration _____ Rhythm name _____

5. Heart rate _____ Regular? _____
   P wave _____ PR interval _____
   QRS duration _____ Rhythm name _____

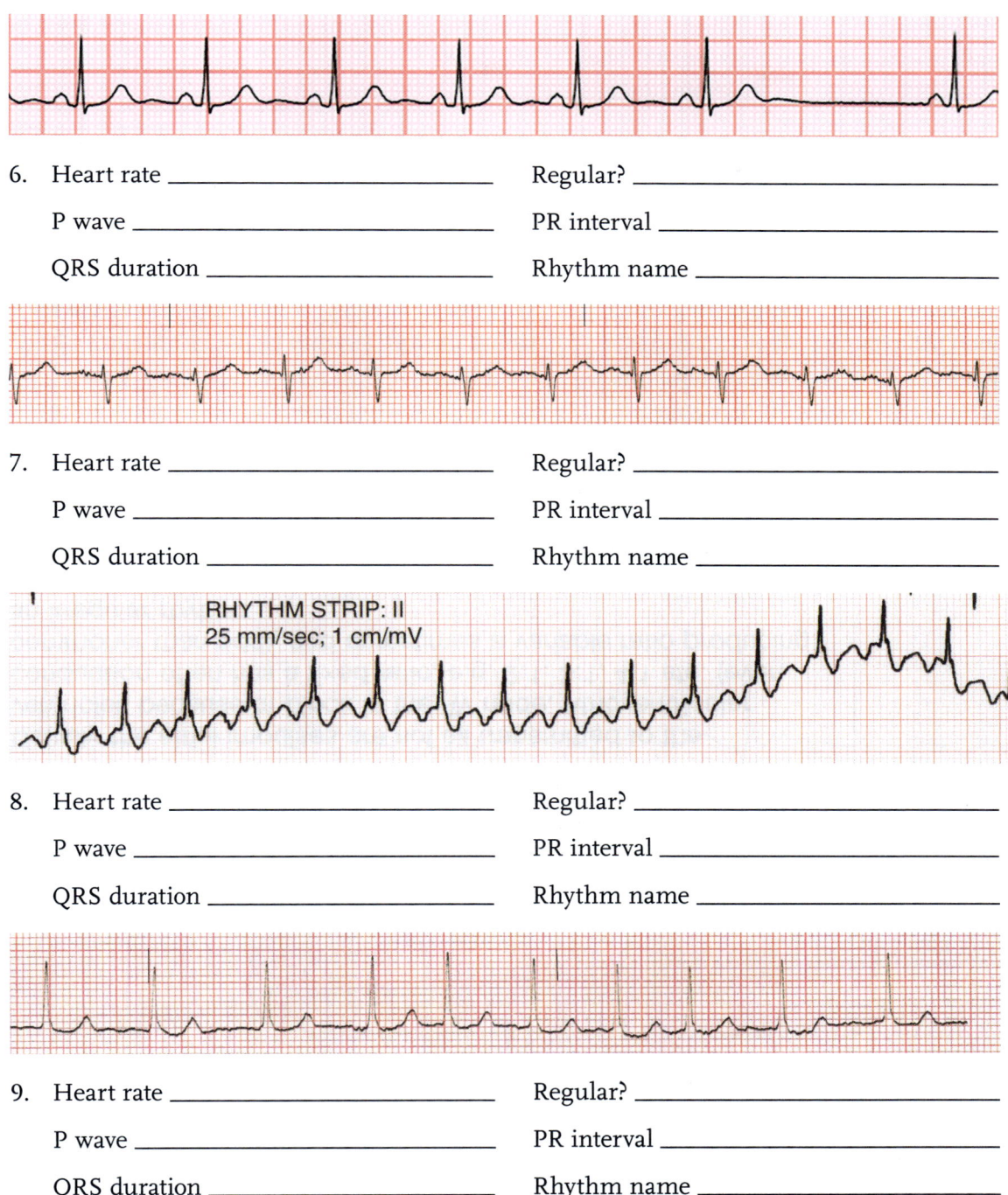

6. Heart rate _____ Regular? _____

   P wave _____ PR interval _____

   QRS duration _____ Rhythm name _____

7. Heart rate _____ Regular? _____

   P wave _____ PR interval _____

   QRS duration _____ Rhythm name _____

8. Heart rate _____ Regular? _____

   P wave _____ PR interval _____

   QRS duration _____ Rhythm name _____

9. Heart rate _____ Regular? _____

   P wave _____ PR interval _____

   QRS duration _____ Rhythm name _____

6. Identify junctional rhythms

Junctional rhythms occur when electrical impulses begin in the AV junction. If the SA node impulse is too slow, is blocked, or is not generated, then cells near the bundle of His will generate an impulse. This area of cells in the AV junction can also become irritable and initiate an impulse that interrupts the sinus rhythm. This impulse travels backward through the atria (the term for this is **retrograde**), so the P wave may be inverted. This means it goes down from the baseline rather than up. The P wave may also be hidden in the QRS complex or appear after the QRS complex. Impulses that start in the junctional area may happen early or late. The duration of the QRS complex in most junctional rhythms is 0.12 seconds or less.

Premature junctional complexes (PJCs) are impulses generated by an irritable area of the AV junction (Fig. 9-15). These beats occur early, meaning that they happen before the next sinus beat would normally occur. These complexes have a normal QRS complex. They can easily be mistaken for PACs. The P wave in a premature junctional complex is inverted. It may appear before the QRS complex. It may also be hidden within the QRS complex, or appear after the QRS complex. It is important to identify the underlying rhythm with PJCs. Examples of possible underlying rhythms include sinus bradycardia and NSR.

If the SA node is very slow or does not generate an impulse at all, the AV junction area may generate an impulse. This causes **junctional escape beats**. PJCs are early beats, and junctional escape beats occur late. This means they come after the next beat should have occurred. A series of junctional escape beats is called **junctional escape rhythm** or *junctional rhythm* (Fig. 9-16). This rhythm can occur if the SA node fails and the atrial tissue does not generate an impulse. The intrinsic rate of the junctional area is only 40–60 BPM, so the rate for a junctional rhythm is usually in this range.

(a) P waves are absent in these premature beats

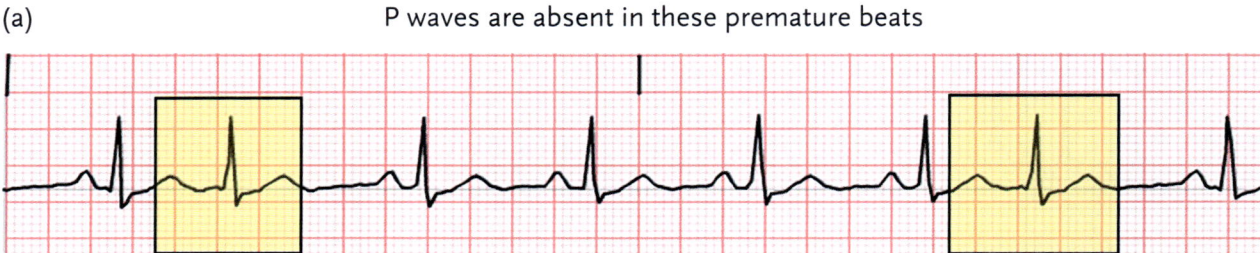

(b) Even in a rapid rhythm the premature beats with missing P waves are easy to recognize

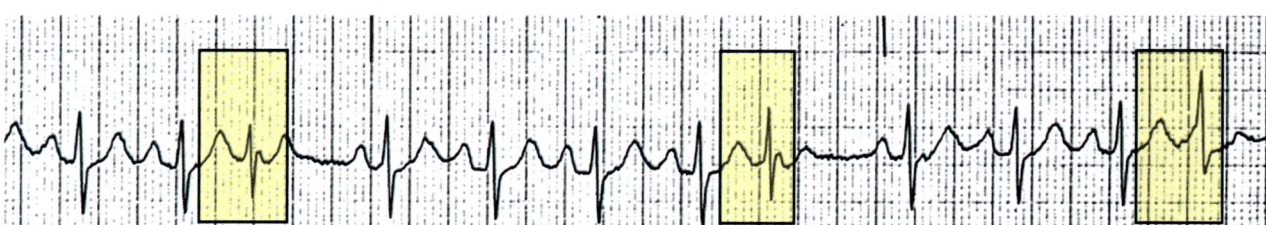

Name of rhythm: Premature junctional complex (PJC) with (a) underlying normal sinus rhythm and (b) underlying sinus tachycardia

Rate: Depends on underlying rhythm [(a) 80 BPM; (b) 115 BPM]

Rhythm pattern: Irregular

P wave characteristics: Inverted or absent; may be before, during, or after QRS

PR interval: <0.12 s or not measurable (not measurable in these premature beats)

QRS duration: <0.12 s (0.08 s in both strips)

Unique identifier: Irregular early beats within underlying rhythm; irregular beats have inverted or absent P wave

Fig. 9-15. *Illustration of premature junctional complexes with (a) underlying normal sinus rhythm and (b) underlying sinus tachycardia.*

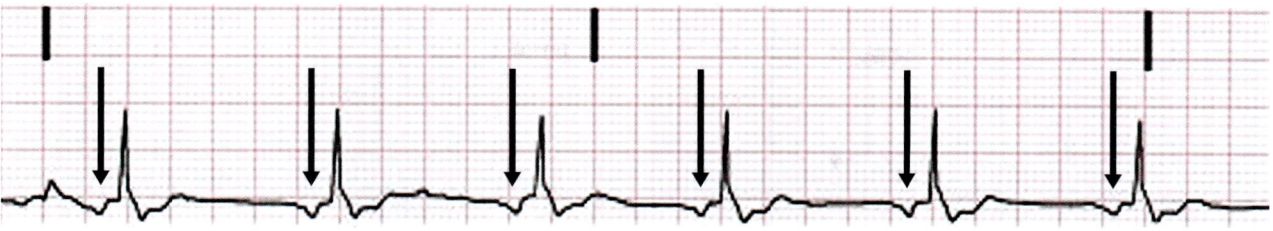

Name of rhythm: Junctional escape rhythm	**PR interval:** Usually <0.12 s or not measurable (0.16 s)
Rate: 40–60 BPM (42 BPM)	
Rhythm pattern: Regular	**QRS duration:** <0.12 s (0.08 s)
P wave characteristics: Inverted or absent; may be before, during, or after QRS	**Unique identifier:** Inverted or absent P wave; normal QRS duration

Fig. 9-16. *Illustration of junctional escape rhythm.*

When the junctional tissue takes over as the heart's pacemaker, the heart does not work as well as it should. Some cardiac output is lost. **Accelerated junctional rhythm** is sometimes seen. It is called *accelerated* because it is faster than the normal intrinsic rate of junctional tissue. In this junctional rhythm, the heart speeds up to make up for the loss of atrial contraction (often referred to as **atrial kick**). An accelerated junctional rhythm allows the body to keep cardiac output high enough to get oxygenated blood to the rest of the body (Fig. 9-17). The normal rate for this rhythm is 60–99 BPM. The P wave characteristics and the QRS width are the same as for other junctional rhythms.

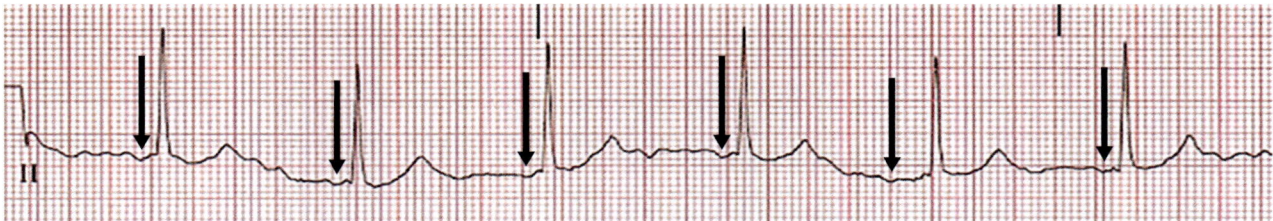

Name of rhythm: Accelerated junctional rhythm	**PR interval:** <0.12 s or not measurable
Rate: 60–99 BPM (62 BPM)	**QRS duration:** <0.12 s (0.06 s)
Rhythm pattern: Regular	**Unique identifier:** Inverted or absent P wave; normal QRS duration
P wave characteristics: Inverted or absent; may be before, during, or after QRS	

Fig. 9-17. *Illustration of accelerated junctional rhythm.*

When the rate of the junctional rhythm is 100 beats per minute or higher, it is called **junctional tachycardia** (Fig. 9-18). This rhythm may be mistaken for some of the other supraventricular tachycardias. They are also fast rhythms with no visible P waves and normal QRS complexes. If the tracing shows a narrow (normal) QRS complex, inverted or no P waves in lead II, and a rate of 100–140 BPM, the rhythm is junctional tachycardia.

P waves are absent or abnormal and rate is 100 BPM or higher

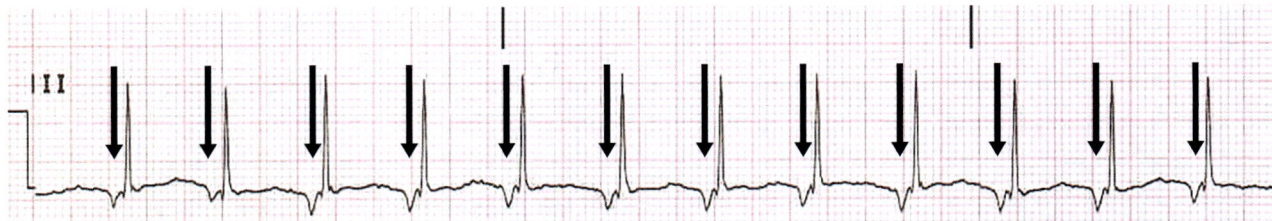

Name of rhythm: Junctional tachycardia

Rate: 100–150 BPM (115 BPM)

Rhythm pattern: Regular

P wave characteristics: Inverted or absent; may be before, during, or after QRS

PR interval: <0.12 s or not measurable (0.08 s)

QRS duration: <0.12 s (0.04 s)

Unique identifier: Inverted or absent P wave; normal QRS duration

Fig. 9-18. Illustration of junctional tachycardia.

7. Discuss what junctional rhythms mean for the patient

Junctional rhythms can be caused by fatigue, stimulants or other medications, heart disease, MI, electrolyte imbalance, hypoxia, or chronic obstructive pulmonary disease (long-lasting lung disorders). A patient with these rhythms may have fatigue or low energy. The patient usually does not realize she has a dysrhythmia until it is seen on an EKG.

When a patient is in a junctional rhythm the usual pattern of atrial contraction and ventricular contraction does not occur. This lack of coordination, along with the slower rate, can result in lower stroke volume. This means less blood is pumped with each heartbeat. It causes lower cardiac output. It may also cause the patient to have confusion, chest discomfort, weakness, or shortness of breath.

Treatment for junctional dysrhythmias includes finding and correcting the cause. It is important for the provider to consider MI as a possible cause. If a patient has junctional escape rhythm with a rate of less than 40 BPM, they may need an artificial pacemaker. This is only done if an underlying cause cannot be found and corrected.

PRACTICE

Analyze the junctional strips below using the 6 steps.

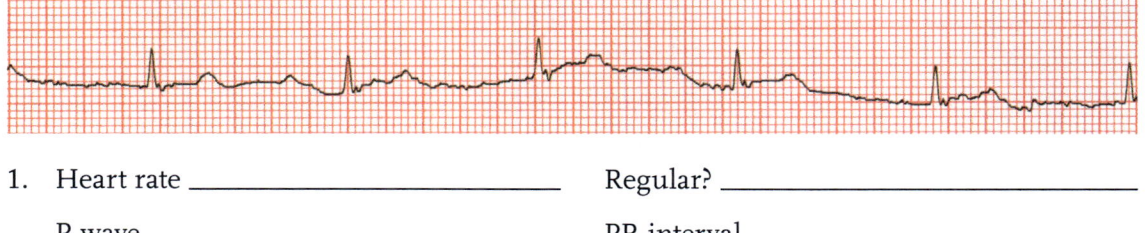

1. Heart rate _____ Regular? _____

   P wave _____ PR interval _____

   QRS duration _____ Rhythm name _____

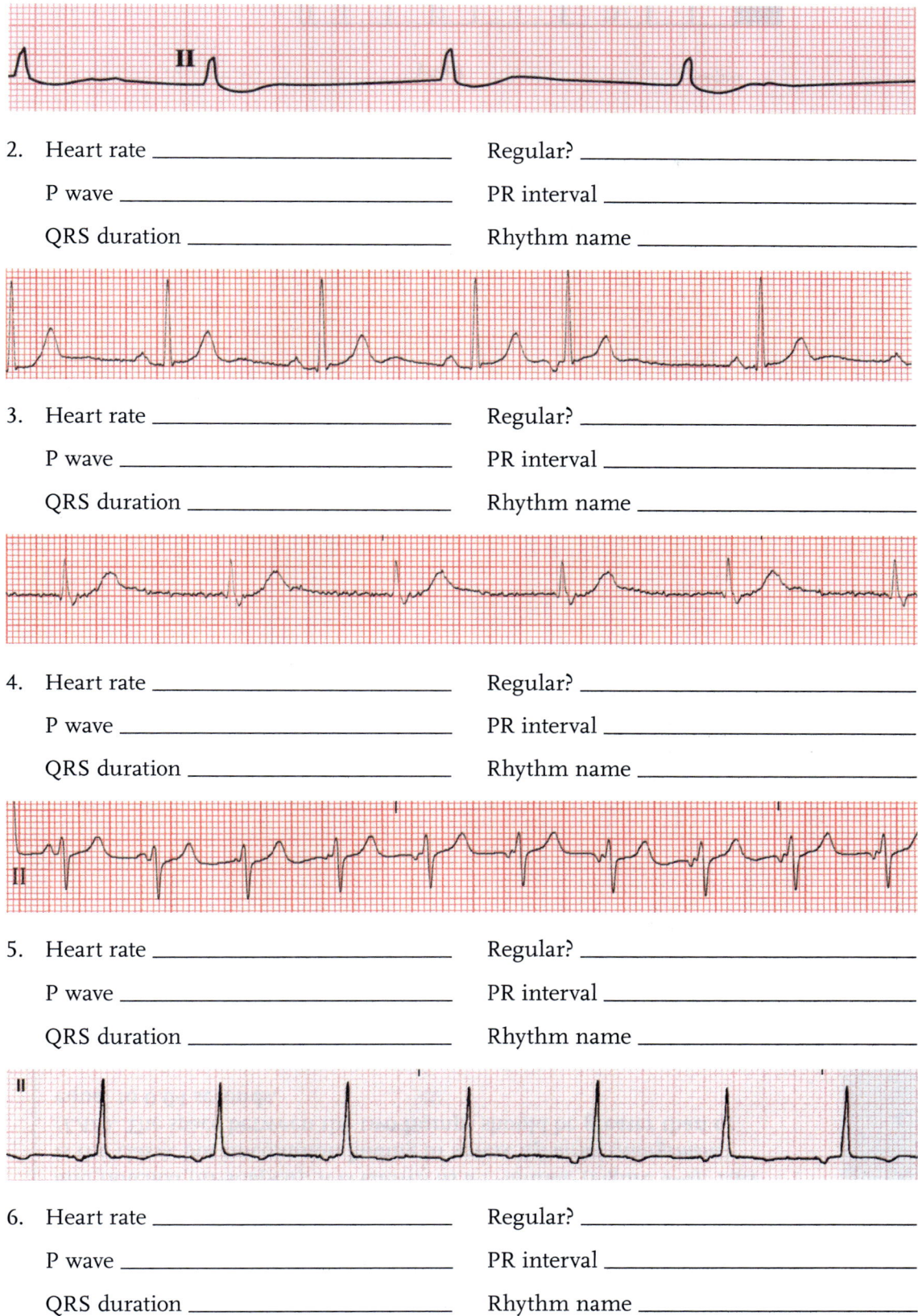

2. Heart rate _____ Regular? _____
   P wave _____ PR interval _____
   QRS duration _____ Rhythm name _____

3. Heart rate _____ Regular? _____
   P wave _____ PR interval _____
   QRS duration _____ Rhythm name _____

4. Heart rate _____ Regular? _____
   P wave _____ PR interval _____
   QRS duration _____ Rhythm name _____

5. Heart rate _____ Regular? _____
   P wave _____ PR interval _____
   QRS duration _____ Rhythm name _____

6. Heart rate _____ Regular? _____
   P wave _____ PR interval _____
   QRS duration _____ Rhythm name _____

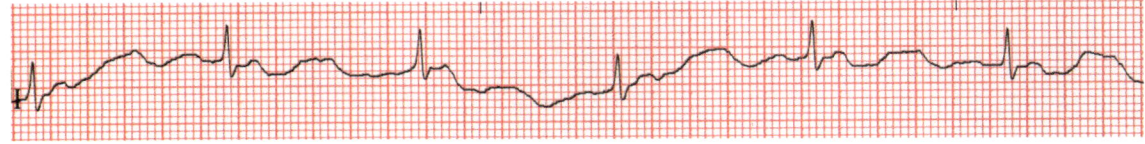

7. Heart rate _____ Regular? _____

   P wave _____ PR interval _____

   QRS duration _____ Rhythm name _____

ADVANCED PRACTICE

Analyze the strips below using the 6 steps. This set of strips includes sinus, atrial, and junctional rhythms. Some rhythms may have both an atrial rate and a ventricular rate. Note both rates when appropriate (mark *A* for *atrial* and *V* for *ventricular*).

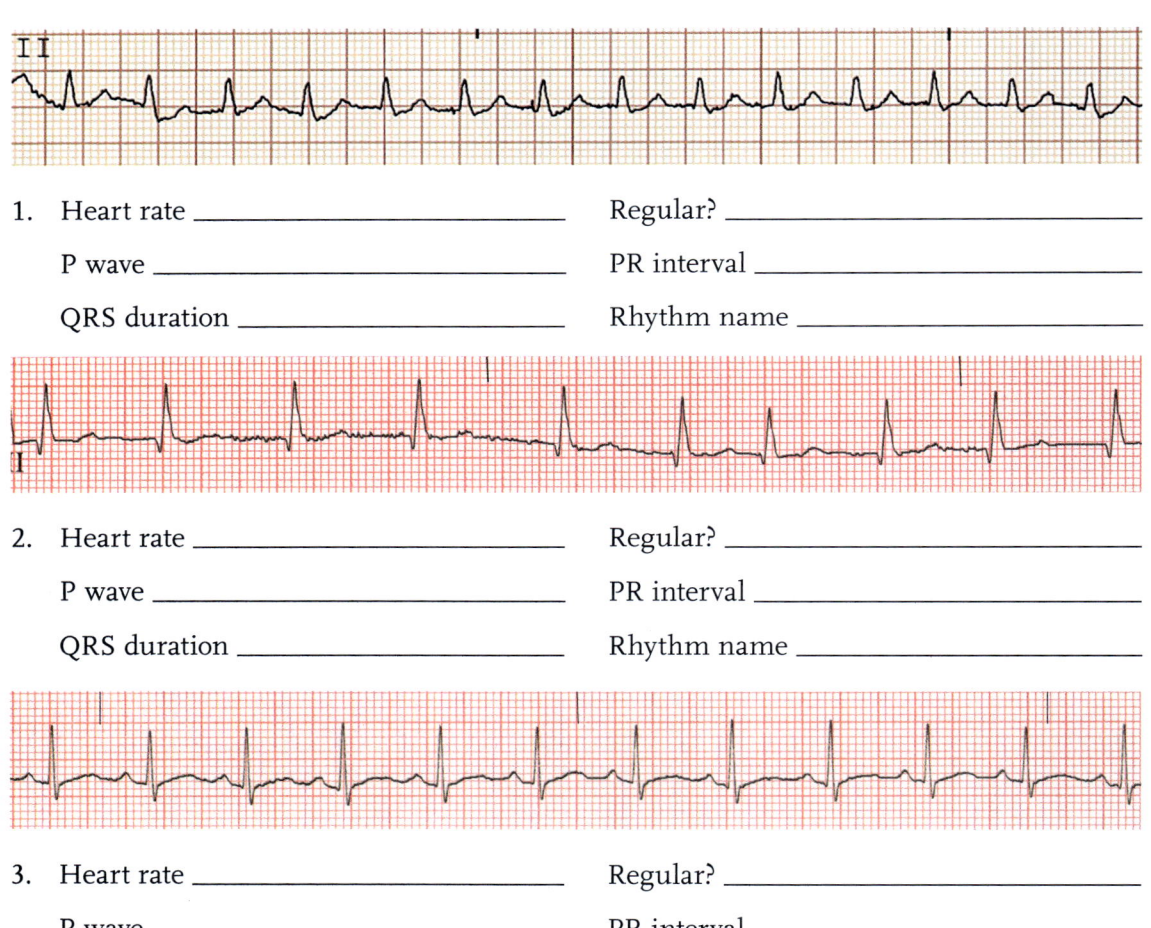

1. Heart rate _____ Regular? _____

   P wave _____ PR interval _____

   QRS duration _____ Rhythm name _____

2. Heart rate _____ Regular? _____

   P wave _____ PR interval _____

   QRS duration _____ Rhythm name _____

3. Heart rate _____ Regular? _____

   P wave _____ PR interval _____

   QRS duration _____ Rhythm name _____

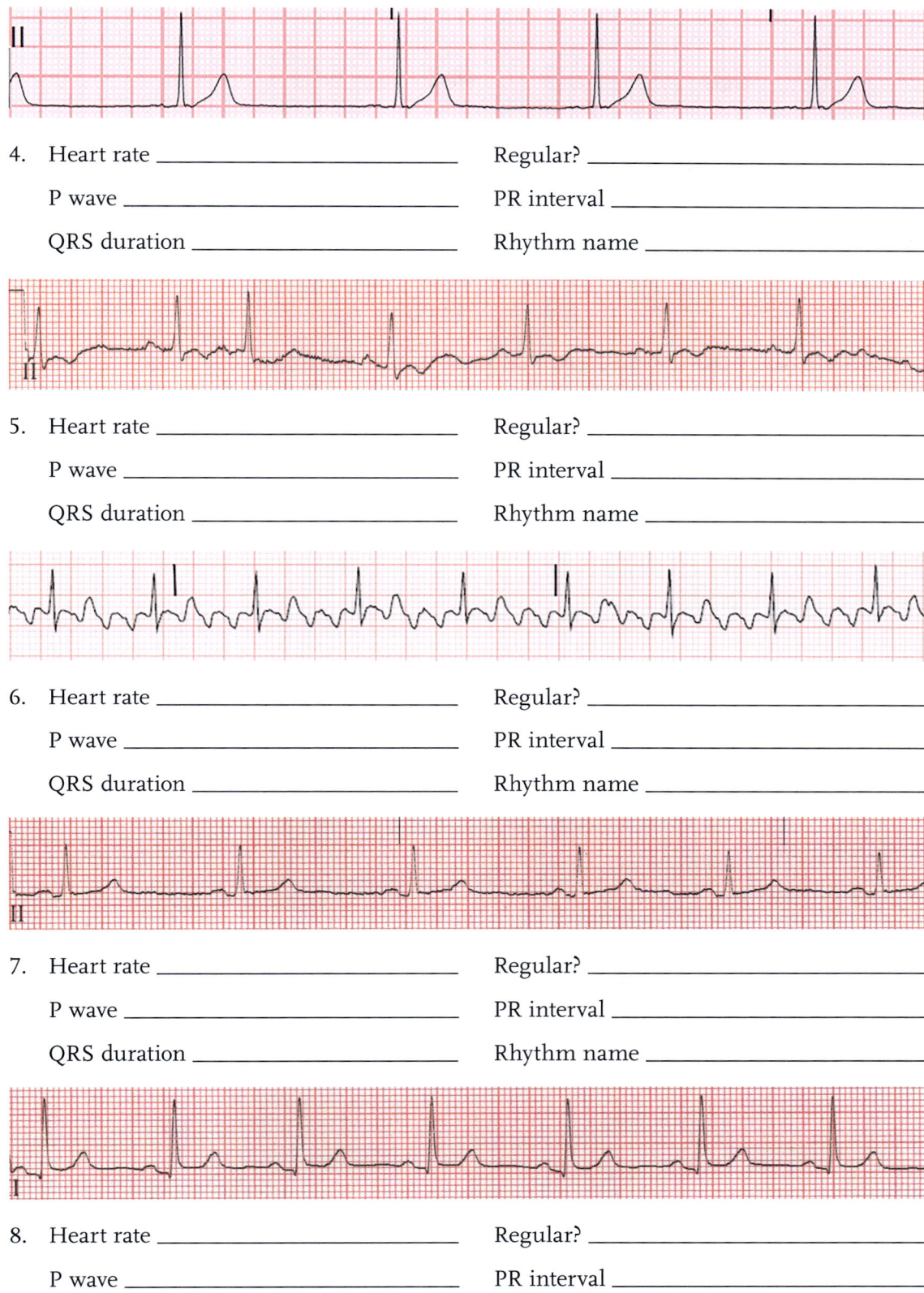

4. Heart rate _____ Regular? _____
   P wave _____ PR interval _____
   QRS duration _____ Rhythm name _____

5. Heart rate _____ Regular? _____
   P wave _____ PR interval _____
   QRS duration _____ Rhythm name _____

6. Heart rate _____ Regular? _____
   P wave _____ PR interval _____
   QRS duration _____ Rhythm name _____

7. Heart rate _____ Regular? _____
   P wave _____ PR interval _____
   QRS duration _____ Rhythm name _____

8. Heart rate _____ Regular? _____
   P wave _____ PR interval _____
   QRS duration _____ Rhythm name _____

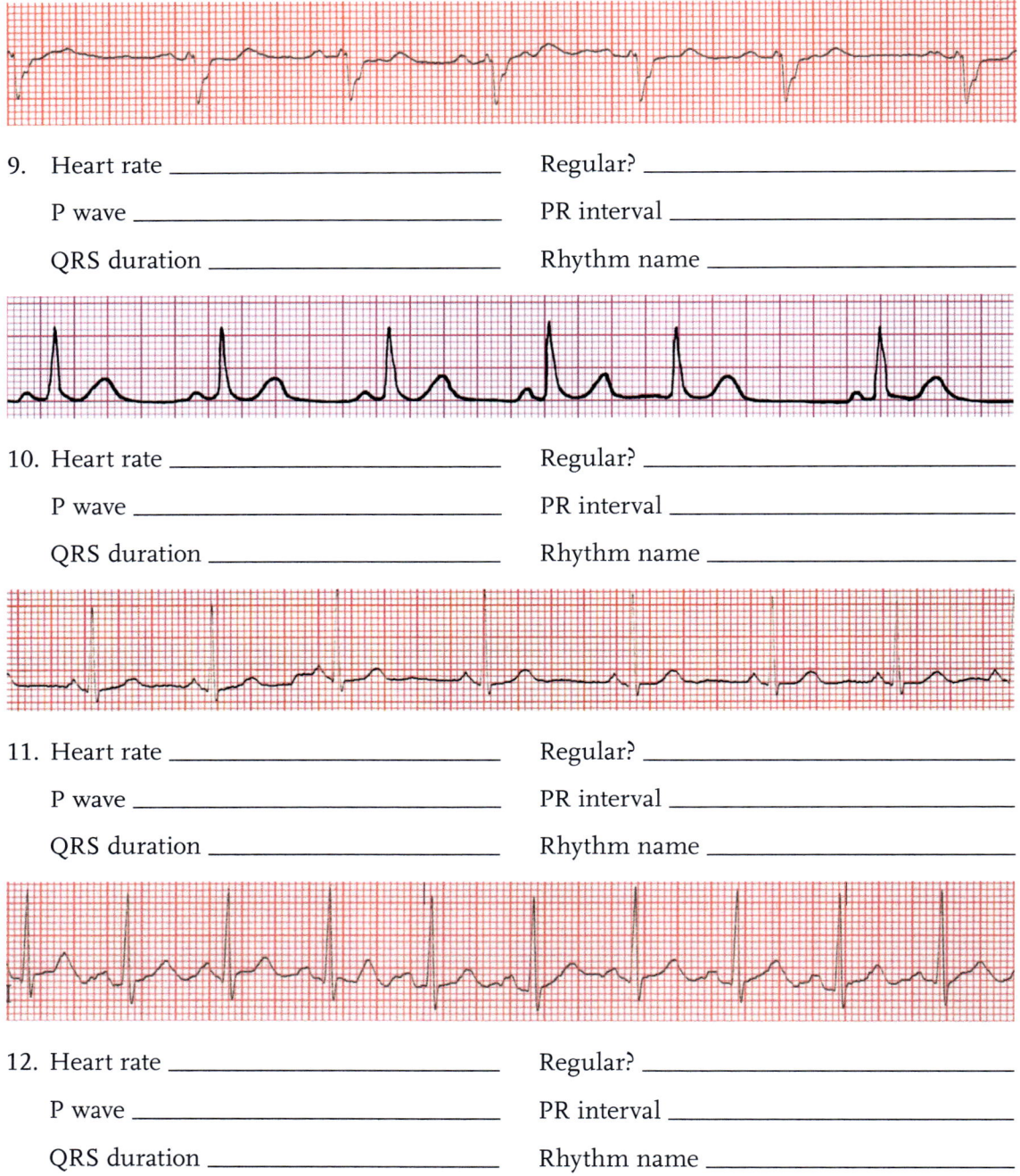

9. Heart rate _____ Regular? _____

   P wave _____ PR interval _____

   QRS duration _____ Rhythm name _____

10. Heart rate _____ Regular? _____

    P wave _____ PR interval _____

    QRS duration _____ Rhythm name _____

11. Heart rate _____ Regular? _____

    P wave _____ PR interval _____

    QRS duration _____ Rhythm name _____

12. Heart rate _____ Regular? _____

    P wave _____ PR interval _____

    QRS duration _____ Rhythm name _____

8. Identify ventricular rhythms

Rhythms that begin in the ventricles are called *ventricular rhythms*. They have a noticeable feature on an EKG tracing. The QRS complex relates to electrical impulses that cause the ventricles to contract. Because the ventricles make up a large part of the heart, the QRS complex is large and is the most easily seen part of an EKG tracing. The QRS complex is even more noticeable in ventricular rhythms. The duration of the QRS is longer than normal. The complex is wider than normal on the EKG tracing.

An irritable area can cause **premature ventricular complexes** (**PVCs**). These premature beats begin low in the cardiac conduction system. They do not travel the normal pathways. This makes the QRS wide and **bizarre** (unusual in appearance). These beats may occur one at a time, in pairs (called couplets), or in short runs of three or more. PVCs may also occur in patterns such as **bigeminy** (every other beat) or **trigeminy** (every third beat) (Fig. 9-19).

(a) Every other beat is early and features a wide, bizarre QRS complex

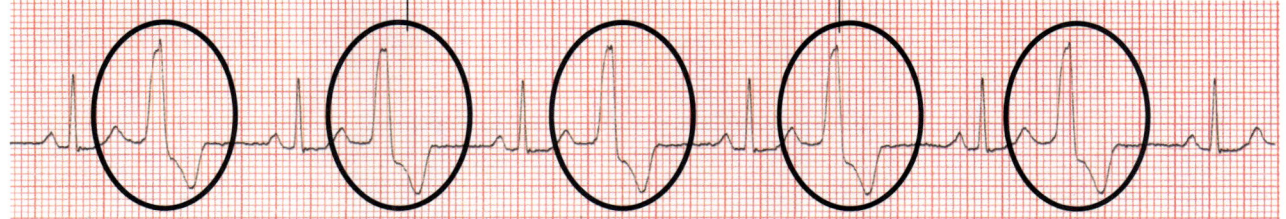

(b) Every third beat is early and QRS in early beats differs from QRS in underlying rhythm

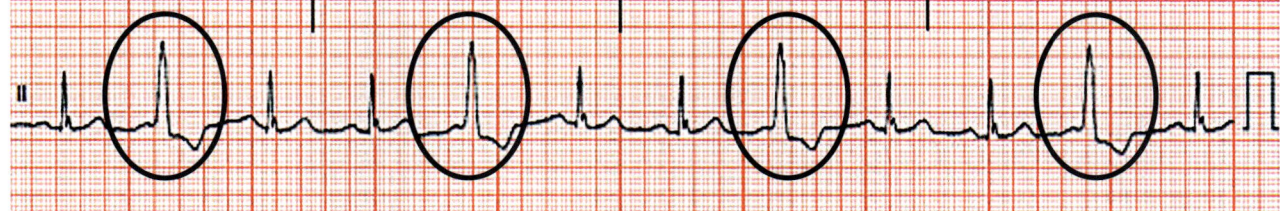

Name of rhythm: Premature ventricular complexes (PVCs): (a) bigeminal with underlying sinus bradycardia; (b) trigeminal with underlying junctional rhythm

Rate: Depends on underlying rhythm

Rhythm pattern: Irregular due to early beats; underlying rhythm may be regular

P wave characteristics: Usually absent in PVC beats

PR interval: Depends on underlying rhythm; no P wave for PVC beats

QRS duration: Depends on underlying rhythm; in PVCs beats, duration is >0.10 s (0.16 s for PVC beats on these strips)

Unique identifier: Early, wide, bizarre beats; QRS deflection may be opposite of QRS of underlying rhythm. Can appear in different patterns, such as the bigeminy and trigeminy illustrated here.

Fig. 9-19. *Illustration of (a) bigeminal PVCs with underlying sinus bradycardia and (b) trigeminal PVCs with underlying junctional rhythm.*

If all of the PVCs on an EKG tracing look the same, they are called **unifocal**. If they look different within the same tracing, they are called **multifocal** (Fig. 9-20). Multifocal PVCs happen when different irritable areas create electrical impulses in the ventricles. The greater the number of PVCs an EKG shows and the greater the variety between the PVCs, the more dangerous the rhythm may be for the patient. It is important to identify and name the underlying rhythm along with the type of PVCs. PVCs often happen when a patient is in sinus bradycardia.

(a) Unifocal PVCs are similar in appearance

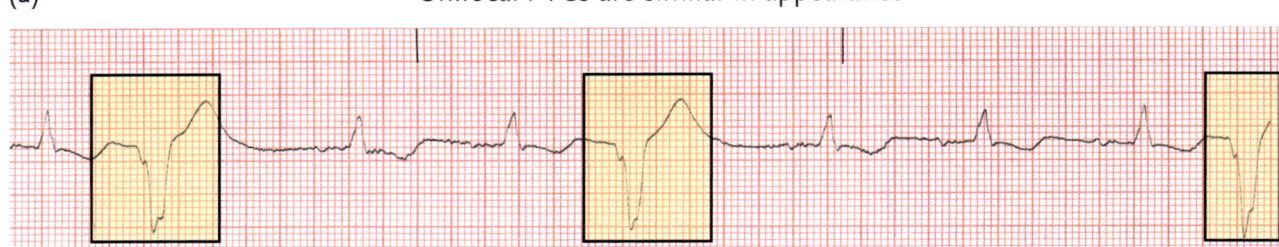

(b) Multifocal PVCs are different in appearance

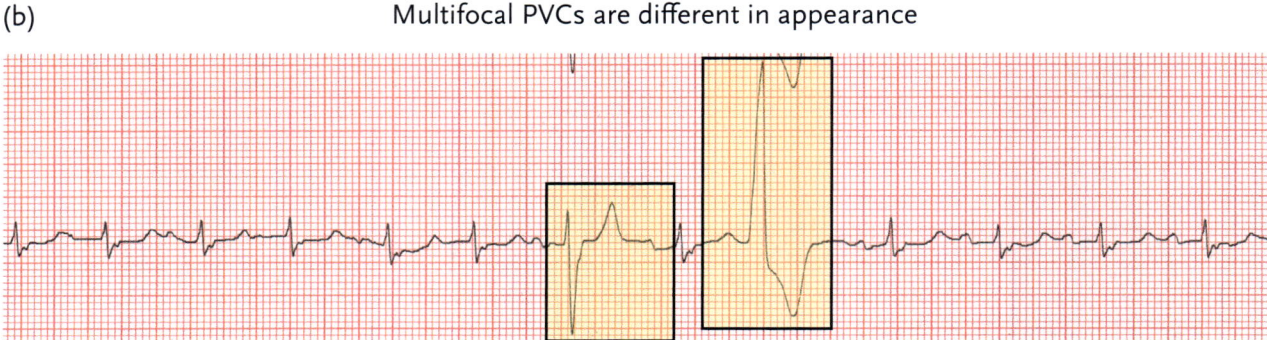

Fig. 9-20. *Illustration of (a) unifocal PVCs with underlying sinus bradycardia and (b) multifocal PVCs with underlying sinus tachycardia.*

Ventricular escape beats may happen when the SA node and other pacemakers above the bundle branches do not initiate an impulse (Fig. 9-21). The difference between a PVC and a ventricular escape beat is their timing. A PVC happens early. A ventricular escape beat happens late. The appearance of the QRS complex in ventricular escape beats is also wide and bizarre. The underlying rhythm, often sinus bradycardia, must also be identified.

The QRS complex in ventricular escape beats is also wide and bizarre

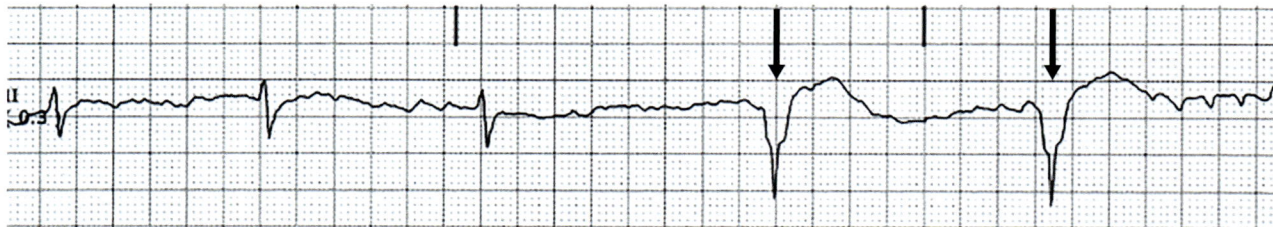

Name of rhythm: Ventricular escape beats with underlying atrial fibrillation (controlled)

Rate: Depends on underlying rhythm (40 BPM)

Rhythm pattern: Irregular due to late beats; underlying rhythm may be regular

P wave characteristics: Generally not visible in ventricular escape beats

PR interval: Not measurable

QRS duration: >0.10 s for ventricular escape beats (0.12 s)

Unique identifier: Late, wide, bizarre beats; QRS deflection may be opposite of QRS in underlying rhythm

Fig. 9-21. *Illustration of ventricular escape beats.*

When three or more ventricular escape beats happen in a row it is called an **idioventricular rhythm** or *ventricular escape rhythm* (Fig. 9-22). Because the intrinsic rate of the Purkinje fibers is only 20–40 BPM, that is the normal rate for this rhythm. The QRS complexes are wide and bizarre. This rhythm is very abnormal but it may not cause lasting damage if it only lasts for a few beats. If this very slow ventricular rhythm continues, however, it can be deadly. A sustained (continued) idioventricular rhythm is called **agonal rhythm**, which means it is associated with the pain of dying.

QRS complexes are wide and bizarre and rate is very slow

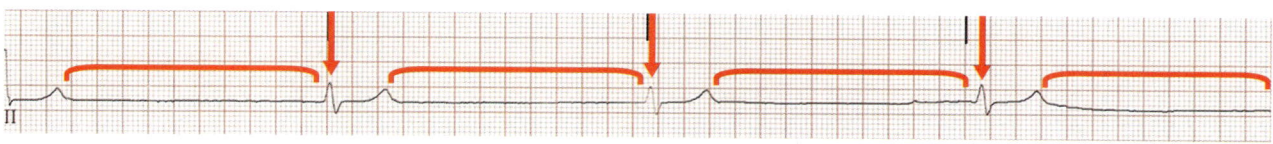

POTENTIALLY LETHAL RHYTHM

Name of rhythm: Idioventricular rhythm
Rate: 20–40 BPM (24 BPM)
Rhythm pattern: Regular
P wave characteristics: Not visible

PR interval: Not measurable
QRS duration: >0.10 s (0.14 s)
Unique identifier: P wave absent; QRS wide and bizarre

Fig. 9-22. *Illustration of idioventricular rhythm.*

Take Action Now!

A slow, sustained idioventricular rhythm is a potentially lethal dysrhythmia. If a patient has this rhythm, the EKG technician should take immediate emergency action, following facility policy.

Accelerated idioventricular rhythm (AIVR) occurs when three or more ventricular escape beats happen in a row with a higher rate, between 40 and 100 BPM (Fig. 9-23). As in other ventricular rhythms, the QRS complexes are wide and bizarre.

QRS complexes are wide and bizarre and rate is rapid

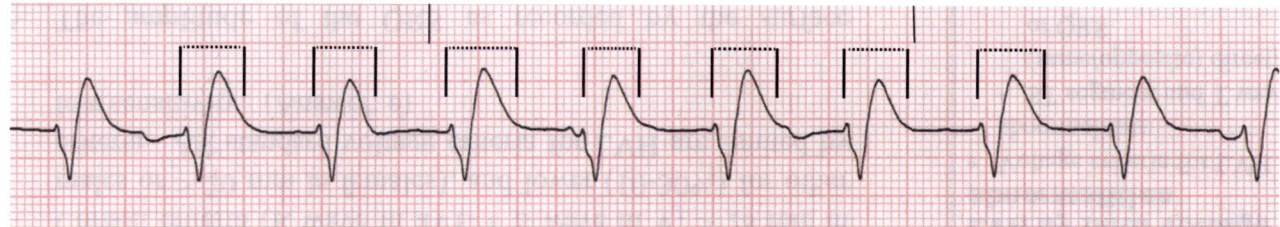

Name of rhythm: Accelerated idioventricular rhythm
Rate: 40–100 BPM (93 BPM)
Rhythm pattern: Regular
P wave characteristics: Not visible

PR interval: Not measurable
QRS duration: >0.12 s (0.36 s)
Unique identifier: P wave absent; QRS wide and bizarre, rate 40–100 BPM

Fig. 9-23. *Illustration of accelerated idioventricular rhythm.*

Ventricular tachycardia (**VT**) is an especially dangerous rhythm. The rate is so fast that it does not allow the coronary arteries to fill. This reduces cardiac output. A patient may or may not have a palpable pulse (a pulse that can be felt) when the VT starts. Without treatment a person with ventricular tachycardia can die. When untreated, ventricular tachycardia can get worse and become a dangerous rhythm called *ventricular fibrillation* (described later in this learning objective).

There are two main categories of ventricular tachycardia: monomorphic and polymorphic (Fig. 9-24). In **monomorphic** VT the QRS complexes are wide and bizarre, but they are uniform in appearance. This means they always look the same. The rate can vary. The usual range is from around 120–250 BPM. In **polymorphic** VT the QRS complexes are not uniform. They vary in amplitude (height), shape, or direction. Polymorphic VT happens in different forms, including **torsades de pointes**. In this rhythm, the QRS complex seems to "twist" from one side of the baseline to the other (Fig. 9-25). Polymorphic VT is less stable than monomorphic VT. The rate for polymorphic VT is 150–300 BPM. It may be irregular. Both monomorphic and polymorphic VT are considered very unstable and potentially lethal dysrhythmias.

Take Action Now!

When three or more premature ventricular contractions occur in a row the rhythm is known as a *run of ventricular tachycardia*. If the EKG technician sees a run of VT, he should tell the provider immediately.

Tip

Bundle Branch Blocks

When a ventricular conduction pathway is damaged, the electrical impulse to part of the ventricles is delayed. That delay is called a **bundle branch block** (**BBB**). It causes recognizable changes on the EKG. All bundle branch blocks have a widened QRS complex (>0.10 s) and leads V1 and V6 show noticeable changes. These changes look different depending on whether a right bundle branch block (RBBB) or left bundle branch block (LBBB) is happening (as shown below). If the EKG technician sees a bundle branch block on an EKG, she should report it to the provider.

RBBB

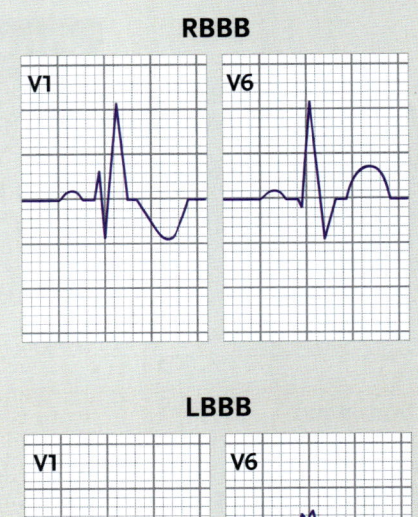

LBBB

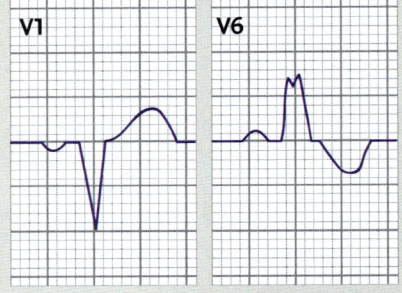

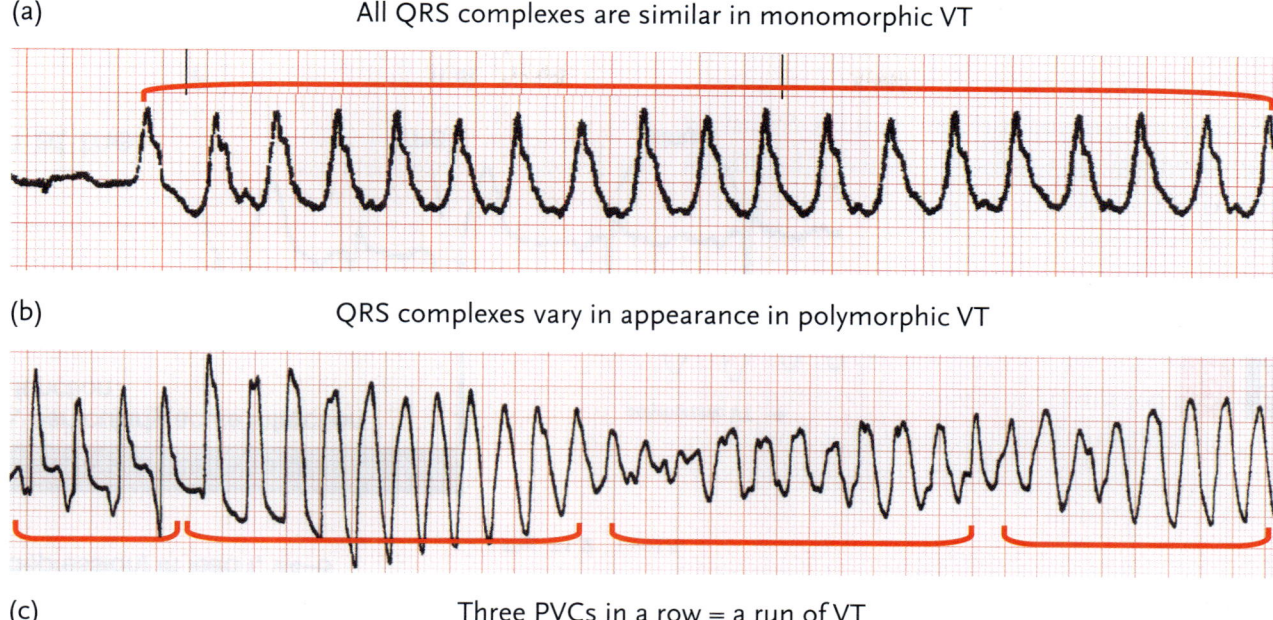

Name of rhythm: Ventricular tachycardia

Rate: 100–200 BPM

Rhythm pattern: Regular

P wave characteristics: Not visible

PR interval: Not measurable

QRS duration: >0.10 s

Unique identifier: Fast rate; P wave absent; QRS wide and bizarre with sawtooth appearance
Be sure to check electrodes/lead wires and clinical condition of patient.

Fig. 9-24. Illustrations of (a) monomorphic ventricular tachycardia, (b) polymorphic ventricular tachycardia, and (c) a run of ventricular tachycardia.

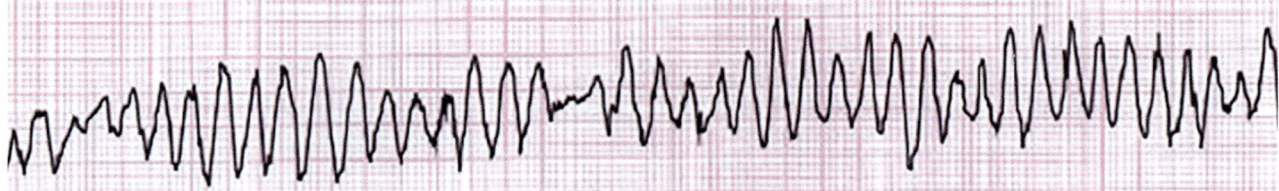

Fig. 9-25. A variation of polymorphic VT called *torsades de pointes* features dramatic movement above and below the isoelectric line.

All the dysrhythmias described so far have an organized but sometimes **aberrant** conduction path. This means the conduction path is different from the normal path but it still works in an organized way. In the case of **ventricular fibrillation** (also known as *VF* or *V-fib*), the conduction path is not organized. Because of this, the heart muscle does not contract in an organized way (Fig. 9-26). In V-fib, multiple sites in the ventricles fire at a very fast rate. The EKG tracing does not show any organized features. It is impossible to analyze rate, regularity, P waves, PR interval, or QRS width. V-fib is considered a lethal dysrhythmia.

> **Take Action Now!**
>
> Ventricular fibrillation may follow untreated ventricular tachycardia. It can also begin after certain types of premature ventricular contractions appear. Couplets of PVCs, multifocal PVCs, and PVCs that show something called **R-on-T phenomenon** are very dangerous. R-on-T phenomenon happens when the QRS complex of a PVC falls on the T wave of the beat before it. This can cause the heart to go into ventricular fibrillation. If an EKG technician sees R-on-T happening in a patient with PVCs, she should notify the provider immediately.
>
>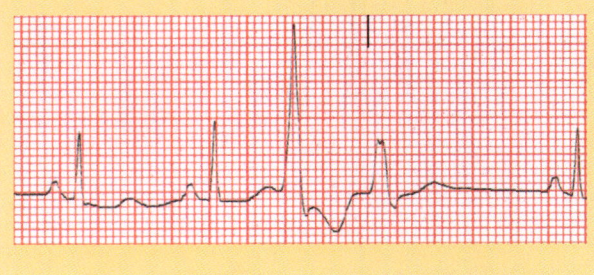

Chaotic and disorganized electrical activity produces no recognizable or measurable features

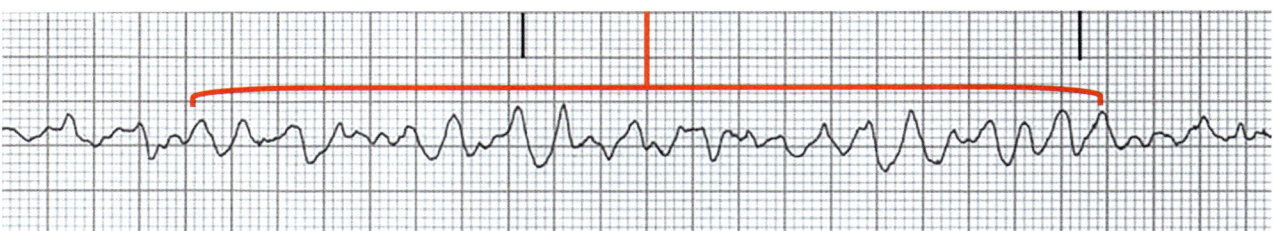

POTENTIALLY LETHAL RHYTHM

Name of rhythm: Ventricular fibrillation

Rate: Not measurable

Rhythm pattern: Chaotic

P wave characteristics: Not visible

PR interval: Not measurable

QRS duration: Not measurable

Unique identifier: Electrical activity chaotic and disorganized; no recognizable waves or complexes
Be sure to check electrodes/lead wires and clinical condition of patient.

Fig. 9-26. *Illustration of ventricular fibrillation.*

The rhythm below is sometimes called *flatline*. Its proper medical name is **asystole**, which means *without contractions* (Fig. 9-27). The EKG tracing may show small changes in the baseline, but there is no cardiac activity. The patient's heart has stopped beating.

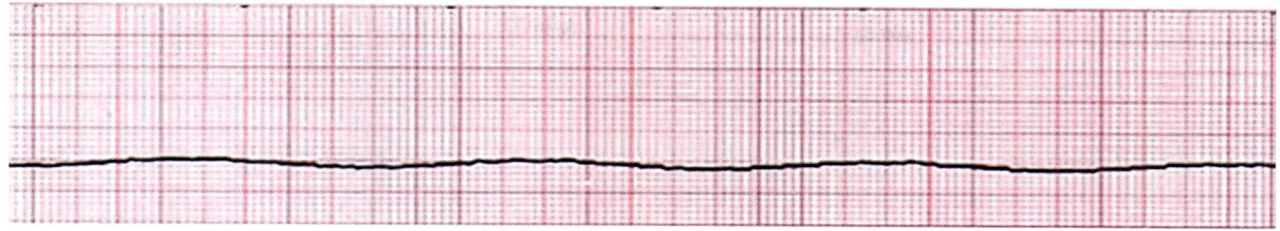

No waves or complexes because there is no electrical activity

POTENTIALLY LETHAL RHYTHM

Name of rhythm: Asystole

Rate: Not measurable

Rhythm pattern: No electrical activity

P wave characteristics: None

PR interval: Not measurable

QRS duration: Not measurable

Unique identifier: Straight line or flat line
Be sure to check electrodes/lead wires and clinical condition of patient.

Fig. 9-27. *Illustration of asystole.*

Tip

Checking the Patient's Condition

It is *very important* for the EKG technician to confirm that a patient's condition matches the patient's EKG. Loose or disconnected lead wires or low gain on the EKG machine can cause errors that look like ventricular fibrillation or asystole.

9. Discuss what ventricular rhythms mean for the patient

Cardiac disease, medication side effects, stimulants, anxiety, or hypoxia can cause premature ventricular contractions. PVCs can also happen normally in some people. Treatment is based on identifying and addressing the cause of the PVCs.

Ventricular escape beats and idioventricular (ventricular escape) rhythm may be caused by MI, electrolyte imbalances, or medication side effects. A patient with idioventricular rhythm may have a pulse but will show signs that result from the slow rhythm. These signs could include a weak or absent pulse, low blood pressure, or blood pressure that cannot be detected. The patient may also have changes in consciousness such as passing out or struggling to stay conscious. A patient with this rhythm must be treated immediately to prevent death.

Take Action Now!

Sometimes a patient may show an organized rhythm on the EKG, but not have a pulse. This condition is called **pulseless electrical activity** (**PEA**). Causes may include electrolyte imbalance, drug overdose, hypothermia (low body temperature), blood clots, hypoxia, or blood loss. PEA is considered a lethal rhythm. CPR should be started immediately and the provider should be notified.

Ischemic heart disease is the most common cause of ventricular tachycardia and other serious ventricular dysrhythmias. VT can also be caused by cardiomyopathy, electrolyte imbalance, medication side effects, or some forms of drug abuse. The patient may have shortness of breath, confusion, lightheadedness, chest pain, or weakness. The intensity of the symptoms depends on the patient's general physical condition, the rate of the tachycardia, and the amount of time the tachycardia has been going on.

VT can also be deadly. It must be treated promptly. This can stop the rhythm from turning into ventricular fibrillation. Depending on the patient's symptoms, VT may be treated with medication and synchronized cardioversion or **defibrillation**. Defibrillation involves using a machine (a defibrillator or an **automated external defibrillator**) to deliver a shock to the patient's heart. The goal of defibrillation is to restore the heart's electrical system to normal function.

Ventricular fibrillation is an unorganized rhythm. It does not generate any cardiac output. The body does not receive the oxygenated blood it needs. Possible causes are similar to those of other ventricular rhythms. Electrocution may also be a cause. Before treating this rhythm it is very important to first make sure that the patient's condition matches the EKG. The EKG technician needs to be certain that the tracing is not the result of an error. Treatment includes prompt CPR and defibrillation.

There is no electrical activity in asystole. Asystole can be caused by all of the factors described in this learning objective. Again, it is very important to be sure that the patient's condition matches the EKG. Loose or disconnected lead wires can create a tracing that looks like asystole. Treatment for asystole includes prompt CPR and medication.

PRACTICE

Analyze the ventricular strips below using the 6 steps. Some rhythms have unmeasurable elements.

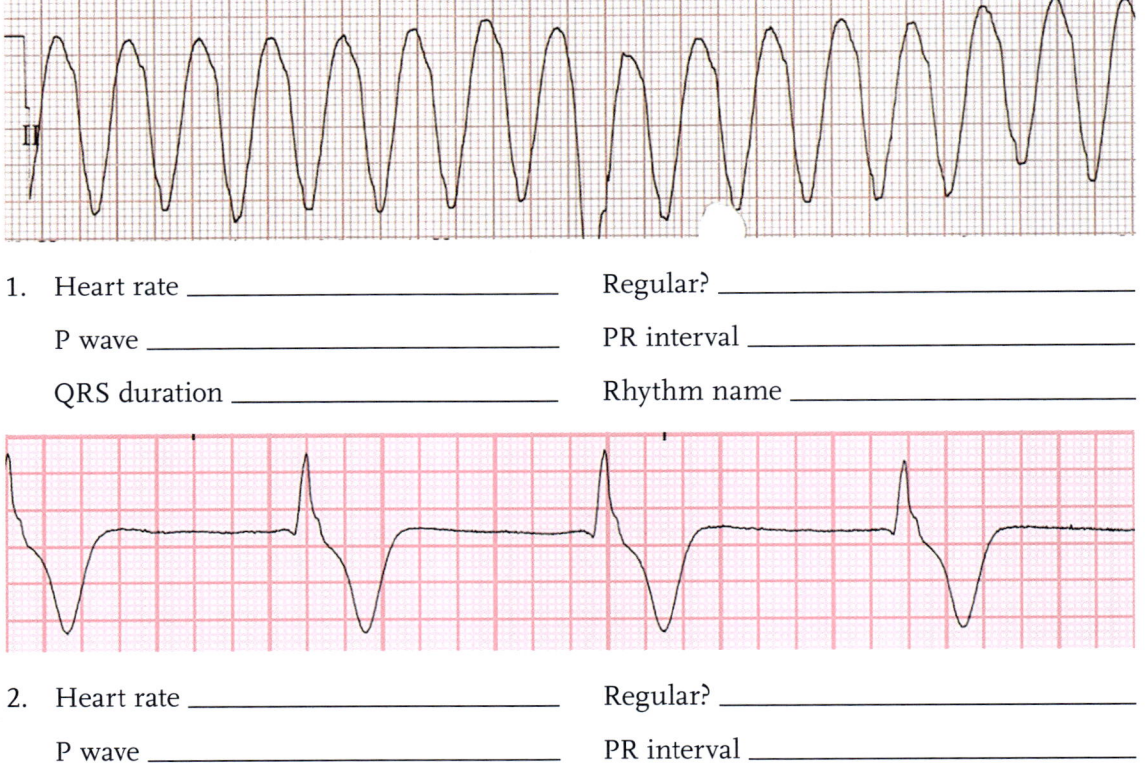

1. Heart rate _____ Regular? _____

   P wave _____ PR interval _____

   QRS duration _____ Rhythm name _____

2. Heart rate _____ Regular? _____

   P wave _____ PR interval _____

   QRS duration _____ Rhythm name _____

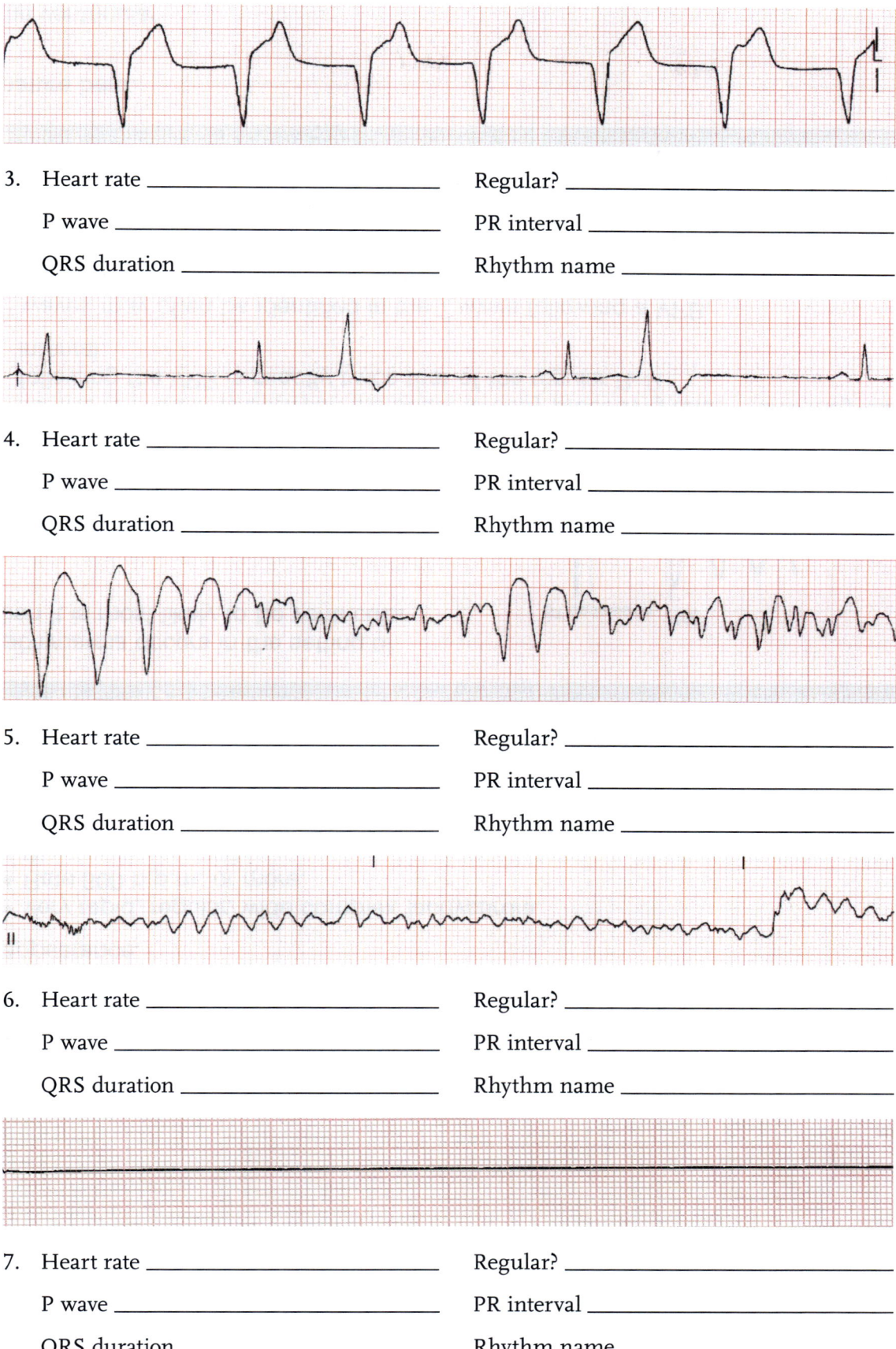

3. Heart rate _____ Regular? _____

   P wave _____ PR interval _____

   QRS duration _____ Rhythm name _____

4. Heart rate _____ Regular? _____

   P wave _____ PR interval _____

   QRS duration _____ Rhythm name _____

5. Heart rate _____ Regular? _____

   P wave _____ PR interval _____

   QRS duration _____ Rhythm name _____

6. Heart rate _____ Regular? _____

   P wave _____ PR interval _____

   QRS duration _____ Rhythm name _____

7. Heart rate _____ Regular? _____

   P wave _____ PR interval _____

   QRS duration _____ Rhythm name _____

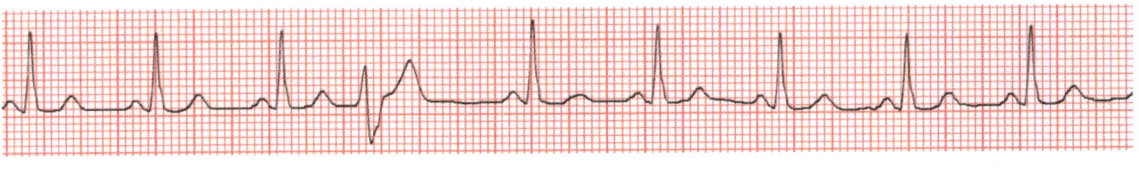

8. Heart rate _____ Regular? _____

   P wave _____ PR interval _____

   QRS duration _____ Rhythm name _____

ADVANCED PRACTICE

Analyze the strips below using the 6 steps. This set of strips includes sinus, atrial, junctional, and ventricular rhythms. Some rhythms may have both an atrial rate and a ventricular rate. Note both rates when appropriate (mark *A* for *atrial* and *V* for *ventricular*).

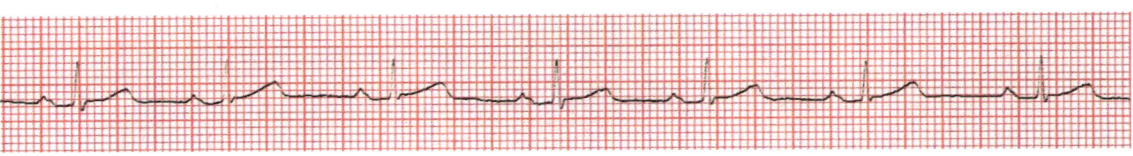

1. Heart rate _____ Regular? _____

   P wave _____ PR interval _____

   QRS duration _____ Rhythm name _____

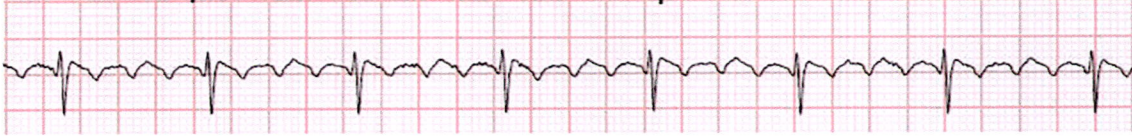

2. Heart rate _____ Regular? _____

   P wave _____ PR interval _____

   QRS duration _____ Rhythm name _____

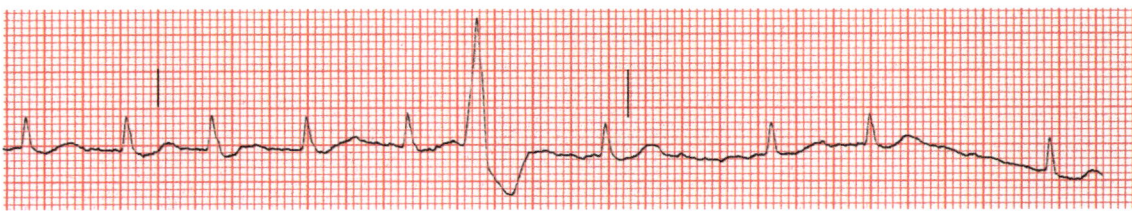

3. Heart rate _____ Regular? _____

   P wave _____ PR interval _____

   QRS duration _____ Rhythm name _____

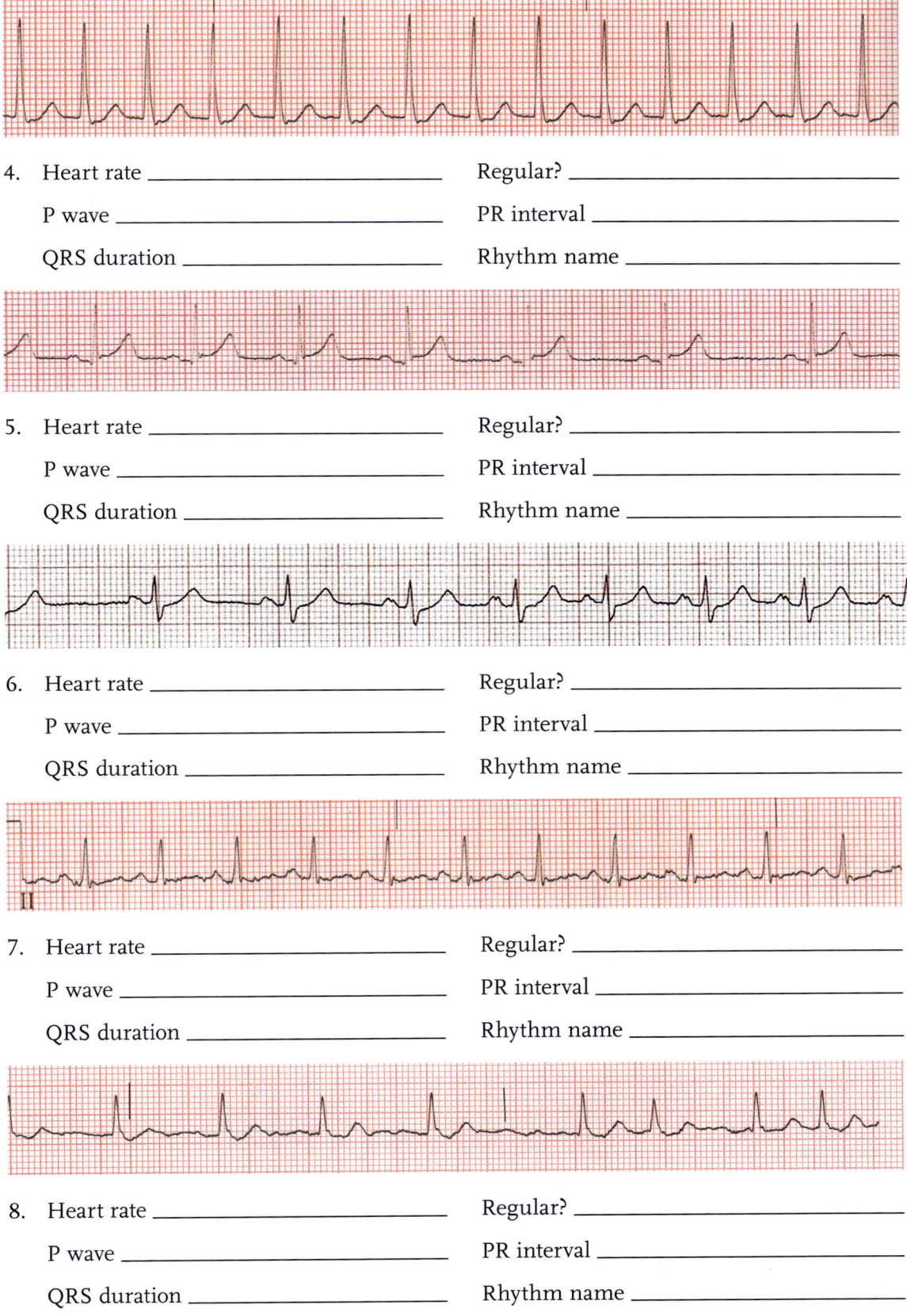

4. Heart rate _____ Regular? _____
   P wave _____ PR interval _____
   QRS duration _____ Rhythm name _____

5. Heart rate _____ Regular? _____
   P wave _____ PR interval _____
   QRS duration _____ Rhythm name _____

6. Heart rate _____ Regular? _____
   P wave _____ PR interval _____
   QRS duration _____ Rhythm name _____

7. Heart rate _____ Regular? _____
   P wave _____ PR interval _____
   QRS duration _____ Rhythm name _____

8. Heart rate _____ Regular? _____
   P wave _____ PR interval _____
   QRS duration _____ Rhythm name _____

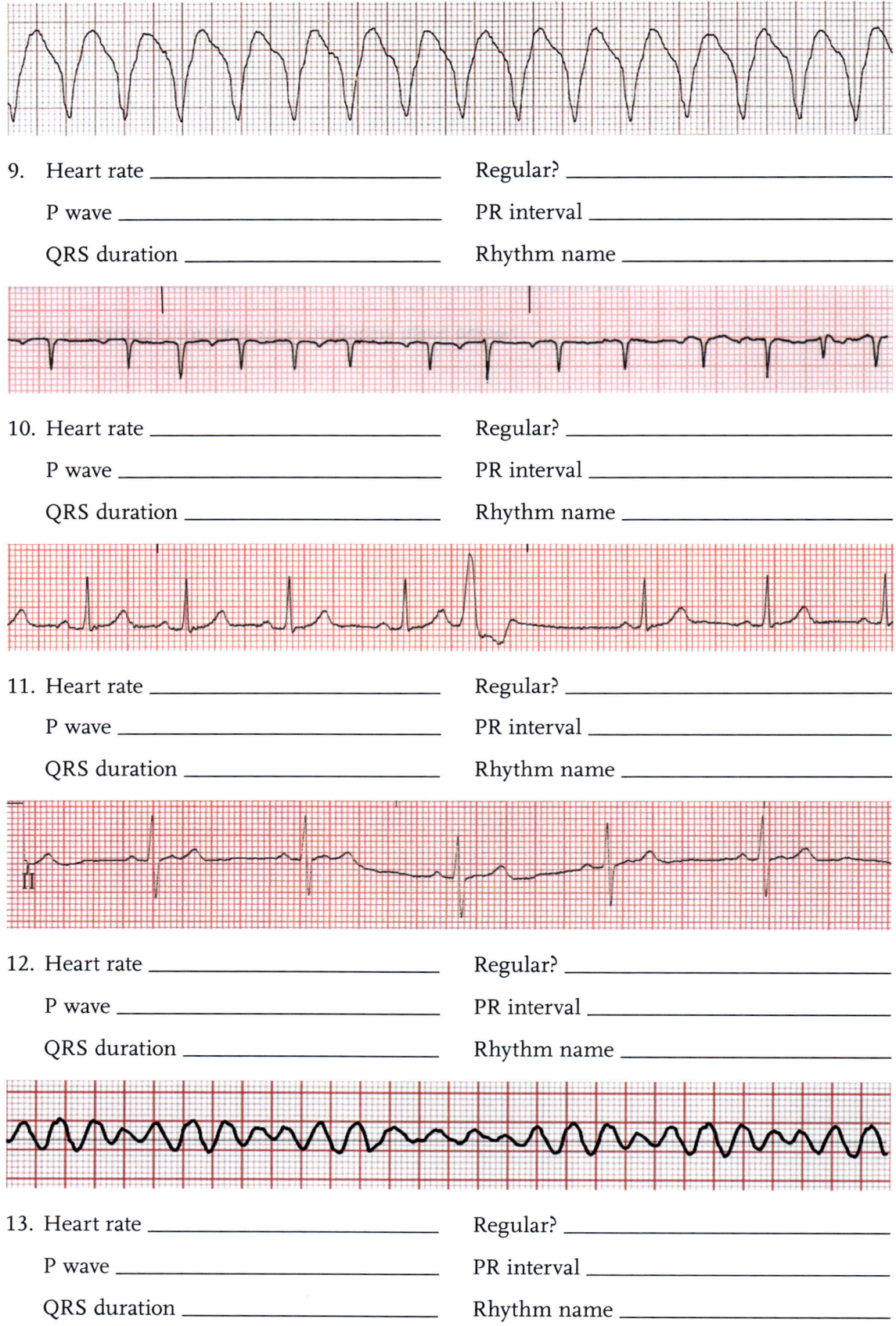

9. Heart rate _____ Regular? _____

   P wave _____ PR interval _____

   QRS duration _____ Rhythm name _____

10. Heart rate _____ Regular? _____

    P wave _____ PR interval _____

    QRS duration _____ Rhythm name _____

11. Heart rate _____ Regular? _____

    P wave _____ PR interval _____

    QRS duration _____ Rhythm name _____

12. Heart rate _____ Regular? _____

    P wave _____ PR interval _____

    QRS duration _____ Rhythm name _____

13. Heart rate _____ Regular? _____

    P wave _____ PR interval _____

    QRS duration _____ Rhythm name _____

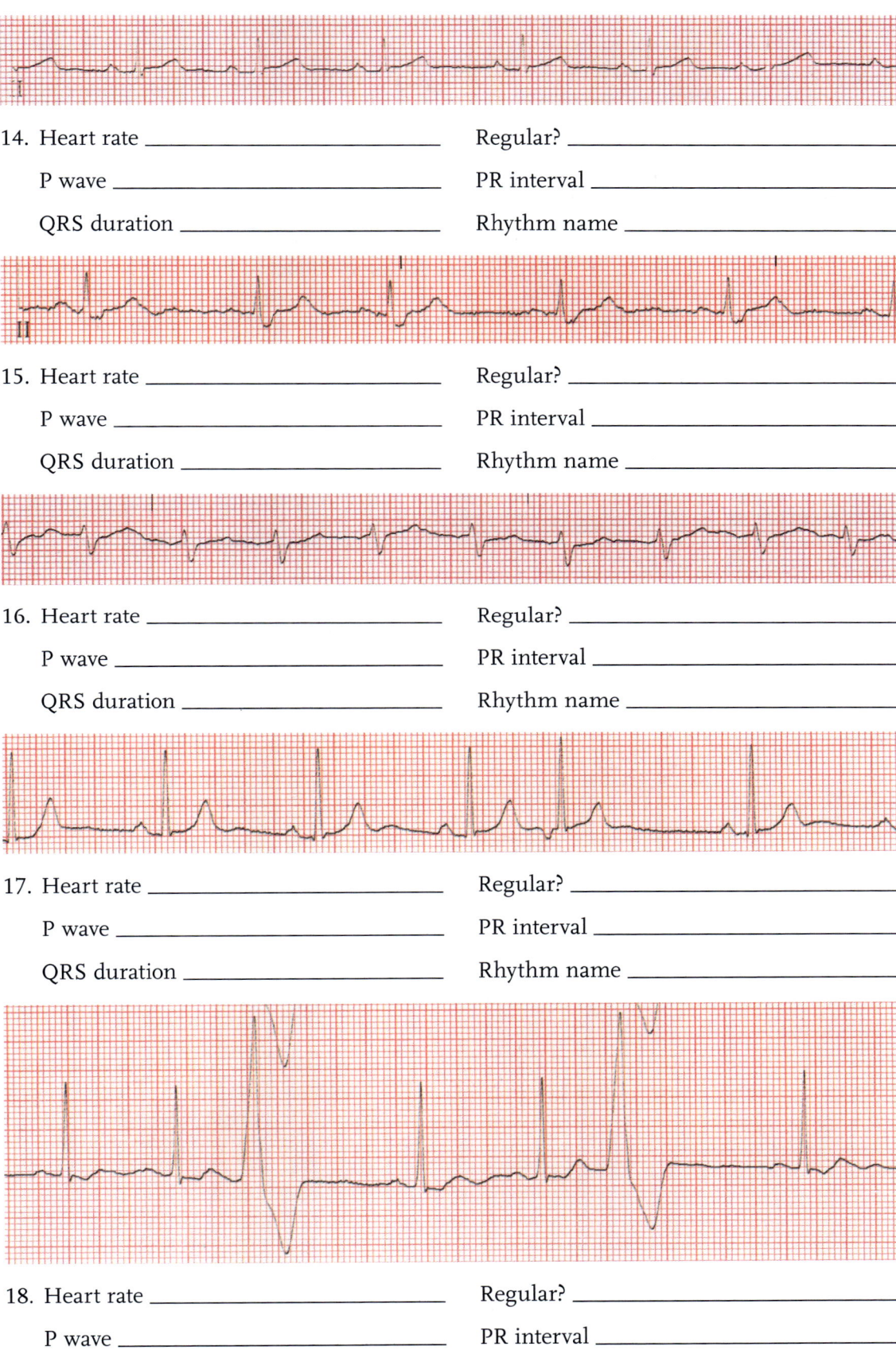

14. Heart rate _____ Regular? _____

    P wave _____ PR interval _____

    QRS duration _____ Rhythm name _____

15. Heart rate _____ Regular? _____

    P wave _____ PR interval _____

    QRS duration _____ Rhythm name _____

16. Heart rate _____ Regular? _____

    P wave _____ PR interval _____

    QRS duration _____ Rhythm name _____

17. Heart rate _____ Regular? _____

    P wave _____ PR interval _____

    QRS duration _____ Rhythm name _____

18. Heart rate _____ Regular? _____

    P wave _____ PR interval _____

    QRS duration _____ Rhythm name _____

10. Identify heart block rhythms

Heart blocks (also called *AV blocks*) happen when an electrical impulse from the SA node is blocked by the AV node or AV bundle. When the heart is working normally, the AV node and AV bundles slow down impulses from the SA node. This allows the ventricles time to fill with blood. Sometimes the delay is too long. The AV node blocks the impulse completely. A block may also happen when impulses are firing too rapidly in the SA node or atrial area. Heart blocks can usually be identified by a prolonged (longer than usual) PR interval. There are three categories of heart block: first-degree; second-degree Mobitz type I; second-degree Mobitz type II; and third-degree.

In **first-degree heart block** the PR interval is longer than 0.20 seconds and the R-R intervals are regular (Fig. 9-28). The beats are conducted, but delayed. In other words, they are not blocked completely. The other parts of the complex are usually within normal range, but it is always important to describe any abnormalities of the underlying rhythm (as in Fig. 9-29).

Tip

Conducted and Blocked Beats

When learning the heart block rhythms, EKG technicians must know the terms **conducted beat** and **blocked beat**. In a *conducted beat*, the electrical impulse continues through the AV node and AV bundles to the ventricles. It may be delayed. In a *blocked beat*, the electrical impulse is stopped completely. When this happens, the EKG tracing shows a P wave without a related QRS complex. The impulse caused the atria to contract but did not continue to the ventricles.

PR intervals are longer than normal, but beats are conducted

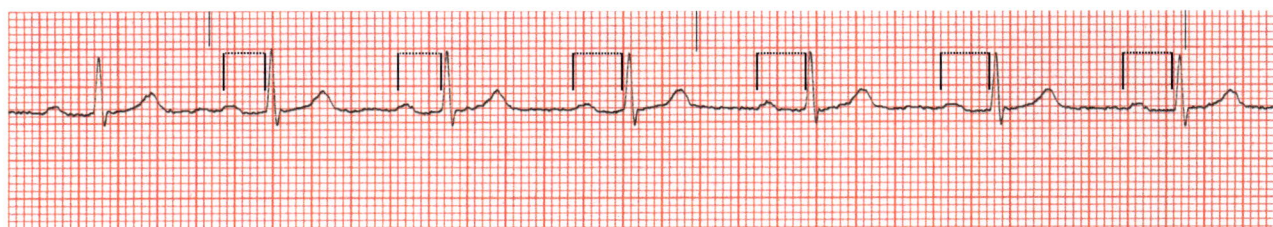

Name of rhythm: First-degree heart block
Rate: 60–100 BPM (68 BPM)
Rhythm pattern: Regular
P wave characteristics: Upright and uniform

PR interval: >0.20 s (0.28 s)
QRS duration: <0.12 s (0.08 s)
Unique identifier: Normal QRS, rate, and rhythm; prolonged PR interval

Fig. 9-28. *Illustration of first-degree heart block.*

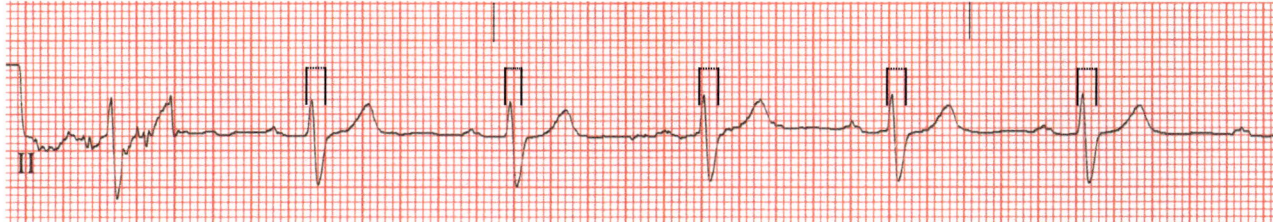

Fig. 9-29. *This strip shows first-degree heart block with a widened QRS complex.*

There are two forms of **second-degree heart block**: **Mobitz type I** (also sometimes called *Wenckebach*) and **Mobitz type II**. Both types have some impulses that are totally blocked by the AV node. The pattern of the block is different in each type.

In Mobitz type I the PR intervals of the conducted beats get longer and longer until a beat is totally blocked. Then the pattern starts again until another beat is totally blocked (Fig. 9-30). This is called a *generally progressive PR interval*. A blocked beat does not move past the AV node to the ventricles, so there is no QRS complex on the tracing. The rhythm of the R-R intervals is regularly irregular. It is irregular, but has a recognizable, repeating pattern.

PR interval gets longer with each conducted beat until a beat is blocked

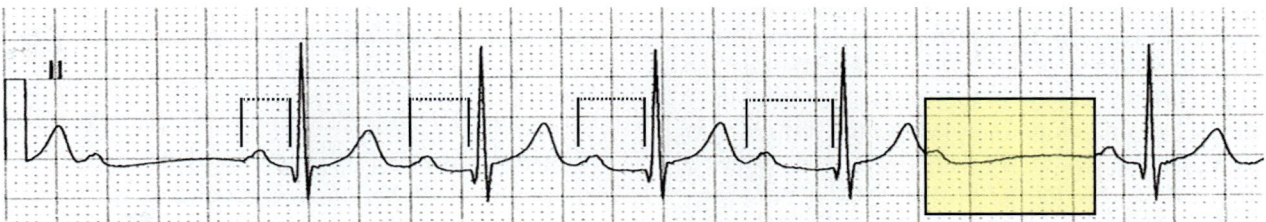

Name of rhythm: Second-degree heart block Mobitz type I

Atrial rate: 60–100 BPM (90 BPM)

Ventricular rate: Slower than atrial rate (70 BPM)

Rhythm pattern: P-P regular for conducted beats; R-R irregular

P wave characteristics: Upright and uniform

PR interval: Variable

QRS duration: <0.12 s (0.08 s)

Unique identifier: PR interval becomes progressively longer until QRS is dropped; occurs cyclically

Fig. 9-30. *Illustration of second-degree, Mobitz type I heart block.*

Mobitz type II heart blocks also show both conducted and blocked beats. The PR intervals in the conducted beats are constant. This means they do not change (Fig. 9-31). The PR intervals may be normal or prolonged. A fixed number of beats is usually blocked for every conducted beat. The P-to-QRS ratio may be 2:1 (two P waves for each QRS complex), 3:1 (three P waves for each QRS), or greater. The ratio may vary. The rhythm of the R-R intervals is regularly irregular if the ratio of blocked to conducted beats stays the same. The rhythm of the R-R intervals is irregular if the ratio changes.

Pairs of conducted beats are followed by a blocked beat

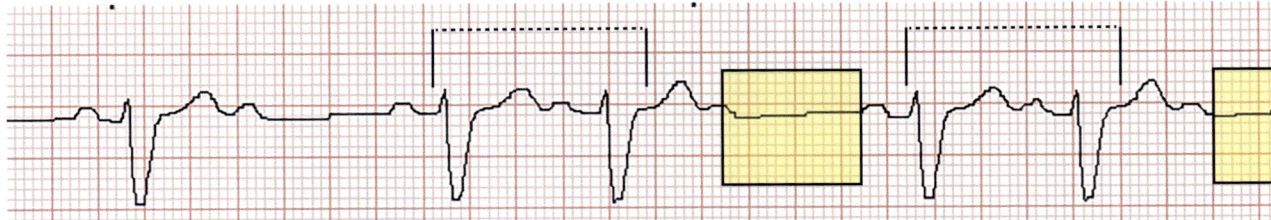

Name of rhythm: Second-degree heart block Mobitz type II

Atrial rate: 60–100 BPM (90 BPM)

Ventricular rate: Slower than atrial rate (50 BPM)

Rhythm pattern: P-P regular for conducted beats, R-R irregular

P wave characteristics: Upright and uniform

PR interval: Variable (0.20 s on conducted beats)

QRS duration: <0.12 s (0.10 s)

Unique identifier: PR intervals remain constant but some QRS complexes are dropped

Fig. 9-31. *Illustration of second-degree, Mobitz type II heart block.*

Heart Block Names

Many of the names for heart rhythms relate to the area of the heart where they start. They can also relate to the type of rhythm involved (e.g., *ventricular tachycardia* is a fast rhythm that starts in the ventricles). Names for heart block rhythms—especially the categories of second-degree heart block—are different. They can be confusing. Late in the 19th century a doctor named Karel Frederik Wenckebach described the pattern of longer and longer PR intervals leading up to a blocked beat. A few decades later another doctor, Woldemar Mobitz, classified the types of second-degree heart block. He called blocks that show the lengthening pattern described by Wenckebach *type I*. He called blocks with a set relationship between the number of blocked to conducted beats *type II*. So second-degree, type I heart block can also be called *Mobitz I* or *Wenckebach*. In most cases, though, the simplest names for second-degree heart blocks are used: *type I* and *type II*.

Third-degree heart block is a potentially lethal rhythm. It must be checked immediately by a provider. In this dysrhythmia, the AV node or bundle areas block all impulses from the SA node. A slower natural pacemaker (called an **escape pacemaker**) in the junctional area or ventricles takes over the job of initiating impulses for the ventricles. The SA node continues to initiate impulses for the atria.

In third-degree heart block, the SA node fires at its intrinsic rate of 60–100 BPM, but the impulse does not continue past the AV node. The QRS is produced by an escape pacemaker area in the ventricles. The intrinsic rate of ventricular tissue is slow. Because of this, ventricular rate in third-degree heart block is usually 40 BPM or less. The QRS duration depends on which pacemaker takes over to stimulate the ventricles. In this rhythm the activity of the atria is not related in any way to the activity of the ventricles. P waves do not match up in any way to the QRS complexes. The P waves look normal, but there will be no measurable PR interval. The P-P interval will be regular and the R-R interval will also be regular. This is because the atria and ventricles have their own distinct rates (Fig. 9-32).

No relationship between P waves and QRS complexes

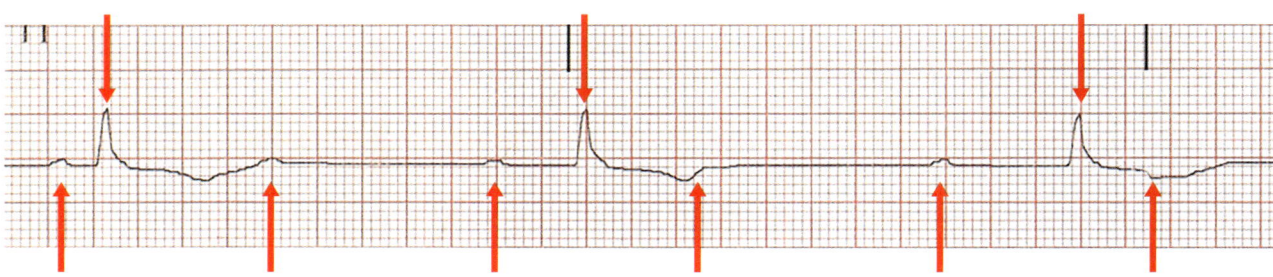

POTENTIALLY LETHAL RHYTHM

Name of rhythm: Third-degree heart block
Atrial rate: 60–100 BPM (60 BPM)
Ventricular rate: 20–60 BPM (25 BPM)
Rhythm pattern: P-P regular, R-R regular, but no relationship between P waves and QRS complexes

P wave characteristics: Normal but may be before, after, or buried in the QRS complex
PR interval: Not measurable
QRS duration: May be normal or widened but will be consistent (0.12 s)
Unique identifier: P waves and QRS complexes are consistent and regular but have no relationship to each other

Fig. 9-32. *Illustration of third-degree heart block.*

11. Discuss what heart block rhythms mean for the patient

First-degree heart block can be caused by certain types of medications. It may also happen in well-conditioned athletes. It does not require treatment.

Second- and third-degree heart blocks can result from aging. Heart disease can also be a factor. These heart blocks can be caused by damage to the conduction system of the heart after an MI. Cardiomyopathy, heart failure, or other forms of heart disease can also be causes.

Wenckebach, or second-degree Mobitz I heart block, is usually harmless. It often resolves without treatment. This condition should be monitored if the patient has a history of heart disease or other serious medical problems. Second-degree Mobitz II heart block may become worse and turn into third-degree heart block.

Third-degree heart block can be deadly because it causes very low cardiac output. The atria and ventricles are not working together. The ventricular rate is very slow. Treatment may include changes to medications and placement of an external pacemaker until a permanent pacemaker can be surgically implanted.

PRACTICE

Analyze the heart block strips below using the 6 steps. Some rhythms may have both an atrial rate and a ventricular rate. Note both rates when appropriate (mark A for *atrial* and V for *ventricular*).

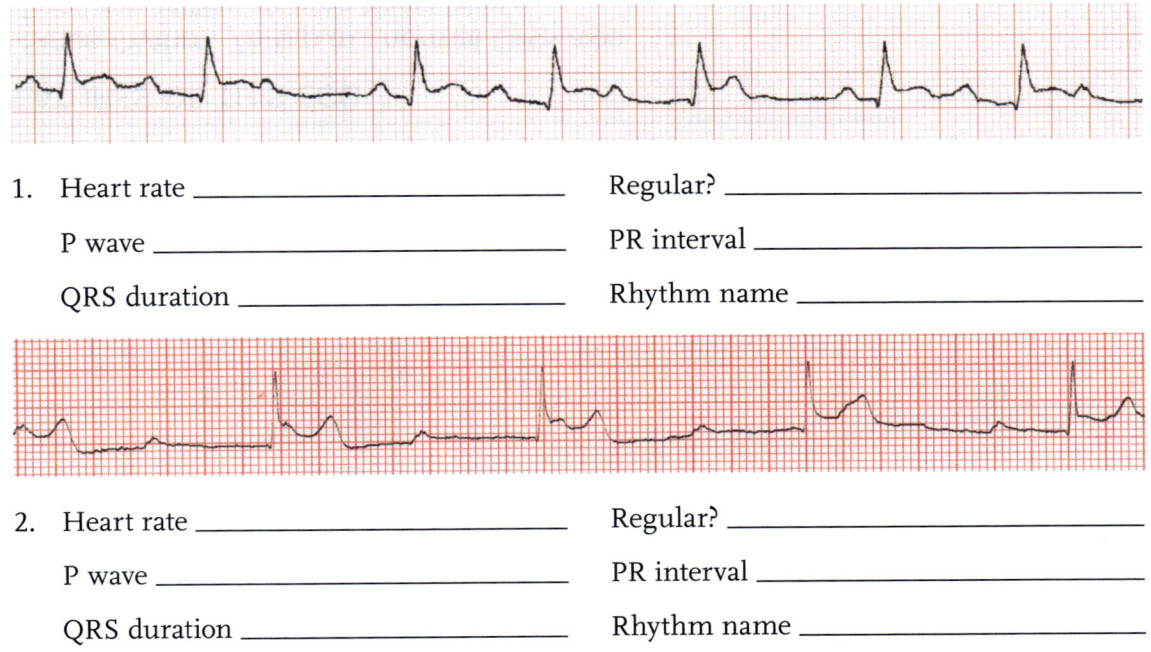

1. Heart rate _____   Regular? _____

   P wave _____   PR interval _____

   QRS duration _____   Rhythm name _____

2. Heart rate _____   Regular? _____

   P wave _____   PR interval _____

   QRS duration _____   Rhythm name _____

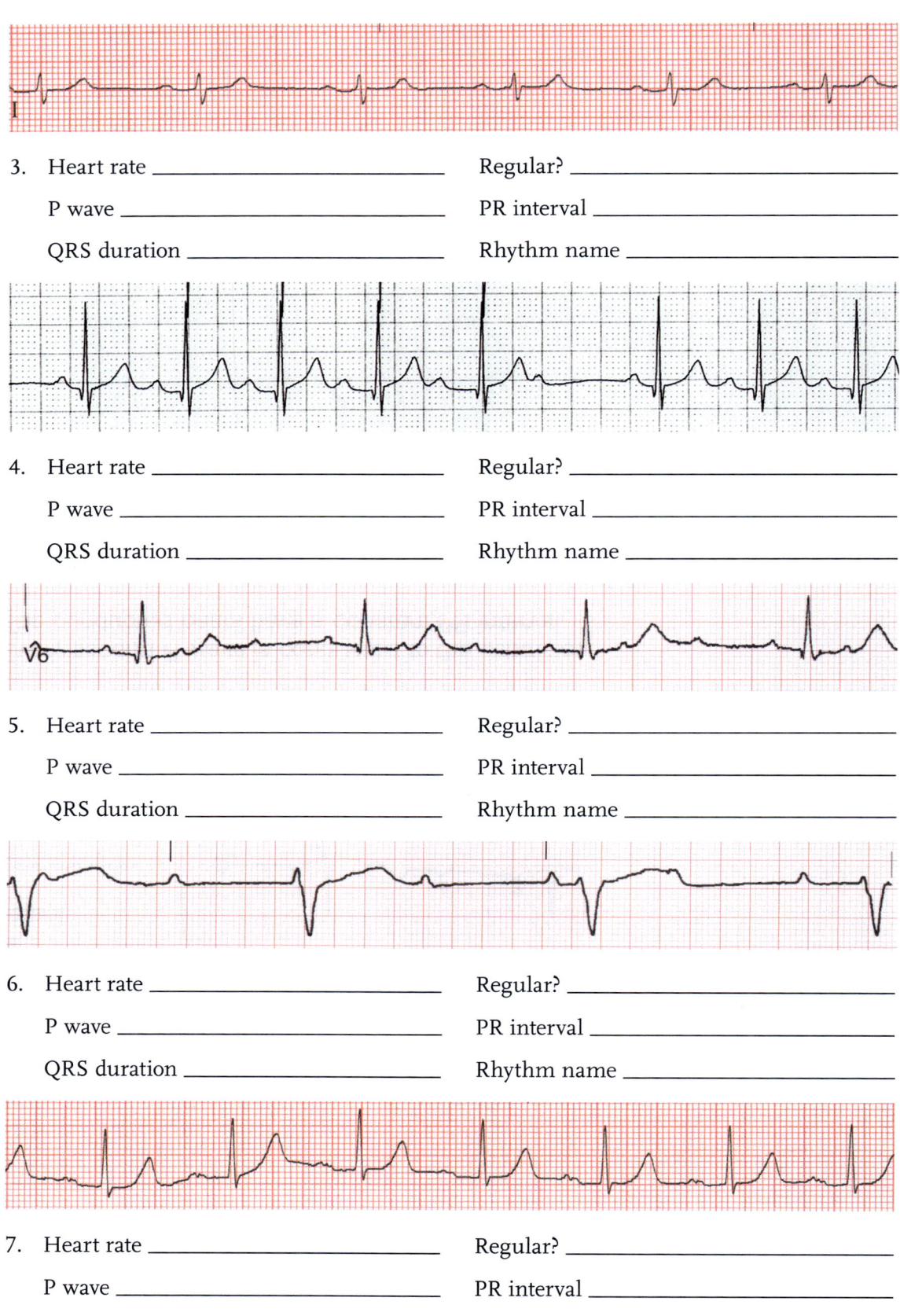

3. Heart rate _____ Regular? _____

   P wave _____ PR interval _____

   QRS duration _____ Rhythm name _____

4. Heart rate _____ Regular? _____

   P wave _____ PR interval _____

   QRS duration _____ Rhythm name _____

5. Heart rate _____ Regular? _____

   P wave _____ PR interval _____

   QRS duration _____ Rhythm name _____

6. Heart rate _____ Regular? _____

   P wave _____ PR interval _____

   QRS duration _____ Rhythm name _____

7. Heart rate _____ Regular? _____

   P wave _____ PR interval _____

   QRS duration _____ Rhythm name _____

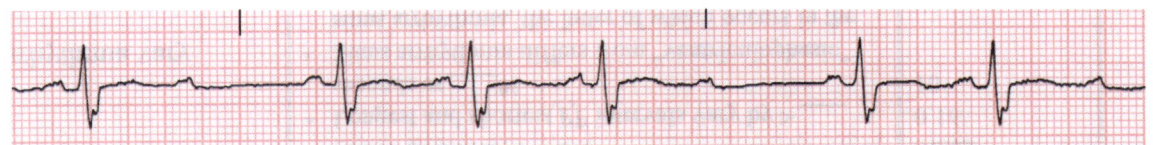

8. Heart rate _____ Regular? _____
   P wave _____ PR interval _____
   QRS duration _____ Rhythm name _____

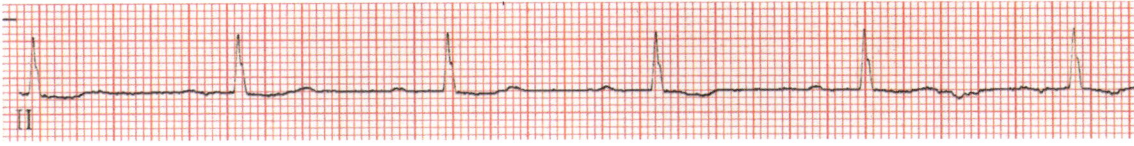

9. Heart rate _____ Regular? _____
   P wave _____ PR interval _____
   QRS duration _____ Rhythm name _____

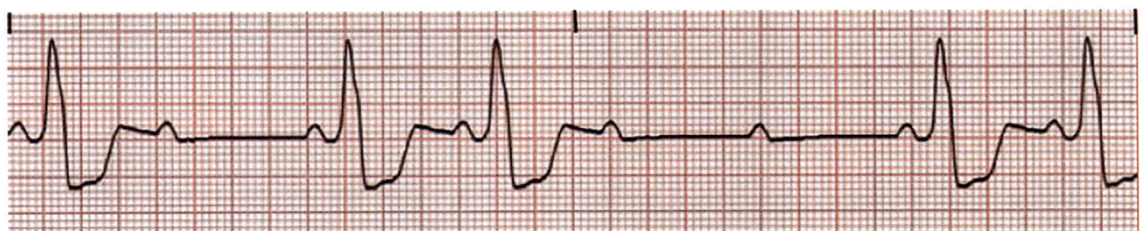

10. Heart rate _____ Regular? _____
    P wave _____ PR interval _____
    QRS duration _____ Rhythm name _____

ADVANCED PRACTICE

Analyze the strips below using the 6 steps. This set of strips includes sinus, atrial, junctional, ventricular, and heart block rhythms.

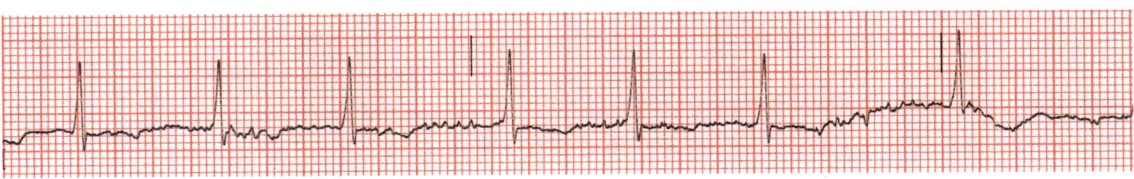

1. Heart rate _____ Regular? _____
   P wave _____ PR interval _____
   QRS duration _____ Rhythm name _____

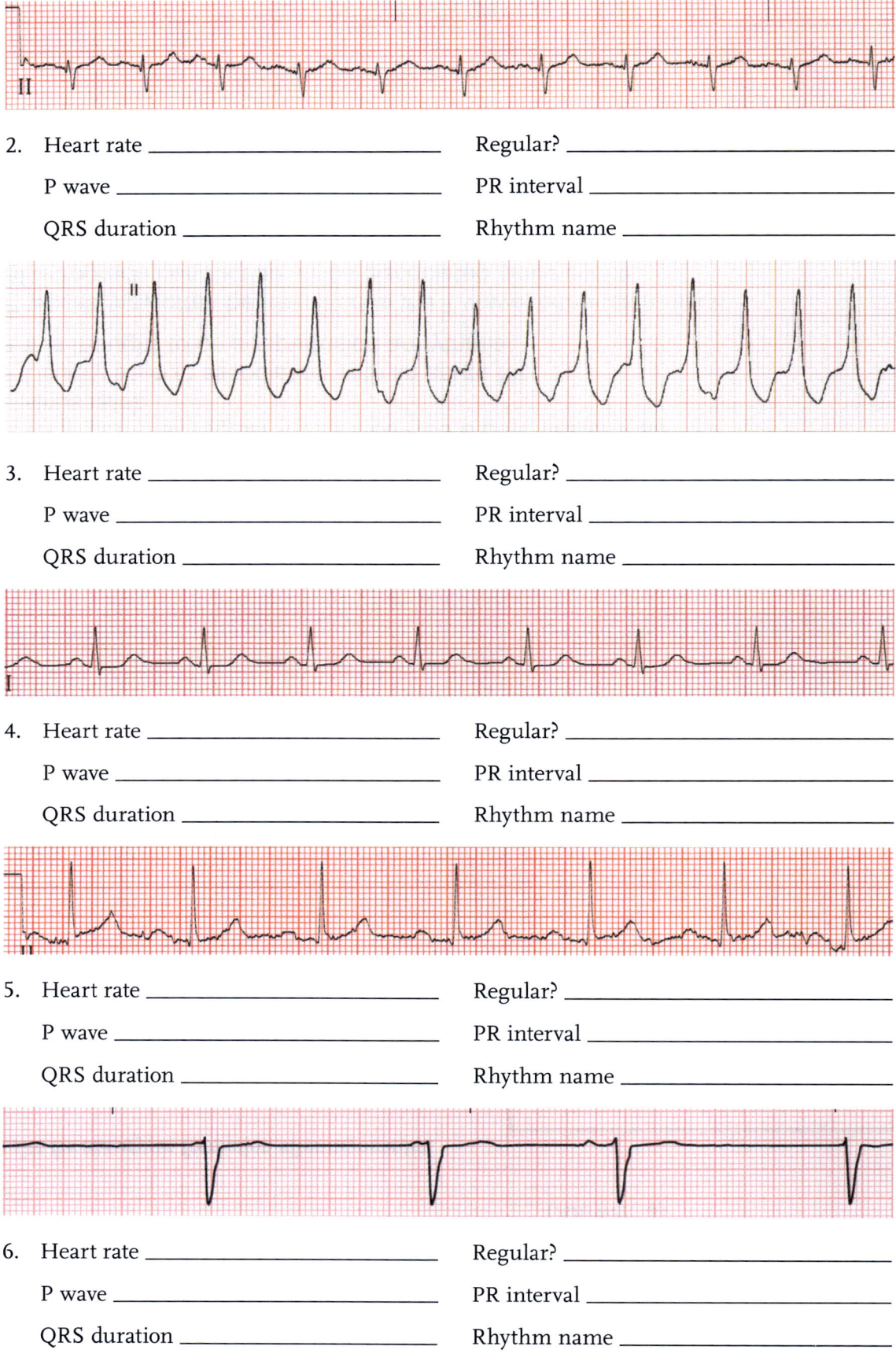

2. Heart rate _____ Regular? _____
   P wave _____ PR interval _____
   QRS duration _____ Rhythm name _____

3. Heart rate _____ Regular? _____
   P wave _____ PR interval _____
   QRS duration _____ Rhythm name _____

4. Heart rate _____ Regular? _____
   P wave _____ PR interval _____
   QRS duration _____ Rhythm name _____

5. Heart rate _____ Regular? _____
   P wave _____ PR interval _____
   QRS duration _____ Rhythm name _____

6. Heart rate _____ Regular? _____
   P wave _____ PR interval _____
   QRS duration _____ Rhythm name _____

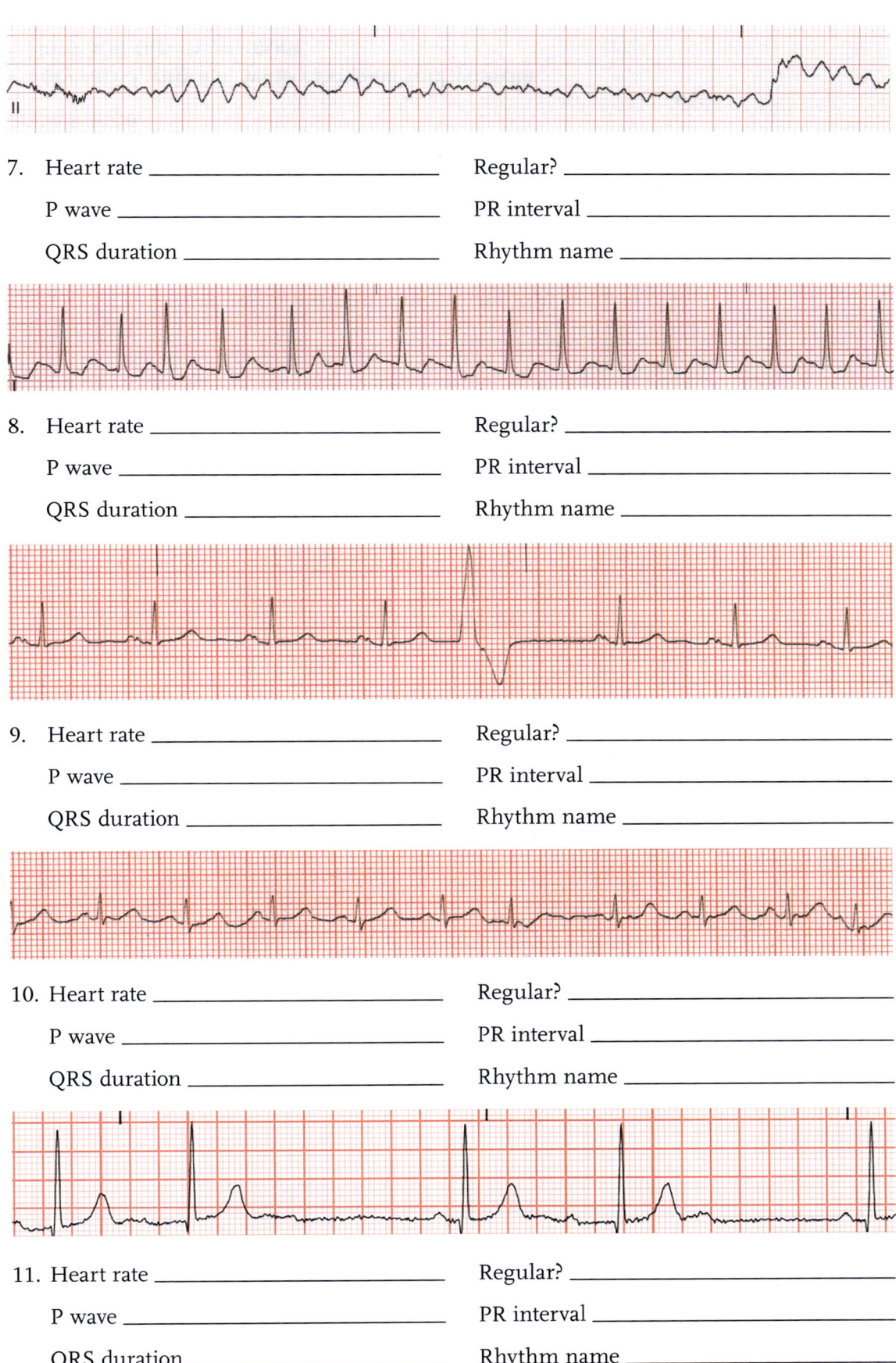

7. Heart rate _____ Regular? _____
   P wave _____ PR interval _____
   QRS duration _____ Rhythm name _____

8. Heart rate _____ Regular? _____
   P wave _____ PR interval _____
   QRS duration _____ Rhythm name _____

9. Heart rate _____ Regular? _____
   P wave _____ PR interval _____
   QRS duration _____ Rhythm name _____

10. Heart rate _____ Regular? _____
    P wave _____ PR interval _____
    QRS duration _____ Rhythm name _____

11. Heart rate _____ Regular? _____
    P wave _____ PR interval _____
    QRS duration _____ Rhythm name _____

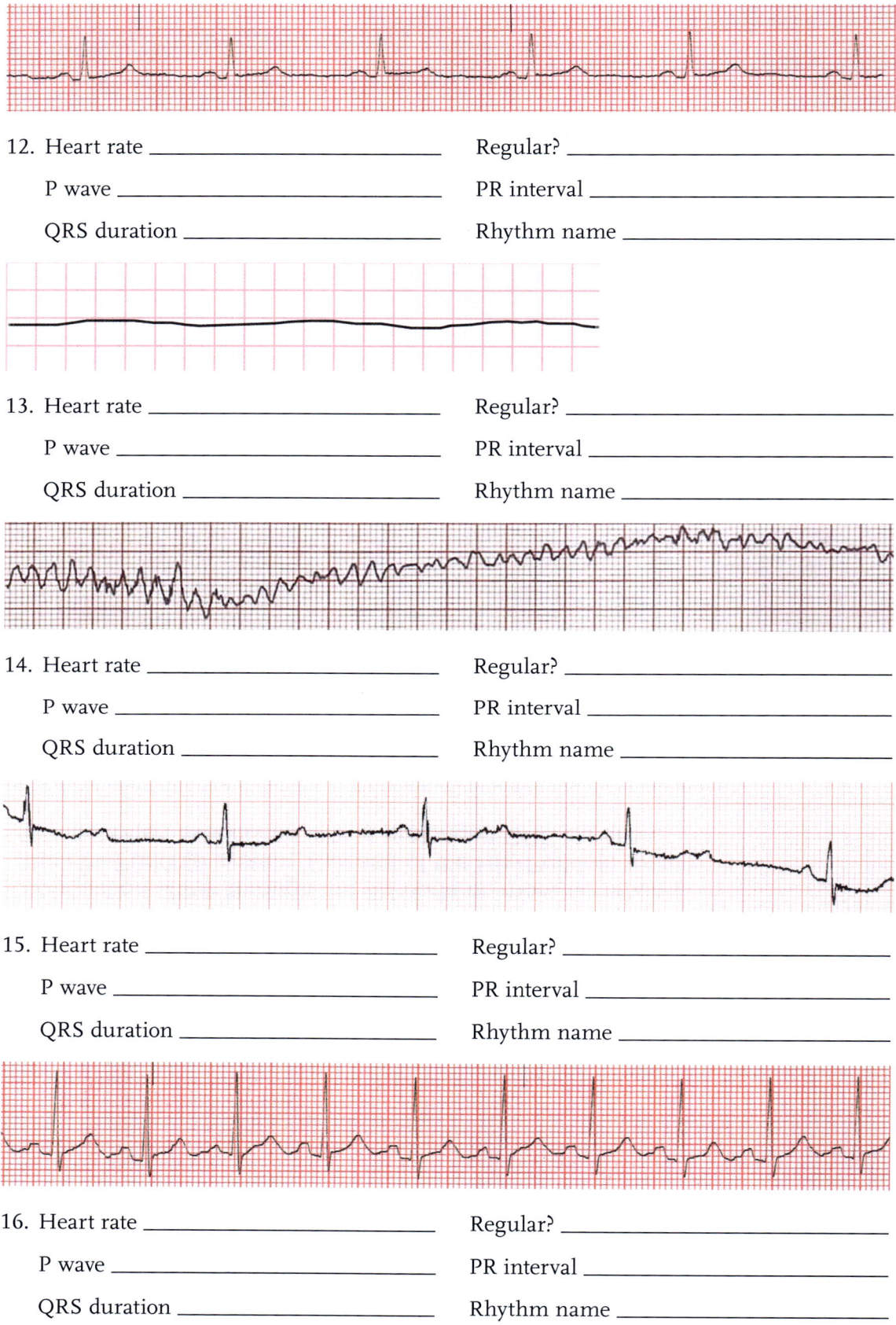

12. Heart rate _____ Regular? _____

    P wave _____ PR interval _____

    QRS duration _____ Rhythm name _____

13. Heart rate _____ Regular? _____

    P wave _____ PR interval _____

    QRS duration _____ Rhythm name _____

14. Heart rate _____ Regular? _____

    P wave _____ PR interval _____

    QRS duration _____ Rhythm name _____

15. Heart rate _____ Regular? _____

    P wave _____ PR interval _____

    QRS duration _____ Rhythm name _____

16. Heart rate _____ Regular? _____

    P wave _____ PR interval _____

    QRS duration _____ Rhythm name _____

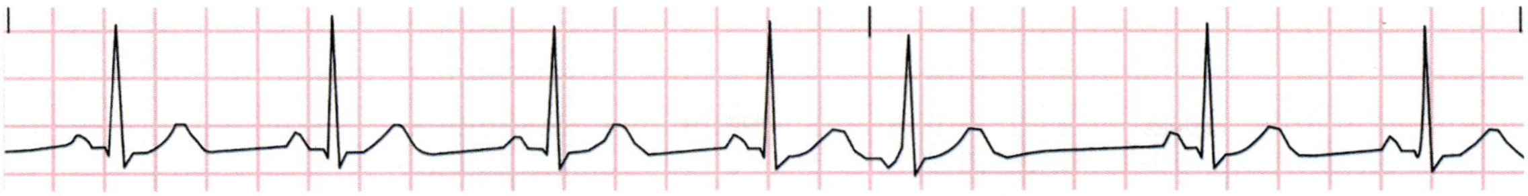

17. Heart rate _____ Regular? _____
    P wave _____ PR interval _____
    QRS duration _____ Rhythm name _____

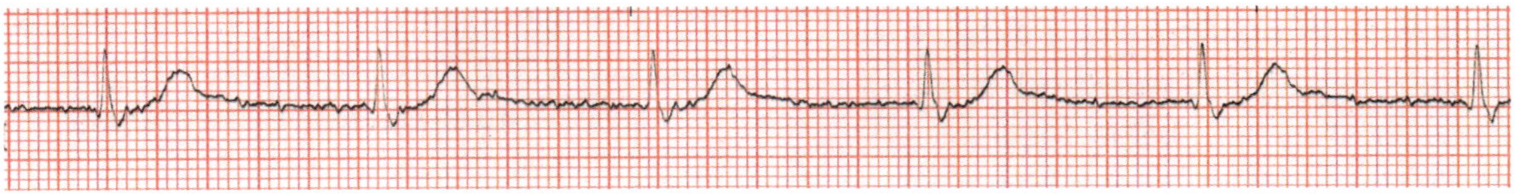

18. Heart rate _____ Regular? _____
    P wave _____ PR interval _____
    QRS duration _____ Rhythm name _____

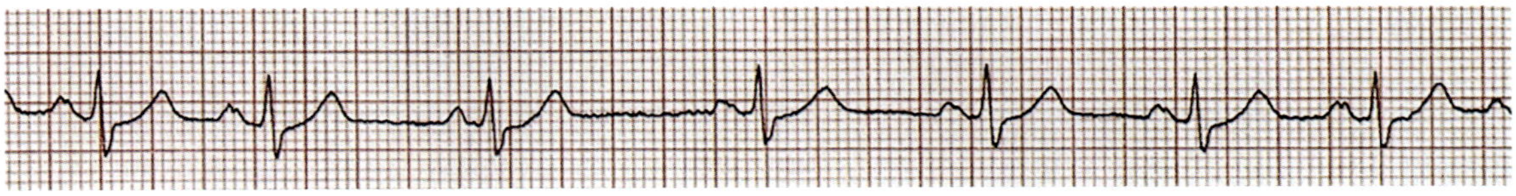

19. Heart rate _____ Regular? _____
    P wave _____ PR interval _____
    QRS duration _____ Rhythm name _____

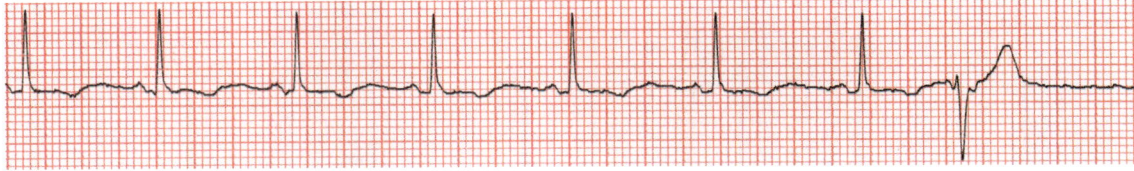
patient has no pulse

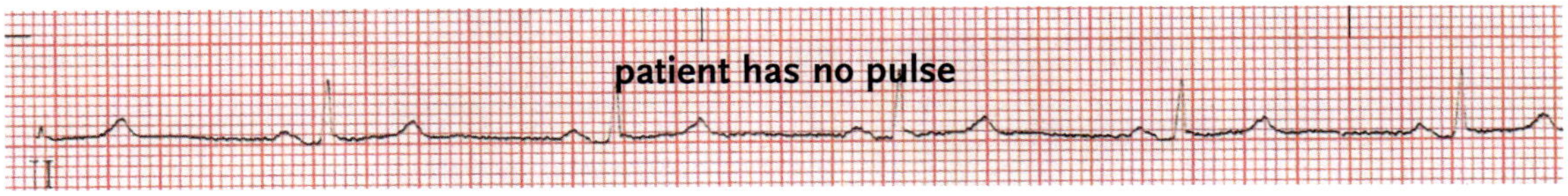

20. Heart rate _____ Regular? _____
    P wave _____ PR interval _____
    QRS duration _____ Rhythm name _____

21. Heart rate _____ Regular? _____
    P wave _____ PR interval _____
    QRS duration _____ Rhythm name _____

12. Recognize artificially paced rhythms on EKG tracings

Artificial pacemakers are implanted surgically when a patient's normal cardiac pacemakers do not work properly (Fig. 9-33). Dysrhythmias (especially very slow rhythms), heart blocks, cardiomyopathy, and heart failure are conditions that may be treated with a pacemaker. Artificial pacemakers have two main parts: a pulse generator, which is usually implanted between the skin and the chest muscle, below the left clavicle; and one or more lead wires, which go through the patient's veins to one or more of the heart's chambers. The device senses the heart's electrical activity.

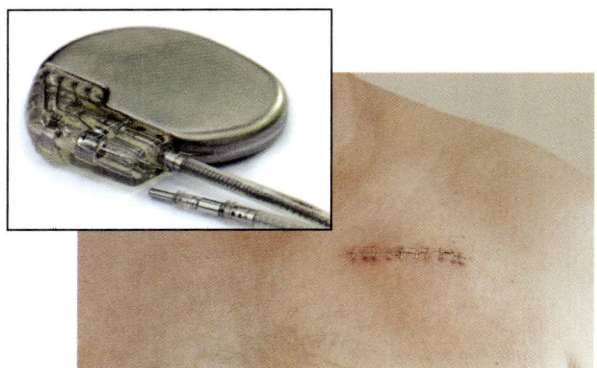

Fig. 9-33. *An artificial pacemaker and a patient with a scar from pacemaker placement.*

The pacemaker stimulates the heart muscle to contract if the patient's own conduction system does not. These artificial impulses make a spike-like wave on EKG tracings. When the patient's natural rhythm is normal, there may be no evidence of a pacemaker spike on the EKG tracing. Most types of pacemakers work as a backup to the patient's own conduction system. They generate impulses only as needed.

A pacemaker may deliver an impulse to stimulate the atria, the ventricles, or both chambers. A **single-chamber pacemaker** can only sense electrical activity and deliver impulses to (or *pace*) one chamber through a single lead wire. It is usually connected to the right atrium or the right ventricle. A **dual-chamber pacemaker** has two lead wires. It can sense and pace in both the atrium and the ventricle.

When an artificial pacemaker is pacing the atria, the EKG shows a pacemaker spike followed by a P wave (Fig. 9-34). If the rest of the patient's conduction system is working normally, the P wave is followed by a normal QRS complex. The PR interval is normal. If the pacemaker is pacing the ventricles, the spike comes just before a wide QRS complex (Fig. 9-35). Some pacemakers pace both chambers. In this case, there are spikes seen before the P wave *and* before the QRS complex (Fig. 9-36).

Since most artificial pacemakers only fire when the patient's conduction system does not, pacing spikes may not be seen for all waves or complexes. Some pacemakers, known as fixed-rate pacemakers, deliver stimulation consistently. An EKG tracing of a patient with a **fixed-rate pacemaker** will show a pacer spike before every complex.

Artificial atrial pacing shows a spike before the P wave

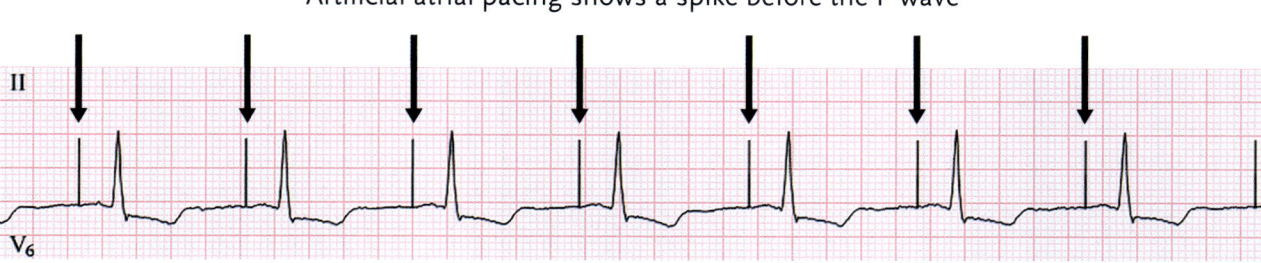

Fig. 9-34. *Pacemaker spikes appear before the P wave when the pacemaker is stimulating the atria.*

Artificial ventricular pacing shows a spike before the QRS complex

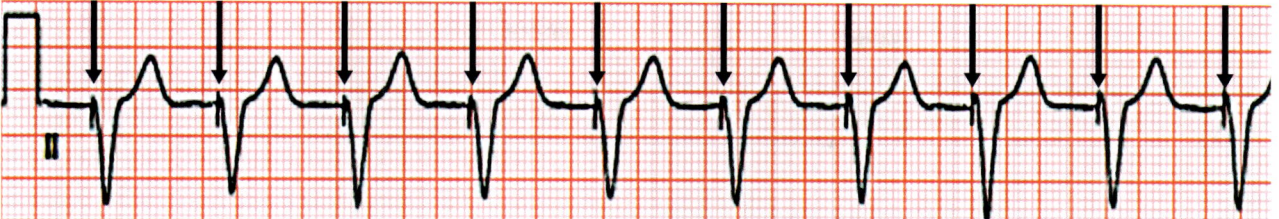

Fig. 9-35. *Pacemaker spikes appear before the QRS complex when the pacemaker is stimulating the ventricles.*

Pacemaker spikes for atrial pacing

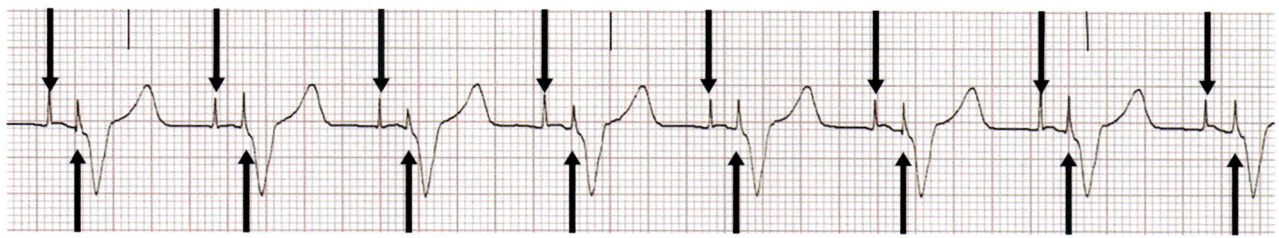

Pacemaker spikes for ventricular pacing

Fig. 9-36. *A patient with a dual-chamber pacemaker may show pacemaker spikes before the P wave and before the QRS complex.*

> **Tip**
>
> **Pacemaker Spikes**
>
> Pacemaker spikes look different in different EKG leads. The spikes are larger in the unipolar leads than in the bipolar leads. Pacemaker spikes are sometimes hard to see in the bipolar leads (leads I, II, and III). It is also important to remember that while *fixed-rate pacemakers* fire for every heartbeat, most pacemakers are *demand pacemakers*. They only fire when the heart's natural pacemakers do not. Some EKG machines automatically mark pacemaker spikes with arrows along the bottom of the strip.

13. Discuss possible complications with artificial pacemakers

Pacemakers can malfunction. When this happens, a patient may have fatigue, shortness of breath, or syncope. EKG technicians do not check or troubleshoot pacemakers. However, an EKG technician may be asked to monitor a patient for problems until the pacemaker can be checked. An EKG tracing may also help the provider determine the source of the problem.

If no pacemaker spikes are shown on the EKG tracing of a patient who has a pacemaker, or if the spikes do not seem to line up with the patient's cardiac activity, the pacemaker may not be sensing properly. This situation has several names: **failure to sense**, *failure to pace*, and *failure to fire* (when the spikes do not appear at all) (Fig. 9-37). **Failure to capture** is another pacemaker malfunction that may be seen on an EKG (Fig. 9-38). Pacemakers are set to deliver the correct amount of electricity needed to generate a contraction in the correct area of the heart. Failure to capture happens when the stimulus does not create a contraction. On the EKG tracing, the pacemaker spike will appear with no other electrical activity after it. The provider should be notified immediately if the EKG tracing shows failure to sense or failure to capture.

No clear relationship between the pacemaker spikes and the patient's cardiac activity

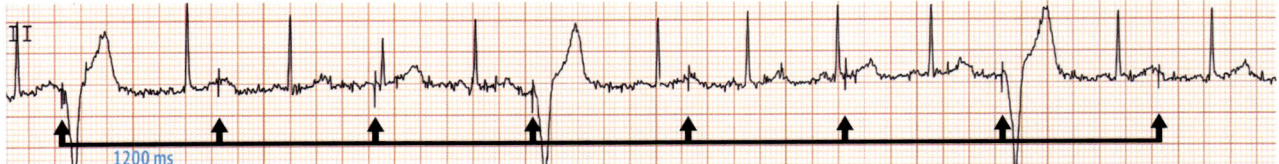

Fig. 9-37. *When an artificial pacemaker fails to sense the patient's cardiac activity properly, the pacemaker spikes do not show a clear relationship to the EKG waveforms.*

Black arrows = pacemaker spikes that do generate electrical activity
Red arrows = pacemaker spikes that do not generate any electrical activity

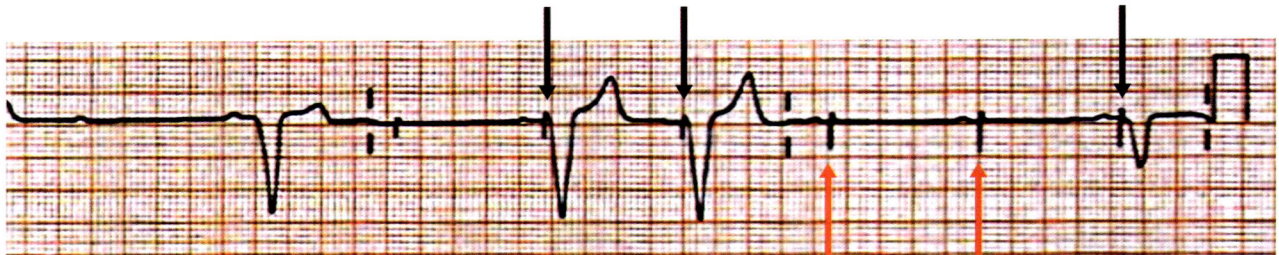

Fig. 9-38. *When pacemaker spikes are not followed by further electrical activity, the patient is experiencing failure to capture.*

Battery failure, broken lead wires, or a malfunction of the pulse generator can also cause problems with an artificial pacemaker. Patients with pacemakers are given a card to carry with information about the type of pacemaker they have. The card includes information about whom to call to have the pacemaker checked in case of problems. If a patient is having trouble with her pacemaker, the provider may call this number or may direct the EKG technician to do so.

Take Action Now!

Interpreting the details of artificially paced rhythms is beyond an EKG technician's scope of practice. EKG technicians do need to be able to recognize an artificially paced rhythm. They should note missing pacing spikes where they should appear or missing electrical activity after a pacing spike. These should be reported to a provider right away.

PRACTICE

Circle the pacemaker spikes in the EKG strips below.

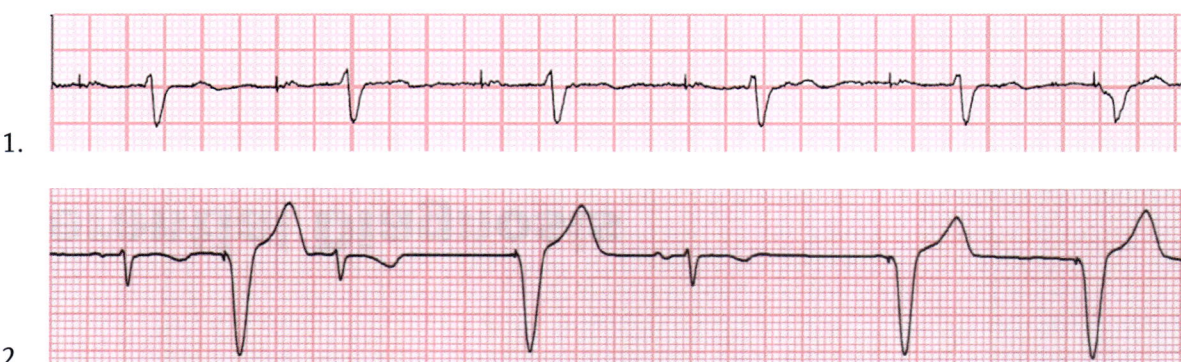

1.

2.

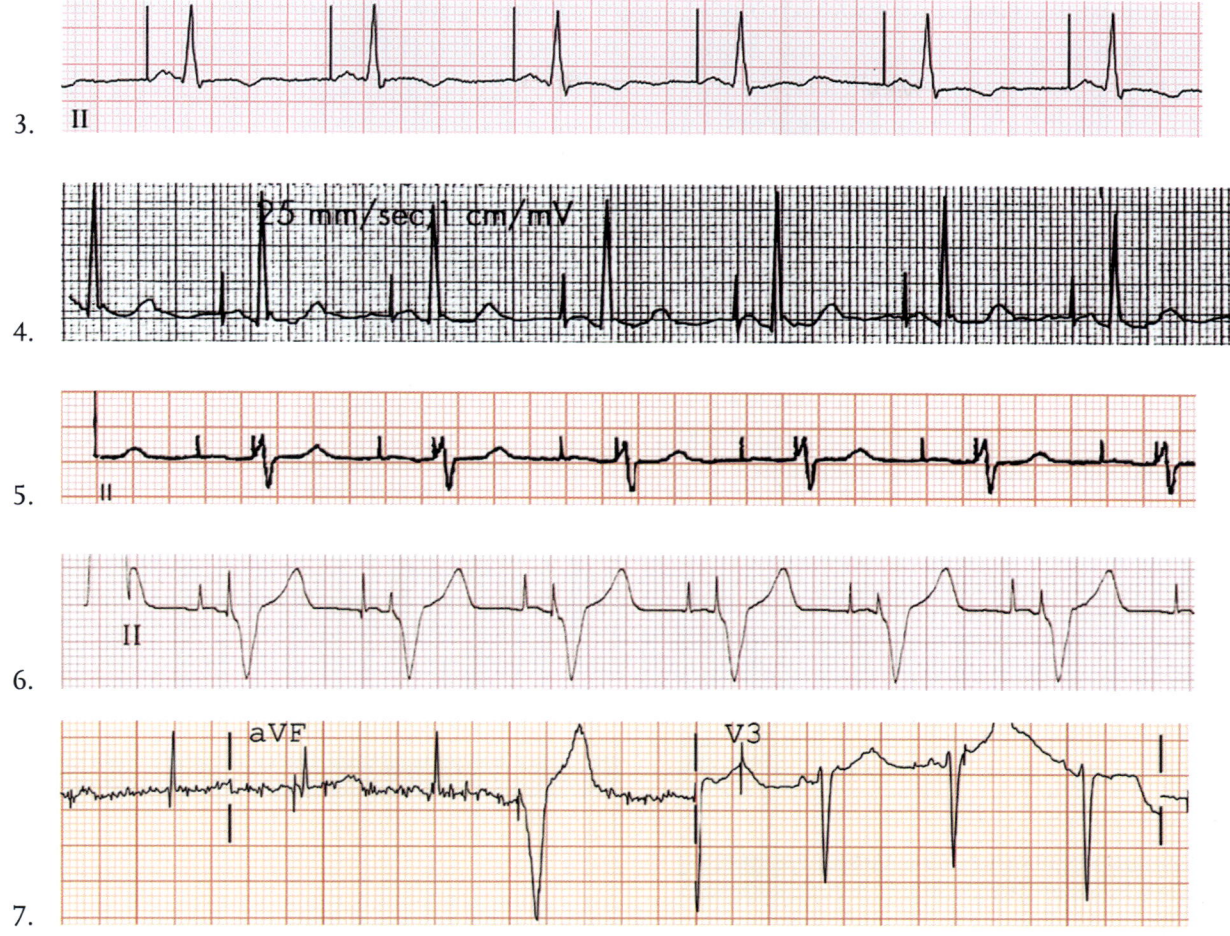

14. Discuss ST segment changes and other indications of injury on the EKG tracing

In addition to identifying abnormal heartbeats and dysrhythmias on EKG tracings, EKG technicians must watch for changes that may be caused by heart problems or injury. Myocardial infarction and cardiac ischemia are some of the conditions that EKGs can detect. Different cardiac conditions and injury can cause changes in different leads, depending on the area of the heart affected.

Chapter 5 introduced the areas of the heart examined by each EKG lead (Figure 5-12 on p. 53). The chart below reviews this information:

Quick Reference

Area	Leads
Inferior wall	II, III, aVF
Lateral wall	I, aVL, V5, V6
Septum	V1, V2
Anterior wall	V3, V4
Posterior wall	V7, V8, V9

Take Action Now!

It can be hard to remember all the possible EKG changes caused by abnormal rhythms or injury. What is most important for an EKG technician is understanding how to identify a *normal* EKG. Anything abnormal is then easier to see and report.

Ischemia can cause recognizable EKG changes. Ischemia happens when there is a lack of blood flow and oxygen to an area of the heart. On the EKG this can result in **ST segment depression**. This means that the ST segment is at least 1 mm below the baseline (Fig. 9-39). It can also cause **T wave inversion**, or a T wave going down, rather than up, from the baseline. When two leads that cover the same area of the heart (two **contiguous leads**) show ST segment depression and T wave inversion, the patient probably has ischemia. If ischemia is not treated immediately, tissue death in the heart will occur.

S wave does not reach the isoelectric line before an inverted T wave begins

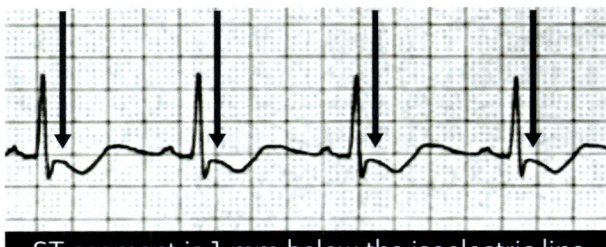

ST segment is 1 mm below the isoelectric line

Fig. 9-39. ST segment depression can indicate that part of the heart is not receiving adequate blood and oxygen.

Untreated ischemia can lead to MI. The shapes of the QRS complex, the T wave, and the ST segment may change during some heart attacks due to heart muscle damage. The ST segment is very important to watch. If the ST segment is elevated at least 1 mm (or one small block) above the baseline, a heart attack has happened recently or was happening during the EKG. This is known as an **ST segment elevation myocardial infarction** (**STEMI**) (Fig. 9-40).

ST segment changes can sometimes help a cardiologist find out when the MI happened or which part of the heart was affected. This is based on which leads show changes. A patient with ST segment elevation must be seen immediately by a provider. A procedure called **cardiac catheterization**, which involves inserting a thin, hollow tube into the body, may be needed to treat coronary artery blockages.

S wave does not return to the isoelectric line before T wave begins

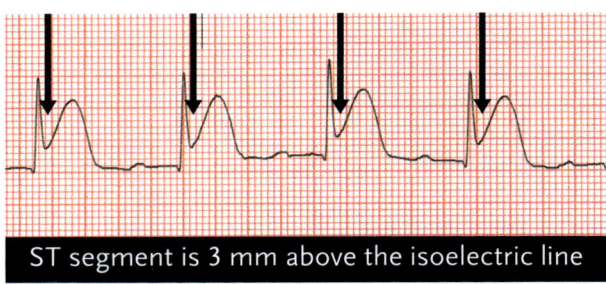

ST segment is 3 mm above the isoelectric line

Fig. 9-40. ST segment elevation is a mark of MI.

Tip

Troponin and MI

A patient with chest pain or other cardiac symptoms may not show ST segment elevation on the EKG. This does not always mean that the patient's symptoms are not related to the heart. In an acute care setting such as a hospital, blood testing is always done along with an EKG in these situations. The blood tests look at a protein in the blood called *troponin*. Blood testing for troponin is usually done three times over a 12-hour period. If troponin is found, the patient is having an NSTEMI, or **non-ST segment elevation myocardial infarction**.

ADVANCED PRACTICE

Analyze the strips below using the 6 steps. This set of strips includes sinus, atrial, junctional, ventricular, heart block, and pacemaker rhythms. Some rhythms may have both an atrial rate and a ventricular rate. Note both rates when appropriate (mark *A* for *atrial* and *V* for *ventricular*). Watch for EKG changes that may indicate heart disease or injury as well.

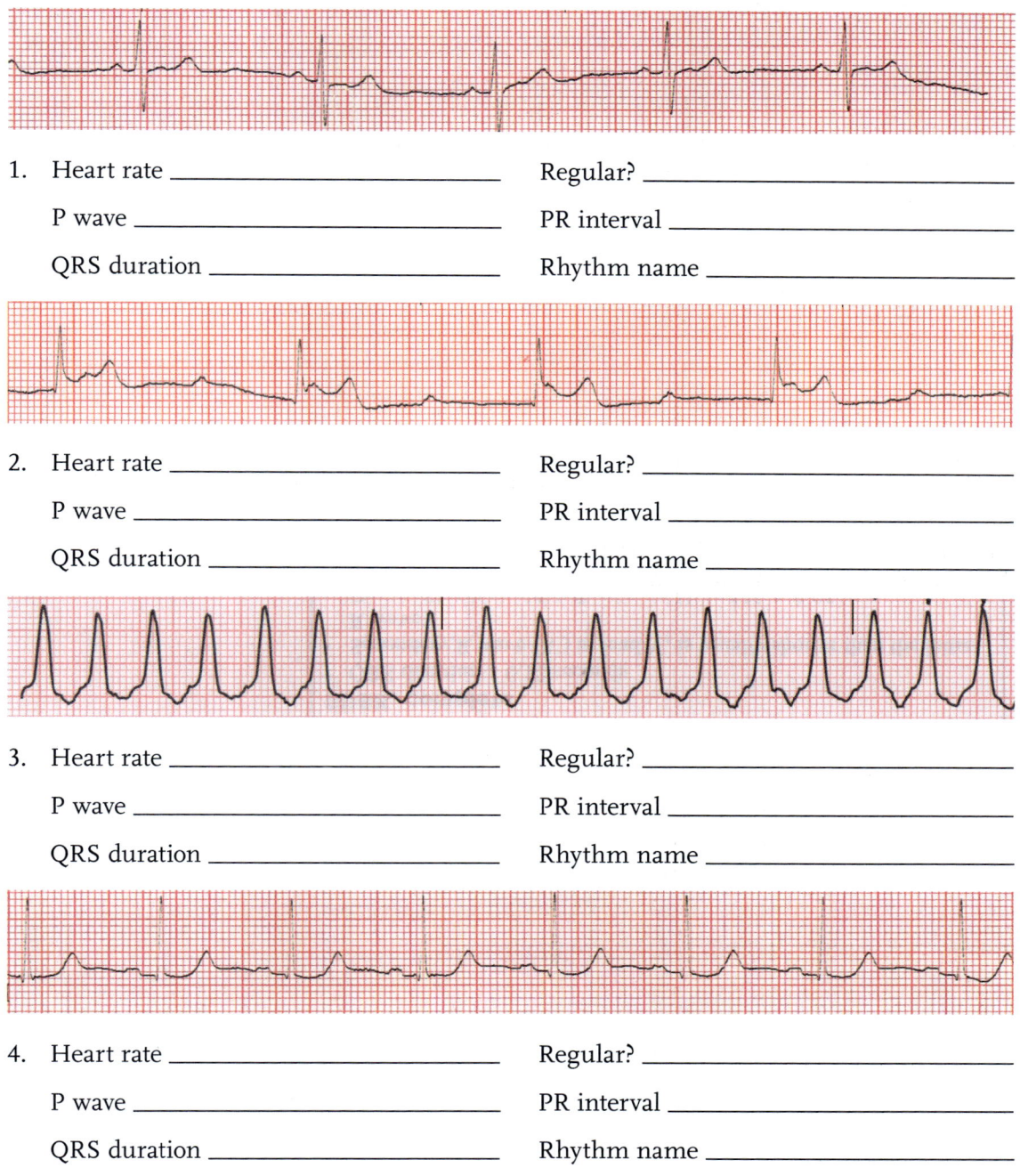

1. Heart rate _____ Regular? _____
   P wave _____ PR interval _____
   QRS duration _____ Rhythm name _____

2. Heart rate _____ Regular? _____
   P wave _____ PR interval _____
   QRS duration _____ Rhythm name _____

3. Heart rate _____ Regular? _____
   P wave _____ PR interval _____
   QRS duration _____ Rhythm name _____

4. Heart rate _____ Regular? _____
   P wave _____ PR interval _____
   QRS duration _____ Rhythm name _____

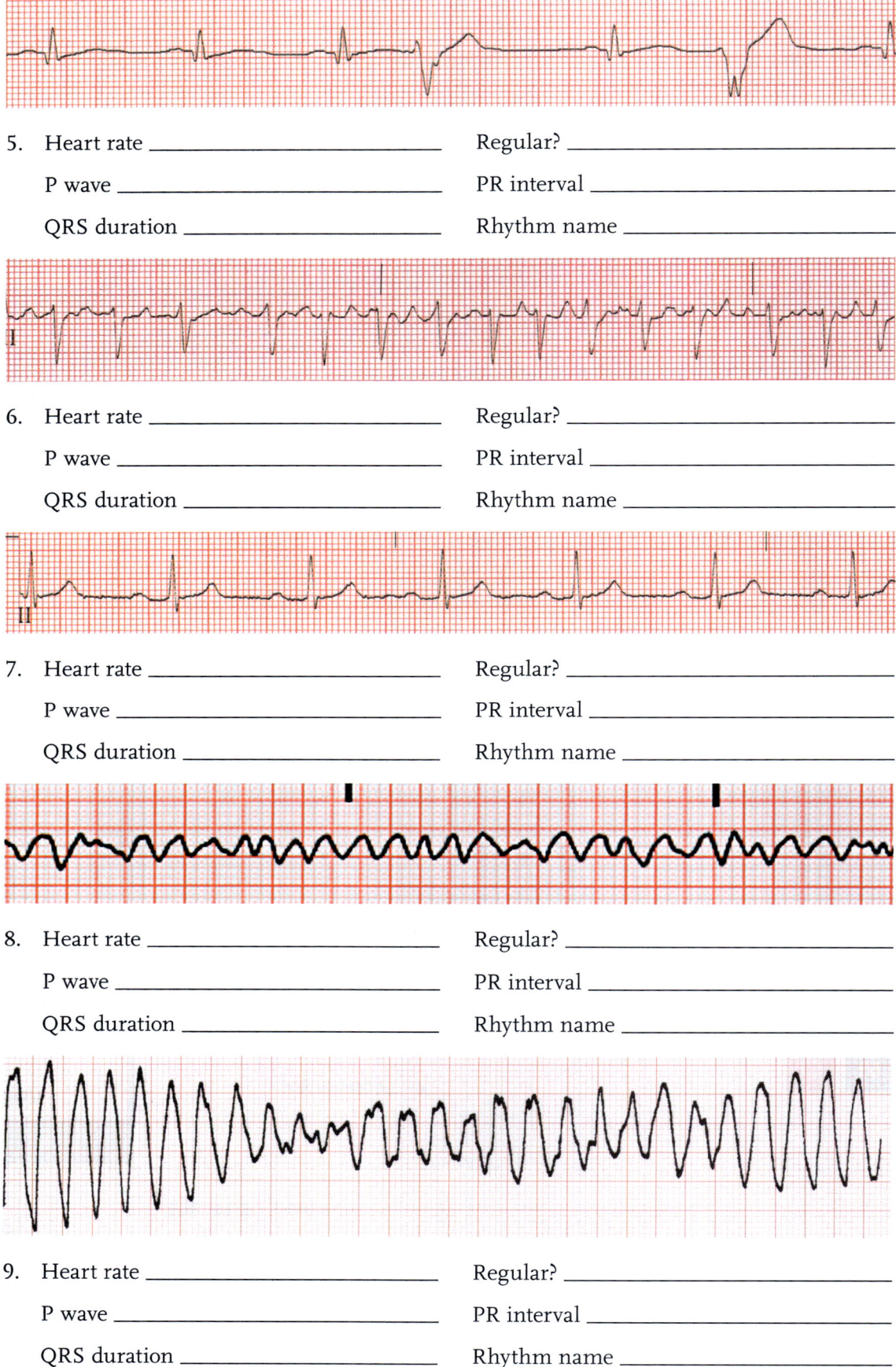

5. Heart rate _____ Regular? _____
   P wave _____ PR interval _____
   QRS duration _____ Rhythm name _____

6. Heart rate _____ Regular? _____
   P wave _____ PR interval _____
   QRS duration _____ Rhythm name _____

7. Heart rate _____ Regular? _____
   P wave _____ PR interval _____
   QRS duration _____ Rhythm name _____

8. Heart rate _____ Regular? _____
   P wave _____ PR interval _____
   QRS duration _____ Rhythm name _____

9. Heart rate _____ Regular? _____
   P wave _____ PR interval _____
   QRS duration _____ Rhythm name _____

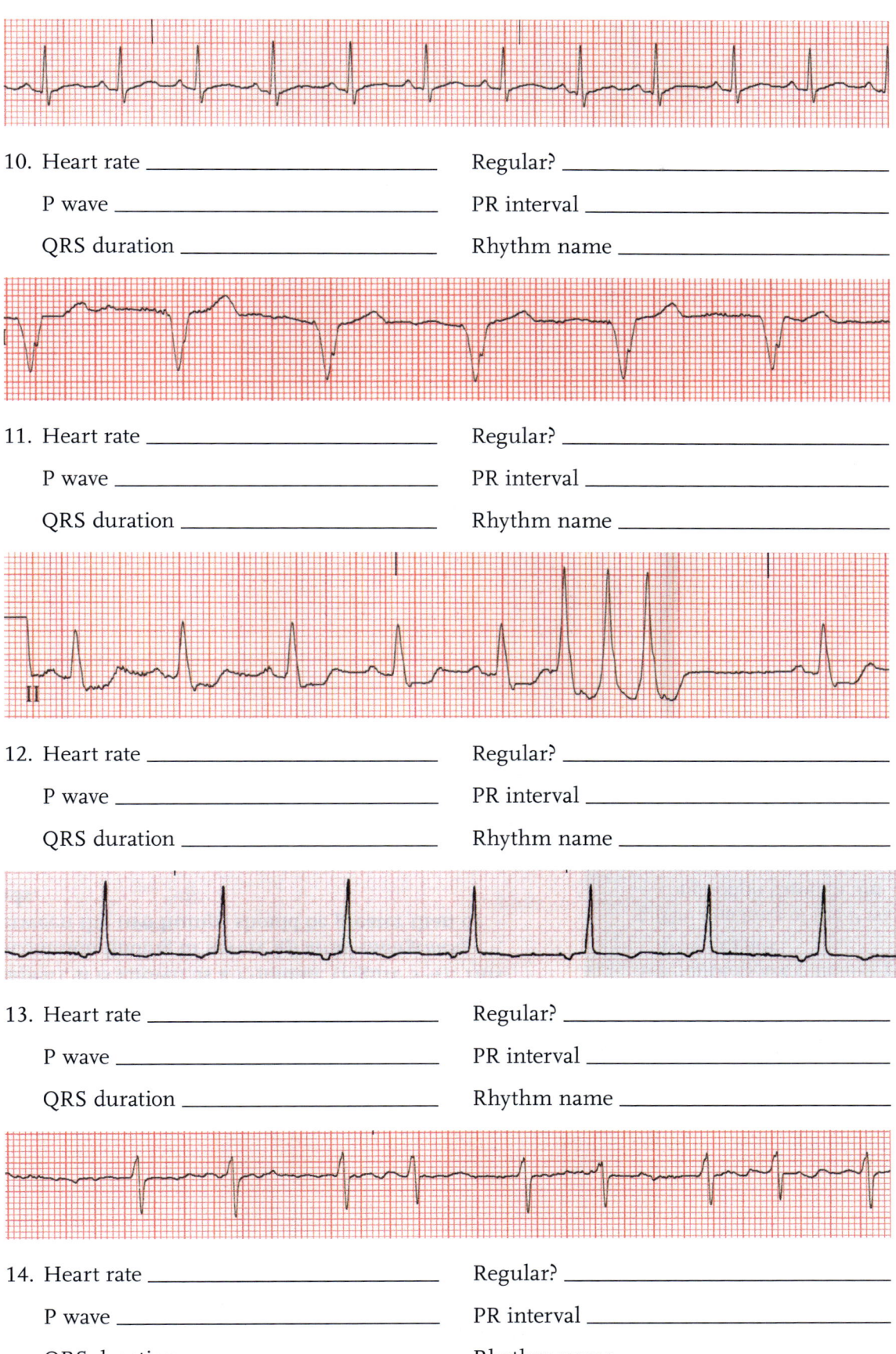

10. Heart rate _____ Regular? _____

    P wave _____ PR interval _____

    QRS duration _____ Rhythm name _____

11. Heart rate _____ Regular? _____

    P wave _____ PR interval _____

    QRS duration _____ Rhythm name _____

12. Heart rate _____ Regular? _____

    P wave _____ PR interval _____

    QRS duration _____ Rhythm name _____

13. Heart rate _____ Regular? _____

    P wave _____ PR interval _____

    QRS duration _____ Rhythm name _____

14. Heart rate _____ Regular? _____

    P wave _____ PR interval _____

    QRS duration _____ Rhythm name _____

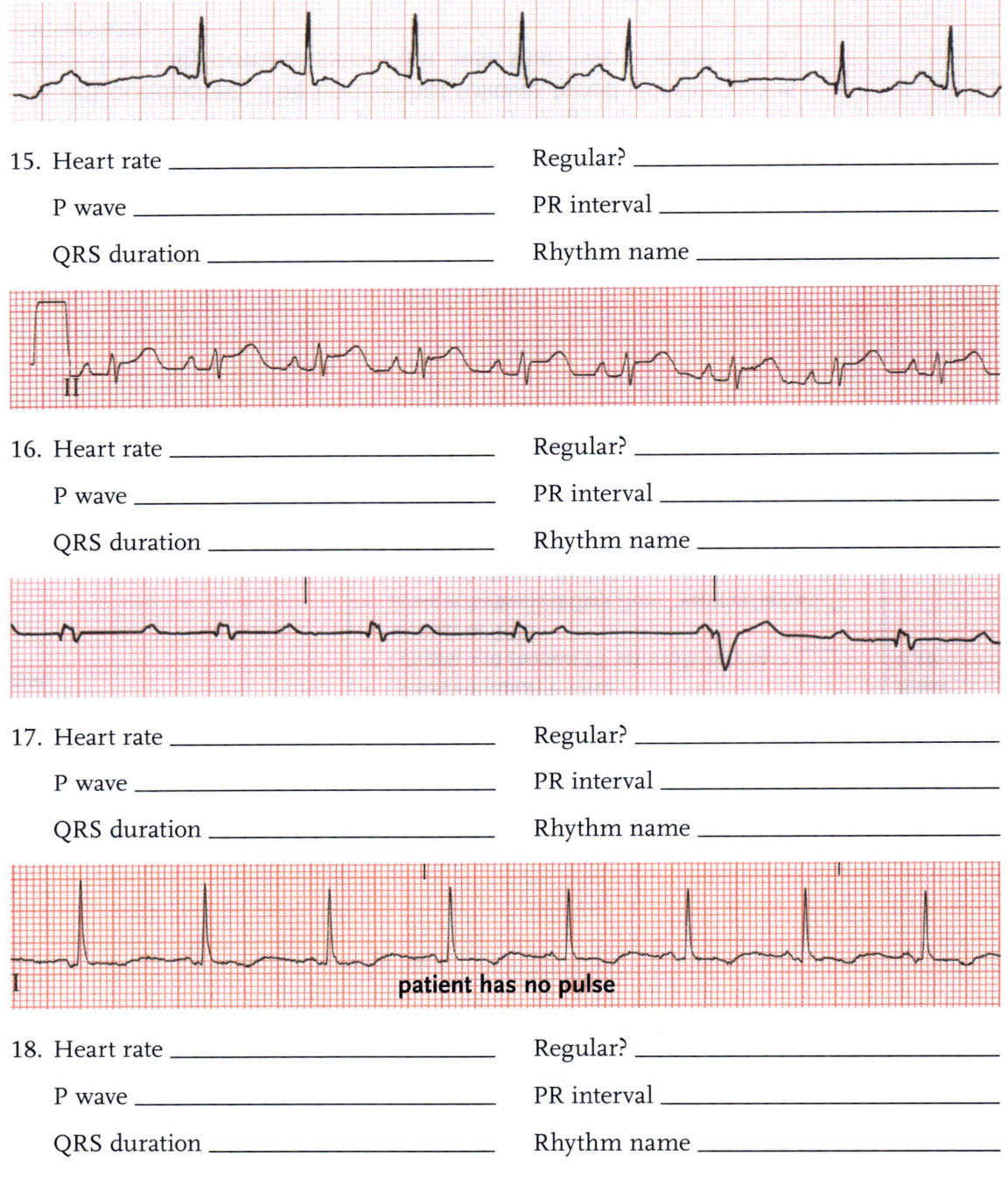

15. Heart rate _____ Regular? _____
    P wave _____ PR interval _____
    QRS duration _____ Rhythm name _____

16. Heart rate _____ Regular? _____
    P wave _____ PR interval _____
    QRS duration _____ Rhythm name _____

17. Heart rate _____ Regular? _____
    P wave _____ PR interval _____
    QRS duration _____ Rhythm name _____

patient has no pulse

18. Heart rate _____ Regular? _____
    P wave _____ PR interval _____
    QRS duration _____ Rhythm name _____

Chapter Review

- It is important for EKG technicians to recognize the most common normal and abnormal cardiac rhythms they will see on EKG tracings.

- Rhythms are named for the areas of the heart where they begin. Sinus rhythms begin in the sinus node, atrial rhythms in the atria, junctional rhythms in the AV junction, and ventricular rhythms in the ventricles. Heart blocks (AV blocks) happen when the AV node delays or completely blocks impulses from the sinus node.

- The steps described in Chapter 8 are applied to interpret all of these types of EKG rhythms.

- Artificial pacemakers change the appearance of EKG tracings. EKG technicians need to be able to recognize these changes.

- Some heart attacks may cause EKG changes. ST elevation is the most common change.

- Other changes to the EKG that are important to note include ST segment depression and no electrical activity after a pacemaker spike.

- A provider will decide whether and what treatment is needed for various heart rhythms. Often, abnormal rhythms have an underlying cause that a provider can diagnose and treat.

- Certain heart rhythms carry a risk of death. These lethal dysrhythmias include the following:
    - Agonal rhythm (very slow idioventricular rhythm)
    - Asystole
    - Pulseless electrical activity
    - Third-degree heart block
    - Ventricular fibrillation
    - Ventricular tachycardia

  Patients with these rhythms need immediate medical attention.

10 Emergency Situations

This chapter provides general information regarding emergency response. Healthcare workers should follow their employers' specific policies and procedures.

1. Recognize emergency situations during cardiac testing

The EKG technician should be able to respond appropriately if an emergency occurs during an EKG procedure. Because emergencies can develop at any time, the EKG technician should continually observe the patient. The EKG technician may be the first to recognize a change that requires urgent intervention.

A change can include increased respiratory rate or shortness of breath. The patient may also complain of weakness and fatigue or pain in the chest, arm, neck, shoulder, or back (Fig. 10-1). The heart rate may increase or decrease compared to baseline measurements (usually vital signs recorded at the beginning of the visit). A patient's blood pressure may increase or decrease. The patient may also become cyanotic (have blue- or gray-tinged skin) or diaphoretic (sweat excessively) as his condition worsens. Decreased oxygen to the brain will result in a change in mental status. When this occurs, the patient may not be able to remember or state simple information such as his name, the date, and where he is. The EKG technician should notify a supervisor immediately if any of these signs or symptoms occur.

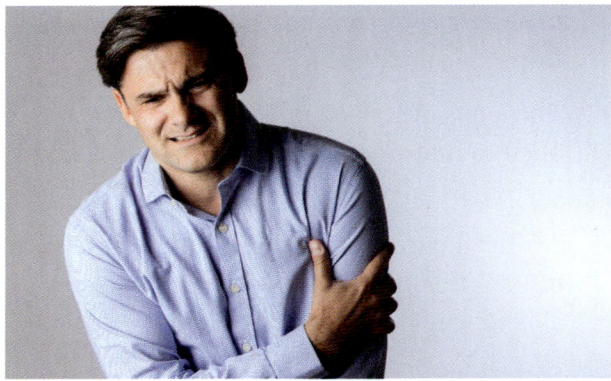

Fig. 10-1. *Pain in the left arm can be related to a cardiac emergency.*

Quick Reference

Symptoms of an emergency to report:
- Increased shortness of breath
- Chest pain or pressure
- Arm, neck, shoulder, or back pain
- Increased weakness or fatigue
- Any other change from baseline

Signs of an emergency to report:
- Increased respiratory rate
- Hypotension (low blood pressure)
- Hypertension (high blood pressure)
- Diaphoresis (excessive sweating)
- Cyanosis (bluish or gray color of skin due to decreased oxygen)
- Bradycardia (heart rate under 60 beats per minute)
- Tachycardia (heart rate over 100 beats per minute)
- Unconsciousness
- Altered mental status
- Any other change from baseline

The first sign of an emergency may be changes in the EKG. A patient having an MI may not experience severe signs or symptoms, or may have signs and symptoms not usually associated with a heart-related emergency. As discussed in Chapter 9, certain EKG changes need to be evaluated by a provider right away.

Two EKG changes requiring immediate attention are ST segment depression or elevation. ST segment depression can indicate ischemia. ST elevation can indicate a type of active MI called an ST elevation myocardial infarction (STEMI). Changes to the ST segment are a sign of decreased oxygen in the heart tissue due to narrowing or blockages of the coronary arteries. Cardiac catheterization may be used to increase blood flow. If catheterization does not help, the cardiologist may recommend open-heart surgery to bypass (go around) the clogged coronary arteries.

Some heart attacks do not cause ST segment changes. If a patient is having severe chest pain or other symptoms of a heart-related emergency, but does not show ST segment changes, the provider may order blood tests for markers of heart muscle damage. An MI diagnosed from these markers, rather than from ST segment abnormalities, is called a non-ST elevation myocardial infarction (NSTEMI). Treatment of NSTEMI may also include cardiac catheterization or open-heart surgery.

In addition to watching for changes in the ST segment, the EKG technician should observe for changes in heart rhythm. These changes can be in the heart rate, the regularity of the rhythm, or the area of the heart's conduction system that is generating an impulse. The EKG technician must know how to recognize a lethal dysrhythmia in case one occurs during testing.

Potentially lethal dysrhythmias include the following:

- Ventricular tachycardia
- Ventricular fibrillation
- Third-degree heart block
- Agonal rhythm
- Pulseless electrical activity
- Asystole

These dysrhythmias prevent the heart from producing adequate blood flow to sustain life. They must be recognized and treated immediately to give the patient the best chance of survival. The EKG technician must always check both the EKG tracing and the patient's condition. Depending on the cause of the dysrhythmia, the patient may not survive despite prompt, proper care.

2. Discuss proper notification of supervisor and 911 in a medical emergency

An EKG technician should know his employer's policies and procedures for patient emergencies. In a hospital, technicians call the operator and ask him to call a special phrase or **code** over the intercom (Table 10-1). *Code blue*, for example, usually means cardiac arrest. The employer's policies and procedures also address the responsibilities of each employee during an emergency. A group including a doctor, nurses, and respiratory therapists, called a **code team** or *rapid response team*, will take over care of the patient until she can be moved to the emergency department or other area of the hospital. EKG technicians should remain calm and professional if an emergency occurs.

CODE	MEANING
Code red	Fire
Code gray	Combative patient/individual
Code pink	Child or infant abduction
Code blue	Cardiac arrest

Table 10-1. Each facility may have its own list of codes. These codes are commonly used in a number of settings.

Quick Reference
EKG changes to report immediately

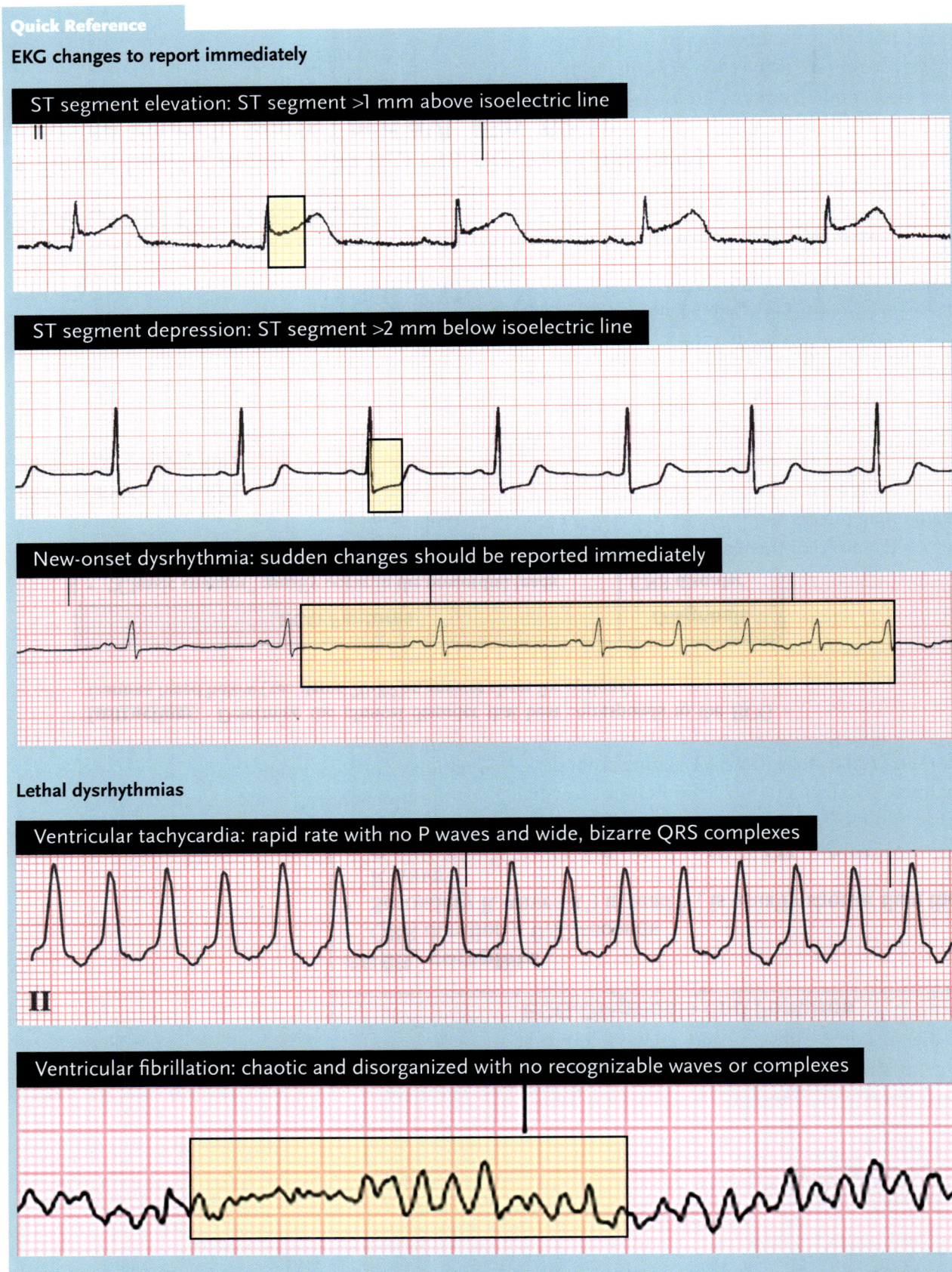

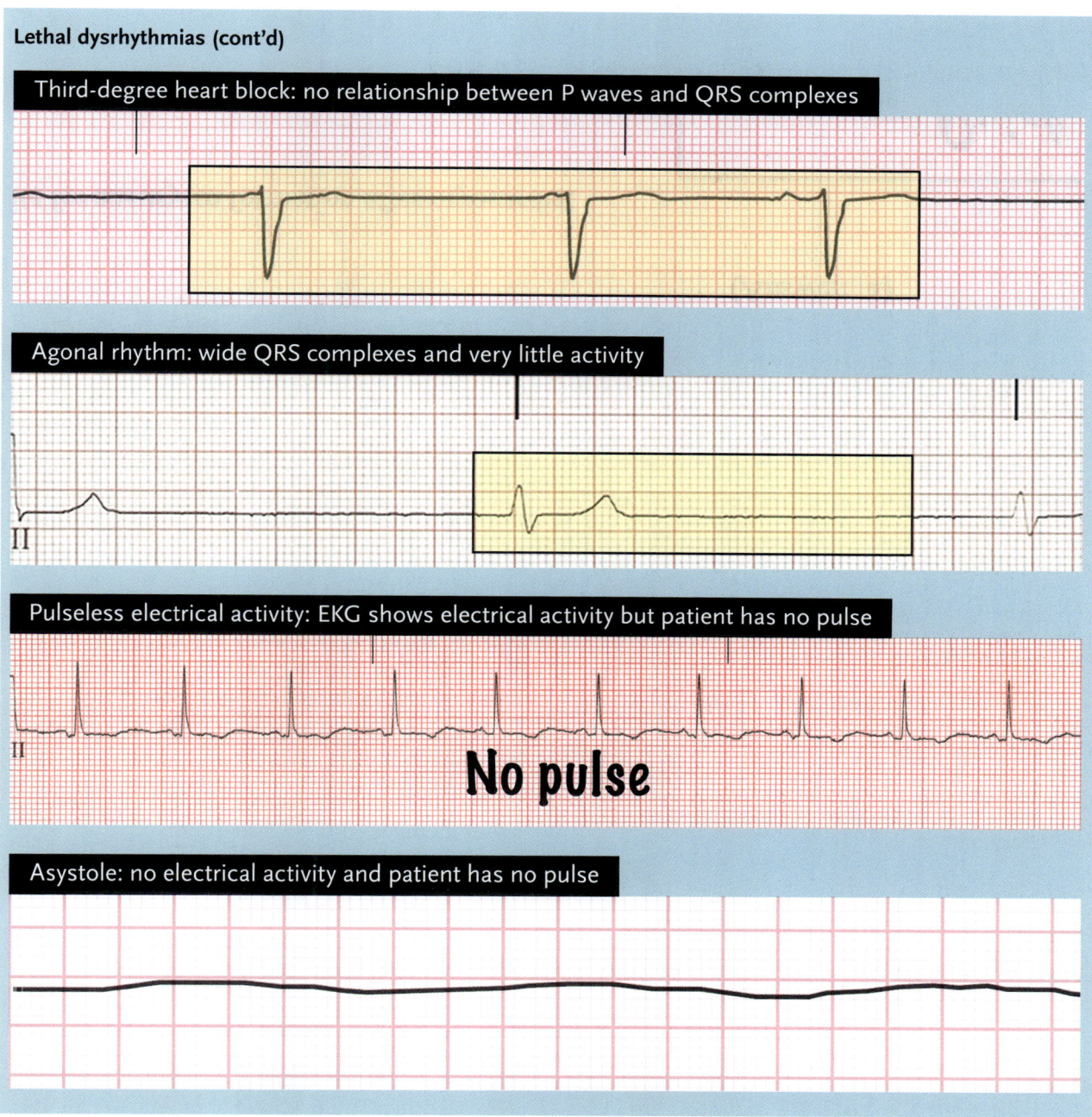

Lethal dysrhythmias (cont'd)

Third-degree heart block: no relationship between P waves and QRS complexes

Agonal rhythm: wide QRS complexes and very little activity

Pulseless electrical activity: EKG shows electrical activity but patient has no pulse

No pulse

Asystole: no electrical activity and patient has no pulse

EKG technicians in a free-standing clinic or doctor's office should notify the nurse or provider and call emergency medical services (EMS) at 911 in an emergency. The person calling 911 should be ready to give information about the illness or injury, the number of patients, any treatment being provided, the address, and a call-back number. In some areas, the emergency services dispatcher may already have some of this information.

The 911 dispatcher should be told if CPR is in progress so he can send enough responders to care for the patient during transport. The person who calls EMS should stay on the line with the dispatcher to answer questions or get instructions on patient care until the dispatcher ends the call. If the facility is large or has many entrances or floors, someone should meet EMS and guide them to the patient.

> **Tip**
>
> **Calling 911 and Assisting with EMS Response**
>
> Be prepared to provide the 911 dispatcher with the following information:
> - Address of emergency
> - Phone number (so dispatcher can call back if the call is disconnected)
> - Description of the emergency situation
> - Any treatment being provided (especially if CPR is in progress)
> - Any information available about the patient's medical history and medications
> - Follow any treatment instructions given by the dispatcher. Be sure someone is at the entrance of the building to guide EMS to the patient.

The EKG technician should help gather patient information to send with the patient. This information should include the following:

- Name
- Date of birth
- Signs and symptoms
- Medical history
- Medications
- Allergies
- Next of kin

If the facility permits, copies of the patient record can be sent with the patient. EMS will assume care of the patient when they arrive.

3. Explain the care of a conscious patient experiencing a cardiac emergency

A conscious patient who is having signs or symptoms of a cardiac emergency should be helped to sit or lie down. After calling for help, the EKG technician should observe the patient closely to be sure his condition does not worsen while waiting for EMS. The patient should be helped into a comfortable position and encouraged to rest and relax (Fig. 10-2). Any activity or stress can increase the heart rate and worsen the patient's situation.

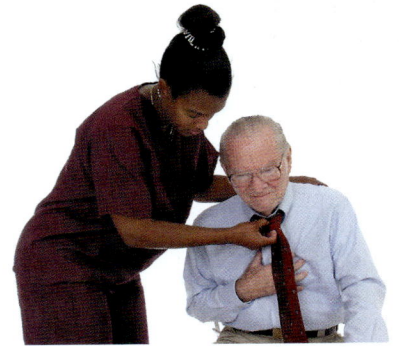

Fig. 10-2. *If a person is thought to be having a cardiac emergency he should be gently helped to sit or lie down.*

The EKG technician may be asked to assist the nurse in administering oxygen to a patient if permitted and trained to do so. The physician or nurse may also give the patient medications to help manage the situation.

The patient should be observed closely until EMS or the code team arrives. The nurse or physician may request that the patient's cardiac rhythm be monitored continuously using 3-lead EKG monitoring to watch for rhythm changes. A 12-lead EKG may also be repeated to give additional information about the heart, especially about changes in the ST segment.

4. Demonstrate the care of an unconscious patient experiencing a cardiac emergency

If the patient loses consciousness (passes out), the EKG technician should immediately call for help and then call or direct someone to call 911. The EKG technician should check the patient for signs of life. First, she should attempt to find a carotid pulse by locating the larynx at the front of the neck and sliding the index and middle finger to the side of the neck. The carotid pulse should be easily felt if the patient's heart is working well enough to provide adequate cardiac output.

If the EKG technician is able to find the pulse, the patient should be placed in the recovery position, as shown in Figure 10-3. In the recovery position the patient is on her side with her head supported by one arm, and her top leg bent to support the body. (This is also called *lateral recumbent* or *three-quarters prone* position.) This position protects the patient from **aspiration**, or inhaling saliva or other material from the mouth into the lungs. The patient should be observed carefully to be sure she continues to breathe.

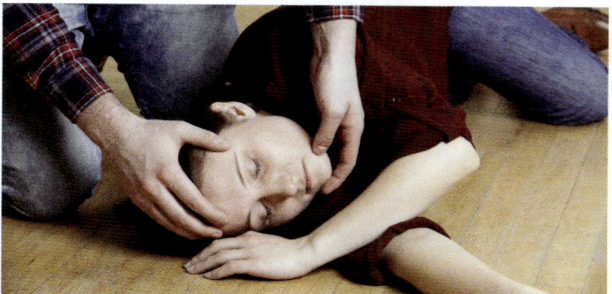

Fig. 10-3. This woman is in the recovery position.

Tip

Vasovagal Syncope

Vasovagal syncope occurs when the nervous system signals the heart to slow and the blood vessels in the lower body to expand. Blood pressure drops, which can cause loss of consciousness due to lack of blood to the brain. Many factors can cause this. Anxiety or strong emotions, standing for long periods of time, overheating, or seeing blood are among the possible triggers. Vasovagal syncope may cause a patient to faint without warning, but often the person will first have symptoms like nausea, pallor, clammy skin, or a dizzy or lightheaded feeling. The patient's pulse may be weak and slow.

If an EKG technician observes these symptoms, he should help the patient to sit and then lie down. Elevating the patient's feet can assist with recovery as well. If the patient loses consciousness, the EKG technician should call for help and make sure the patient is out of harm's way. Most people begin to recover from vasovagal syncope within seconds or minutes, but they should take care getting up. Vasovagal syncope is not, in itself, dangerous. It does not usually signal a serious underlying problem, but if it occurs it should be noted in the patient's record and the supervisor should be informed.

If the patient stops breathing (also referred to as being *apneic*), he will need to be ventilated, or actively assisted to breathe. This is done with a device called a bag valve mask (BVM). The patient must be supine, or lying flat on his back, and the EKG technician must be standing at the head of the patient to use the BVM. The mask should cover both the mouth and nose and seal easily on the patient's face (Fig. 10-4). Masks come in many sizes. The EKG technician may have to change masks to ensure a proper seal.

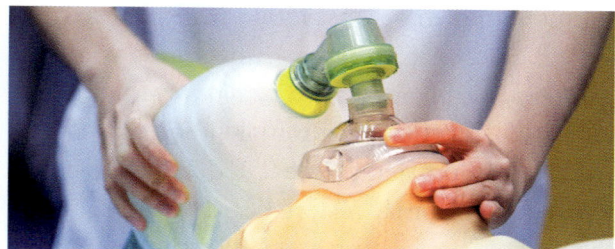

Fig. 10-4. A bag valve mask can assist with breathing for a patient who has stopped breathing on his own.

When using a BVM, the bag should be squeezed evenly. Breaths should be delivered over 1 second at a rate of 10–12 breaths per minute. The technician should watch the patient's chest to be sure it rises with each breath and air is not leaking around the mask. The mask should be attached to supplemental oxygen as soon as possible using the tubing connected to the bag. Many medical facilities have outlets on the wall to supply medical oxygen (Fig. 10-5). The correct setting for using oxygen with a BVM is 15 liters per minute (LPM).

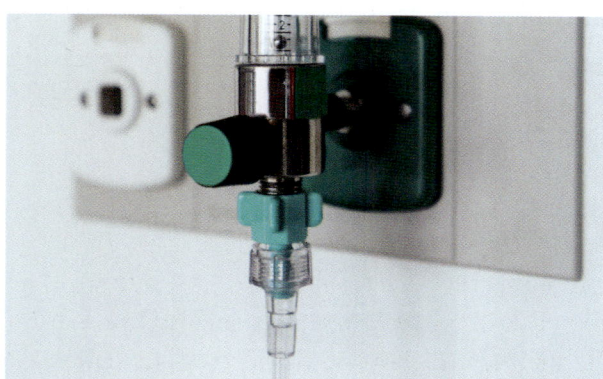

Fig. 10-5. Supplemental oxygen can be connected to the bag valve mask if it is available.

If the patient does not have a pulse or show signs of life, the EKG technician will need to begin CPR. The technician should not spend more than 5–10 seconds attempting to find a pulse. Beginning CPR promptly is a priority.

5. Describe cardiopulmonary resuscitation (CPR) and defibrillation using an automated external defibrillator (AED)

Cardiopulmonary resuscitation (CPR) is used to keep the heart and lungs functioning when a person's heart stops (called *cardiac arrest*) or is in ventricular fibrillation. Prompt CPR followed by use of an automated external defibrillator (AED), when available, may restore heart function. If the heart is not beating and CPR is not being performed effectively, blood is not circulating and cells are not receiving oxygen. Brain death will occur in less than 10 minutes.

The most common cause of death from MI is ventricular fibrillation. AEDs deliver an electric shock that can correct ventricular fibrillation. AEDs can be found in healthcare facilities as well as many public areas, such as schools, airports, malls, and stadiums. The AED attaches to the patient and analyzes heart rhythm, delivering a shock if needed. It is designed for use by the public, first responders, and healthcare workers. Depending on facility policy, an EKG technician may use an AED in some emergency situations (Fig. 10-6).

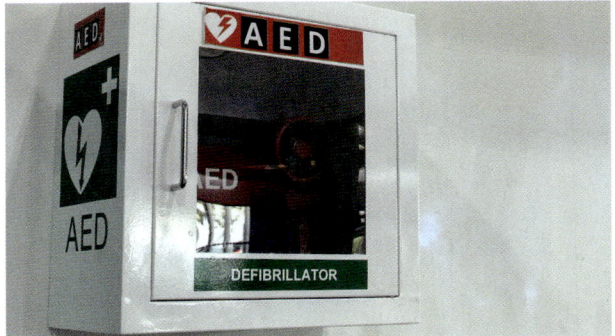

Fig. 10-6. AEDs are often available in public places.

AEDs vary, but all are designed to guide even an inexperienced person through the process of using the device. This includes when to start or stop CPR. Visual and verbal prompts from the machine direct the process. The AED attaches to the patient with two adhesive pads placed on the patient's bare chest. Directions for placing the pads are shown on the back of the pads or on the pad packaging (Fig. 10-7).

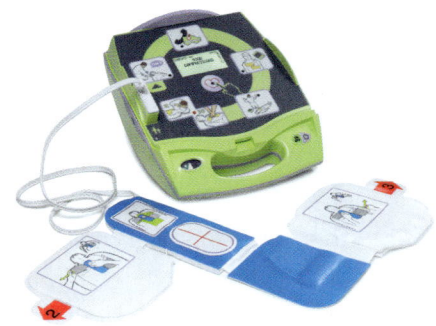

Fig. 10-7. AEDs are designed to be used easily by healthcare workers or members of the public. (PHOTO COURTESY OF ZOLL MEDICAL CORPORATION, 978-421-9637, WWW.ZOLL.COM.)

When the AED is on and the pads are properly placed, a prompt tells the rescuer that the heart rhythm is being analyzed and the patient should not be touched. After the heart rhythm is analyzed, the prompt will state either "shock advised" or "no shock advised, continue CPR." If the prompt states "shock advised," the rescuer will be instructed to deliver the shock once the AED has charged. Before delivering the shock, the rescuer should always check that no one is in contact with the patient and loudly state, "Everyone clear!"

The AED will prompt the rescuer to resume CPR after the shock has been delivered. It will not deliver a shock unless it determines that the patient is in pulseless ventricular tachycardia or ventricular fibrillation. It will not shock asystole (flatline) or any other heart rhythm. If the prompt states "no shock advised, continue CPR," then the rescuer should resume CPR. The AED should be left on and the pads left in place during CPR so the AED can reanalyze the heart rhythm every two minutes. Some AEDs also make a rhythmic sound to help the rescuer perform CPR compressions at a rate of at least 100 per minute.

> **Tip**
>
> **AEDs**
>
> Although AEDs all operate in the same basic manner, EKG technicians should know the specific brand, location, and policies regarding the AED at his facility. Knowing this information could help save a patient's life.

6. Describe the care of a patient experiencing a stroke

Any patient with a cardiovascular disorder is also at risk for a cerebrovascular accident (CVA) (also called a *stroke*). This is especially true for patients with atrial fibrillation, high blood pressure, diabetes, or high cholesterol. Atrial fibrillation can allow blood to pool in the heart, where it can clot and then travel to the brain. CVA can occur when a vessel in the brain becomes blocked by a clot, causing brain tissue to die, or when a blood vessel in the brain ruptures.

A patient may experience one or more ministrokes, called **transient ischemic attacks (TIAs)**, before having a CVA. The signs and symptoms of TIA resolve completely within hours, unlike those of CVA. The signs and symptoms of a CVA include facial drooping on one side, arm weakness on one side, and slurred speech (described in Chapter 4). The EKG technician should notify the supervisor immediately if he suspects a patient is having a CVA. He should carefully note the time when symptoms began. The patient must be treated at a hospital and prompt treatment is critical.

> **Take Action Now!**
>
> **F.A.S.T.**
>
> The American Heart Association recommends the use of the acronym F.A.S.T. to remember stroke symptoms and necessary actions.
>
> **F**ace: Is one side of the face drooping? Is it numb? Ask the person to smile. Is the smile uneven?
>
> **A**rms: Is one arm numb or weak? Ask the person to raise both arms. Check to see if one arm drifts downward.
>
> **S**peech: Is the person's speech slurred? Is the person unable to speak? Can the person be understood? Ask the person to repeat a simple sentence and see if the sentence is repeated correctly.
>
> **T**ime: Time is of the utmost importance when responding to a stroke. If the person shows any of the symptoms listed above, report to the provider immediately.

7. Discuss drugs that may be used in a cardiac emergency

The EKG technician should know common drugs used in a cardiac emergency. The EKG technician's scope of practice does not include giving medications. Some facilities, however, may train EKG technicians to administer oxygen in specific situations. They may also allow technicians to assist a patient to take his own medication (Fig. 10-8).

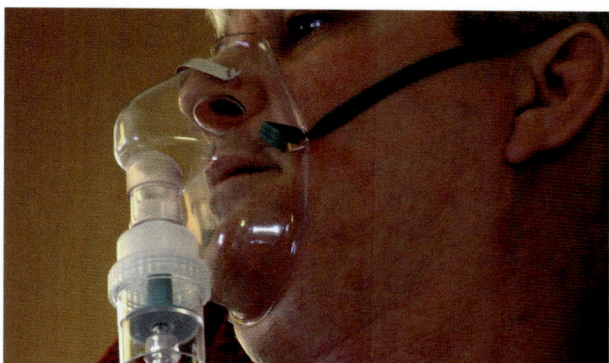

Fig. 10-8. *Oxygen may be administered in a cardiac emergency.*

> **Tip**
>
> **EKG Technicians and Medications**
>
> Administering medications is not within the scope of practice of the EKG technician. However, understanding cardiac medications and their actions makes the technician a valuable member of the healthcare team, especially during cardiac emergencies.

During a cardiac emergency drugs must be administered in a specific way. This is done to make sure the patient receives the effects quickly and efficiently. If the patient is having difficulty breathing, oxygen can be administered by nasal cannula or face mask. This increases the amount of oxygen in the blood. Increasing the amount of oxygen in the blood increases the amount of oxygen available to the heart muscle.

The provider may give the patient aspirin if MI is suspected. Aspirin reduces the ability of blood to clot, and blood clotting in a coronary artery can be the cause of MI. The patient should chew and swallow the aspirin tablets to increase the speed of their effect.

Patients having chest pain may be given a medication called **nitroglycerin**. This medication relaxes and dilates, or expands, the coronary arteries and improves blood flow to the heart muscle. Nitroglycerin is available as a pill that is dissolved under the tongue or as a spray that can be sprayed onto or under the tongue. The patient should be carefully monitored after he has received medication.

Quick Reference

Drug	Indications	Effects	Comments
Oxygen (O_2)	Shortness of breath, cyanosis, chest pain or pressure, fatigue, weakness	Provides additional oxygen for the body's tissues	Given by nasal cannula, simple face mask, or non-rebreather mask.
Aspirin	Chest pain or pressure or suspicion of MI	Decreases blood clotting	Patient should chew aspirin before swallowing.
Nitroglycerin	Chest pain or pressure	Dilates arteries to improve blood flow to heart muscle	Patients who have angina may carry this drug with them to treat episodes of chest pain. May drop blood pressure quickly, so patient should be seated or supine before administration; blood pressure should be monitored.

8. Describe response to nonmedical emergencies

Nonmedical emergencies can include weather-related events such as a tornado, earthquake, or flood, or human-created events such as acts of terrorism or active shooter situations. Each healthcare facility should have a disaster plan that outlines the role of each team member in a disaster. Facilities usually have regular training on the disaster plan, often including drills on disasters. Area emergency agencies such as EMS, fire departments, and police may attend these drills. EKG technicians should pay close attention to this training so they understand how to respond if disasters occur.

Guidelines: Disasters

The following guidelines apply to many disaster situations:

G Remain calm.

G Know the locations of all exits and stairways.

G Know where the fire alarms and extinguishers are located.

G Know the appropriate action to take in various situations based on facility training.

G Use the internet to stay informed, or keep the radio or television tuned to a local station to get the latest information.

In addition, you should also know specific guidelines for the area in which you work. For example, an EKG technician working where hurricanes occur needs to know the guidelines for hurricane preparedness. The following general guidelines are separated by the type of disaster:

Fire

G Know the location of fire extinguishers, alarms, and exit doors.

G Follow the RACE acronym:

- **R**emove anyone in danger if you are not in danger.
- **A**ctivate alarm or call 911.
- **C**ontain the fire if possible by closing all doors and windows.
- **E**xtinguish the fire, or the fire department will extinguish it. Evacuate the area if instructed to do so.
- If operating a fire extinguisher, remember the PASS acronym:
  - **P**ull the pin.
  - **A**im at the base of the fire when spraying.
  - **S**queeze the handle.
  - **S**weep back and forth at the base of the fire.

Tornadoes

- Seek shelter inside, ideally in a steel-framed or concrete building.
- Stay away from windows.
- Stand in the hallway or in a basement, or take cover under heavy furniture.
- Lie as flat as possible and protect your head with your hands.

Power Outages

- Keep calm and take prompt action to provide light.
- Use a backup pack for electrical medical equipment, such as a cardiac monitor. Backup packs do not last more than 24 hours, so contact emergency services when instructed.

Hurricanes

- Know the hurricane's category and track its expected path.
- Evacuate if advised to do so.

Earthquakes

- Drop to the ground.
- Get under a sturdy piece of furniture, such as a heavy table, if possible. Hold on until the shaking stops.
- If no table or desk is available, stay crouched down in the inside corner of a building. Cover your face and head with your arms.
- Stay away from windows, outside walls, and anything that might fall over or fall down.
- Do not exit a building during the shaking.
- Do not use elevators.
- If trapped under debris after an earthquake, do not light a match or ignite a lighter. Avoid kicking up dust. Breathe through a handkerchief or clothing. Make tapping noises or use a whistle, if available, to get rescuers' attention. Do not shout. Shouting could cause you to inhale dangerous amounts of dust.

Active Shooter

- Follow the facility's emergency notification procedures.
- If there is an escape path, try to evacuate. If the area cannot be safely evacuated, stay where you are.
- Turn off the lights, secure the door, and stay hidden from outside view.
- Turn off phone ringers.
- If safe to do so, call 911 and notify the operator of your exact location in the building.
- Provide information on the number and description of the shooter(s), the number of victims and nature of their injuries, and their locations, if known.
- Move heavy furniture to barricade the door and cover any openings or windows in the door.

- When police arrive on the scene, do not move toward any police vehicle until directed to do so by the officers. Move with your hands on top of your head and follow all directions given by police.
- Remain in the area until released by police.

Chapter Review

- Because of their close contact with patients during cardiac testing, EKG technicians are able to observe for signs of a developing cardiac emergency.

- EKG technicians observe closely for the signs, symptoms, and EKG changes that might signal a cardiac emergency. If an EKG technician observes these signs, he should call for help right away.

- ST segment elevation or depression, a lethal dysrhythmia, and a newly developing dysrhythmia are all EKG changes that must be reported immediately. Ventricular tachycardia, ventricular fibrillation, third-degree heart block, agonal rhythm, pulseless electrical activity, and asystole are the lethal dysrhythmias.

- Every facility has standard procedures for responding to medical emergencies. EKG technicians should know these procedures and follow them at all times.

- Some emergencies may require that the EKG technician start CPR and/or use an automated external defibrillator (AED). Technicians will be trained to do this.

- Some cardiac conditions are closely connected to stroke (also known as cerebrovascular accident or CVA). EKG technicians should know the signs and symptoms of stroke and be prepared to respond quickly.

- Medications may be given to patients having cardiac emergencies. While it is outside the scope of practice for EKG technicians to give medications, they may be trained to assist with medications or oxygen administration.

- All healthcare workers need to know how to respond to nonmedical emergencies such as fire, natural disasters, and acts of terrorism or violence in the workplace. EKG technicians should know facility policies and procedures for responding to emergencies. They should actively participate in drills and training sessions.

Glossary

aberrant: in reference to the cardiac conduction system, an adjective used to describe a path of electrical impulses that differs from the normal path.

abrade: in electrocardiography, to lightly scrub the outer layer of the skin to remove debris that can interfere with electrode contact.

accelerated idioventricular rhythm: a faster ventricular rhythm consisting of three or more ventricular escape beats, with a rate of 40–100 BPM.

accelerated junctional rhythm: a cardiac rhythm with a rate of 60–100 BPM; this rhythm has a higher rate than what is usually associated with rates generated by junctional tissue, and the increased rate represents the body's attempt to compensate for the lack of atrial contractions.

acute care: care provided in an inpatient setting such as a hospital where the emphasis is on providing short-term, immediate care for illnesses and injuries.

age-predicted maximal heart rate: a calculation determined by subtracting a patient's age from 220; 85% of this rate is the target rate for stress testing.

agonal rhythm: a variation of idioventricular rhythm with a rate of 20 BPM or less. Requires immediate intervention to prevent death.

alveoli: the air sacs in the lungs where oxygen and carbon dioxide are exchanged.

ambulatory care: care provided in an outpatient setting such as a doctor's office or urgent care center.

ambulatory monitoring: a type of EKG technology that can record or monitor a patient's heart rate and rhythm over an extended period while the patient continues with normal life; Holter, event, and mobile telemetry monitors are examples.

anatomy: the study of the structures of the body.

angina: chest pain, pressure, or discomfort.

aorta: the body's largest artery, which branches off into the body's smaller arteries to distribute oxygen-rich blood.

aortic valve: the heart valve located between the left ventricle and the aorta; also called the *aortic semilunar valve*.

apex: the tip of the heart, formed by the left ventricle.

aphasia: difficulty speaking.

apical pulse: the pulse located on the left side of the chest, just below the nipple.

apnea: the absence of breathing.

arteries: blood vessels that carry blood away from the heart.

arteriosclerosis: a condition in which one or more of the coronary arteries becomes blocked, hardened, or narrowed by fatty deposits (plaque).

artifact: in electrocardiography, interference or distortion that appears on a tracing.

ascites: abnormal fluid in the abdominal cavity.

aspiration: inhaling oral secretions into the lungs.

asymptomatic: not experiencing symptoms.

asystole: a rhythm in which there are no contractions and no cardiac activity; also sometimes called *flatline*.

atria: the two upper chambers of the heart (singular *atrium*).

atrial fibrillation: a common dysrhythmia that occurs when multiple irritable sites fire in the atria; considered *controlled* if the ventricular rate is under 100 BPM and *uncontrolled* if the ventricular rate is above 100 BPM.

atrial flutter: an atrial rhythm that occurs when an irritable site in the atria fires at a very rapid rate.

atrial kick: a common term used to describe the force of atrial contractions.

atrial rate: the rate at which the atria contract (in normal rhythms, it is the same as the ventricular rate).

atrial rhythm: a cardiac rhythm originating in the atria instead of the SA node.

atrial tachycardia: a fast atrial rhythm caused by irritability in the atria, with a rate of 160–250 BPM.

atrioventricular (AV) junction: part of the electrical conduction system of the heart, located between the AV node and the bundle of His.

atrioventricular (AV) node: part of the electrical conduction system of the heart, located at the bottom of the right atrium, behind the tricuspid valve, with an intrinsic rate of 40–50 BPM.

augmented limb leads: in electrocardiography, the collective name for leads aVR, aVL, and aVF.

auscultation: use of a stethoscope to listen to the body's internal sounds.

automated external defibrillator (AED): a device attached to a patient to analyze heart rhythm and deliver a shock, if needed, to restore a normal heart rhythm.

autonomic nervous system (ANS): the part of the nervous system that controls body functions that are not consciously directed (for example, breathing and heartbeat).

baseline: what is considered normal for a particular patient; what her initial vital sign readings are and how she normally responds and acts.

bicuspid valve: the heart valve located between the left atrium and the left ventricle; also called the *mitral valve*.

bigeminy: a word used to describe premature ventricular complexes that occur every other beat.

bipolar leads: in electrocardiography, leads that measure voltage between an electrically positive and electrically negative pole; the limb leads are bipolar leads.

bizarre: in EKG interpretation, a word used to describe a wave or complex with an abnormal appearance.

blocked beat: a heartbeat in which the electrical impulse that begins in the SA node is prevented from continuing through the cardiac conduction system to the ventricles.

blood clot: blood that has become solid within the body.

blood pressure: the force put on the walls of the blood vessels by blood as it is pumped through the body.

brachial pulse: the pulse located inside the elbow, about one to one-and-a-half inches above the elbow.

broken recording: an EKG artifact that occurs when the signal is compromised by frayed or faulty lead wires.

bronchi: the two tubes that take air to the lungs; (singular: *bronchus*).

bronchioles: smaller branches from the bronchi; tubes that carry air farther into the lungs, reaching the air sacs (alveoli).

bundle branch block (BBB): a slowing down of the electrical impulse within the ventricles, either in the left or right bundle branches, which causes the ventricles to depolarize one after another, rather than at the same time.

bundle branches: part of the electrical conduction system of the heart; they divide from the bundle of His and carry the electrical impulse to the walls of the ventricles.

bundle of His: part of the electrical conduction system of the heart, located in the upper part of the interventricular septum, with an intrinsic rate of 40–50 BPM; also called *AV bundle*.

calipers: a tool with adjustable points, used to measure intervals on EKG tracings.

capillaries: the smallest blood vessels; they carry oxygen and nutrients to and remove carbon dioxide and wastes from cells throughout the body.

cardiac arrest: a total loss of heart function.

cardiac catheterization: a procedure that involves inserting a tube into a blood vessel and into the heart for testing or treatment of heart conditions.

cardiac conduction system: the pathway of electrical impulses that controls the heart's pumping action.

cardiac output: the amount of blood pumped by the heart.

cardiologist: a doctor specializing in the health of the heart.

cardiomyopathy: a condition in which the muscular layer of the heart is enlarged, making the heart unable to pump effectively.

cardiopulmonary resuscitation (CPR): medical procedures used when a person's heart or lungs have stopped working.

carotid pulse: the pulse located on the side of the neck, just below the jaw.

Centers for Disease Control and Prevention (CDC): a federal government agency that issues guidelines to protect and improve the health of individuals and communities.

central nervous system: the part of the nervous system that is composed of the brain and the spinal cord.

cerebrovascular accident (CVA): a condition that occurs when blood supply to part of the brain is blocked or a blood vessel leaks or ruptures within the brain; also called *stroke*.

certification: a credential issued by a school, a facility, or an organization verifying that a person has met certain standards and/or completed a certain course of study.

chain of command: the line of authority within a facility or agency.

Cheyne-Stokes: alternating periods of slow, irregular breathing and rapid, shallow breathing.

clinical experience: experience working with patients in a healthcare facility.

code: an emergency signal used in healthcare settings to alert staff to a needed response while preventing panic and stress among patients and visitors; *code blue* usually means cardiac arrest.

code of ethics: a list outlining behavior that is considered morally right or wrong in a particular setting.

code team: a group of healthcare workers designated to respond to emergency codes in a medical facility.

complex: several EKG waves considered together.

conducted beat: a heartbeat in which the electrical impulse that begins in the SA node continues through the cardiac conduction system to the ventricles.

confidentiality: the legal and ethical principle of keeping information private.

congenital defect: an abnormality that occurred before birth.

congestive heart failure: a condition in which the heart muscle is damaged and is no longer able to pump effectively; causes blood to back up in various parts of the body.

contiguous leads: in electrocardiography, two or more leads that record activity in the same area of the heart.

coronary arteries: the arteries that provide oxygen and nutrients to the tissues of the heart.

crash cart: a cart containing supplies needed immediately in the case of a medical emergency.

cyanosis: a situation in which the nail beds and the skin around the mouth become blue or gray; indication of lack of oxygen.

deep vein thrombosis (DVT): a condition in which a blood clot forms deep under the skin, usually in the legs.

defibrillation: delivery of a shock to a patient's heart with the goal of stopping a dangerous cardiac rhythm and restoring a healthy rhythm.

depolarization: an electrical change in the heart in which the voltage of the cells becomes more positive and the cells contract.

dextrocardia: a rare heart condition that causes the heart to develop pointing to the right side of the chest instead of the left side.

diagnosis: determination of medical condition by a doctor or other qualified healthcare provider.

diaphoresis: profuse sweating.

diaphragm: a muscle that divides the thoracic cavity from the abdomen.

diastole: the phase when the heart relaxes or rests.

diastolic: blood pressure reading associated with the phase when the ventricles relax or rest; the bottom, smaller number in the blood pressure measurement.

dual-chamber pacemaker: an artificial pacemaker that stimulates both the atria and the ventricles.

dyspnea: shortness of breath or difficulty breathing.

dysrhythmia: a difficult or abnormal heart rhythm; includes rhythms that are too fast, too slow, or originate in an area of the heart other than the SA node; sometimes called *arrhythmia*.

echocardiogram: a test that uses sound waves to visualize the heart; provides information about the mechanical function of the heart.

ectopic focus: a situation in which an irritable area in the cardiac conduction system begins to generate an impulse even though the SA node may be working normally.

Einthoven's triangle: the imaginary triangle formed by the placement of the electrodes that record the limb leads.

EKG technician: a healthcare worker who performs or assists with different types of EKG tests.

EKG tracing: a record of the electrical activity of a patient's heart during an electrocardiogram (EKG) as recorded by an EKG machine; also called *EKG strip* or *rhythm strip*.

electrical interference: in electrocardiography, a type of artifact caused by the presence of other appliances or equipment in the area surrounding the EKG machine.

electrocardiogram (EKG): a recording in visible form of the electrical activity of a patient's heart; also called *ECG*.

electrode: in EKG technology, a pad that conducts electricity and is connected to the patient's body and to electrode cables to conduct electrical signals from the heart to the EKG machine.

embolus: a blood clot or loosened plaque that travels from its original site and can block blood flow.

empathy: the ability to understand and experience the feelings of another person.

endocardium: the thin, innermost layer of the heart; forms a smooth, elastic surface that allows blood to flow without stopping or clotting.

epicardium: the outermost layer of the heart; a thin layer of connective tissue and fat that protects the heart and also contains the blood vessels that supply oxygen and nutrients to the heart (coronary arteries).

erythrocytes: red blood cells; contain the protein (hemoglobin) that carries oxygen in the blood.

escape beat: a heartbeat created when a part of the heart's electrical conduction system other than the SA node initiates the electrical impulse that causes the heart to beat.

escape pacemaker: in the cardiac conduction system, a natural pacemaker below the SA node that takes over generating electrical impulses when the SA node fails to generate them or when impulses from the SA node are blocked.

escape rhythm: a rhythm in which a part of the heart's electrical conduction system other than the SA node initiates all electrical impulses that cause the heart to beat (i.e., acts as the heart's primary pacemaker).

event monitor: a type of ambulatory monitor that records heart rate and rhythm when the patient indicates that she is experiencing symptoms.

exchange sites: places in the body where oxygen and substances needed by the cells are delivered and waste products removed.

F waves: short for *flutter waves*; waves displayed on the EKG tracing of a patient with atrial flutter, representing the distortion of the P wave as the AV node blocks impulses that exceed 180 per minute; also called *sawtooth* or *picket fence waves*.

failure to capture: a situation in which the electrical stimulation generated by an artificial pacemaker does not result in contraction of the heart muscle.

failure to sense: a situation in which an artificial pacemaker does not appropriately sense the heart's electrical activity and does not create electrical stimulation when it should; also called *failure to pace* or *failure to fire*.

first-degree heart block: a heart block rhythm marked by a PR interval greater than 0.20 seconds.

fixed-rate pacemaker: an artificial pacemaker that delivers stimulation consistently.

formed elements: the solid portion of blood.

Fowler's position: a body position in which a person's upper body is elevated 45 to 60 degrees; in *semi-Fowler's* position the elevation is 45 degrees or lower.

gain control: the mechanism on an EKG machine that allows adjustment of the height of the markings shown on the tracing.

hand hygiene: washing hands with either plain or antiseptic soap and water and using alcohol-based hand rubs.

hard skills: skills that involve performing specific tasks, such as measuring blood pressure, applying electrodes, and operating EKG machines.

heart block: a type of cardiac rhythm caused when the AV node or AV bundle delays the electrical impulse from the SA node too long; also called *AV block*.

heart rate: the speed at which the heart is beating.

heart rhythm: the overall pattern of the heartbeat.

hemiparesis: paralysis on one side of the body.

hemiplegia: weakness on one side of the body.

hemoglobin: a protein that transports oxygen and carbon dioxide in the blood.

Holter monitor: a type of ambulatory monitor that allows a provider to evaluate heart rate and rhythm over an extended period of time (usually 24–48 hours) while the patient continues with normal life.

homeostasis: a state of balance and stability within the systems of the body.

hypertension: high blood pressure; diagnosed when systolic pressure is consistently 130 or higher and/or diastolic pressure 80 or higher.

hypoxia: inadequate (not enough) oxygen supply to the tissues of the body.

idioventricular rhythm: a potentially lethal ventricular rhythm consisting of three or more ventricular escape beats in a row, with a rate of 20–40 BPM; also known as *ventricular escape rhythm*. Related to *agonal rhythm* (see separate entry).

infection prevention: the set of methods practiced in healthcare facilities to prevent and control the spread of disease.

inferior vena cava: one of the largest veins in the body; returns oxygen-depleted blood from the lower body to the heart.

inpatient treatment: care provided to a patient who has been admitted to a hospital.

interval: on an EKG tracing, a wave and a segment taken together.

intrinsic rate: the normal firing rate (expressed in beats per minute) associated with a part of the heart's electrical conduction system.

irregular rhythm: a general category of heart rhythm in which QRS complexes may look alike or different from each other, and do not repeat with consistent timing.

irritable: in reference to the cardiac conduction system, more likely to initiate an electrical impulse at the wrong time or in the wrong location.

ischemia: a condition in which an embolus blocks a coronary artery, resulting in a lack of oxygen to the heart muscle supplied by that vessel.

isoelectric line: on an EKG tracing, the straight line between upward and downward movements (also sometimes called the *baseline*).

junctional escape beats: a cardiac rhythm in which the AV junction area generates an impulse because the SA node is either slow to generate an impulse or does not generate one at all; as in premature junctional complexes, the P wave is abnormal, but these beats are late while PJCs are early.

junctional escape rhythm: a cardiac rhythm created by a series of junctional escape beats; rate is usually 40–60 BPM.

junctional rhythm: a cardiac rhythm originating in the cells near the bundle of His or in the area of the AV junction rather than in the SA node.

junctional tachycardia: a junctional cardiac rhythm with a rate above 100 BPM.

large block method: a method used to determine heart rate from an EKG tracing that involves counting the numbers of large blocks between two consecutive R waves and dividing that number into 300, which is the number of large blocks in a one-minute EKG strip; also called the *300 method*.

larynx: an organ that includes the vocal cords and allows air to pass into the trachea.

lead: in an EKG, the imaginary line between two electrodes attached to the patient; each lead can produce a different EKG tracing and a different view of the heart's electrical activity.

lead wire: wire that connects an electrode placed on a patient's body to an EKG machine; also called *leadwire* or *electrode wire*.

leukocytes: white blood cells; capable of producing antibodies and destroying pathogens.

liability: a legal term that means a person can be held responsible for her actions if someone is harmed.

licensure: a legally required process that involves completing an approved course of education, passing a written exam, and, in some cases, completing a skills test in order to practice a medical profession.

limb leads: in electrocardiography, the lead group made up of leads I, II, and III; also known as the *bipolar leads*.

metabolism: the physical and chemical processes carried out by the body systems to maintain homeostasis.

Methicillin-resistant *Staphylococcus aureus* (MRSA): bacteria that have developed resistance to the antibiotic methicillin.

microorganism: a living thing so small it is only visible under a microscope.

mobile cardiac telemetry: a type of ambulatory monitor that detects heart rate or rhythm irregularities automatically and transmits data to a healthcare professional when an irregularity occurs.

monomorphic: in EKG interpretation, a word used to describe identical EKG features (e.g., premature ventricular complexes that look the same each time they occur).

morphology: the shape and direction of waves, complexes, and segments on an EKG tracing.

multifocal: in electrocardiography, originating from multiple irritable sites in the heart's conduction system, as in *multifocal premature ventricular contractions*.

multifocal atrial tachycardia: a rhythm related to wandering atrial pacemaker, but with a ventricular rate greater than 100 BPM.

myocardial infarction (MI): a condition that occurs when the heart muscle does not receive enough oxygen because blood flow is blocked; also called *heart attack*.

myocardium: the middle and thickest layer of the heart; made up of cells capable of continuous rhythmic contraction.

nitroglycerin: a medication sometimes given during cardiac emergencies to relax or dilate the coronary arteries.

non-ST segment elevation myocardial infarction (NSTEMI): a heart attack that does not show elevation of the ST segment on an EKG tracing.

normal sinus rhythm (NSR): the cardiac rhythm produced when the electrical system of the heart is functioning normally.

nuclear stress test: a variation of stress testing in which a harmless radioactive substance is injected into the patient's bloodstream and traced during exercise, giving the provider more detailed information about possible blockages in coronary arteries.

objective information: information based on what a person sees, hears, touches, or smells; also called *signs*.

occlude: to block or plug up.

Occupational Safety and Health Administration (OSHA): a federal government agency that makes rules to protect workers from hazards on the job.

orthopnea: difficulty breathing when lying flat.

outpatient treatment: care provided without the patient being admitted to a hospital.

oxygen-depleted blood: blood that is returned to the heart through the veins after supplying oxygen to the rest of the body and is then pumped to the lungs to receive oxygen again; also called *deoxygenated blood*.

oxygen-rich blood: blood that returns to the heart from the lungs after receiving oxygen and is then pumped throughout the body; also called *oxygenated blood*.

oxygen saturation: the amount of oxygen in the blood.

pacemaker: something that regulates the heart's contractions; natural pacemakers are part of the cardiac conduction system, with the SA node acting as the primary pacemaker when the heart is functioning normally. An artificial pacemaker is a battery-powered device that creates electrical impulses to stimulate the heart.

palpation: feeling with the fingers, as in the method normally used to measure radial pulse.

palpitations: a feeling of the heart fluttering or beating in the chest.

parasympathetic nervous system: part of the autonomic nervous system that works to slow heart rate.

pathogens: microorganisms that are capable of causing infection and disease.

peripheral edema: fluid buildup in the body; can cause swelling in the lower legs, ankles, feet, and, in severe cases, the abdomen.

peripheral nervous system: part of the nervous system made up of the nerves that extend throughout the body.

personal protective equipment (PPE): equipment that helps protect employees from serious workplace injuries or illnesses resulting from contact with workplace hazards.

pharynx: the area of the throat behind the mouth and nasal cavity.

physiology: the study of how various systems of the body work.

plaque: in cardiology, fatty deposits in the coronary arteries.

plasma: the liquid part of blood.

policy: a course of action that should be taken every time a certain situation occurs.

polymorphic: in EKG interpretation, a word used to describe EKG features that correspond to the same thing but have differing appearances (e.g., premature ventricular complexes that look different each time they occur); also called *multifocal*.

precordial leads: in electrocardiography, the unipolar lead group composed of leads V1, V2, V3, V4, V5, and V6; also known as the *chest leads*.

prejudice: an unfavorable opinion of a person or group of people based on race, religion, etc., that is without basis.

premature atrial complex (PAC): an atrial rhythm featuring obvious premature beats; other aspects of the rhythm are often normal.

premature junctional complex (PJC): a cardiac rhythm in which an early impulse is generated by an irritable area of the AV junction; characterized by an abnormal P wave.

premature ventricular complex (PVC): a premature beat originating in the ventricles.

PR interval: on an EKG tracing, the interval from the beginning of the P wave to the beginning of the QRS complex.

procedure: a method or way of doing something.

protected health information (PHI): a person's private health information, which includes name, address, telephone number, social security number, email address, and medical record number.

pulmonary circuit: the circulation of blood between the heart and the lungs.

pulmonary edema: fluid buildup in the lungs; can interfere with gas exchange.

pulmonary embolism: a blood clot or other blockage found in the lungs.

pulmonary valve: the heart valve located between the right ventricle and the pulmonary artery; also called the *pulmonary semilunar valve*.

pulse: the beat that is felt at different points of the body when the heart contracts and pumps blood through the arteries.

pulseless electrical activity: a situation in which a patient shows organized electrical activity but does not have a pulse; considered a lethal rhythm and requires prompt CPR and notification of the doctor or healthcare provider.

pulse oximeter: a noninvasive device that uses a light to determine the amount of oxygen in the blood.

Purkinje fibers: part of the electrical conduction system of the heart; they divide from the bundle branches and have an intrinsic rate of 20–40 BPM.

P wave: in normal sinus rhythm, the first positive deflection (upward movement) seen on an EKG tracing; corresponds to the contraction of the atria.

QRS complex: an EKG complex that includes the Q, R, and S waves and corresponds to the contraction of the ventricles; appearance in EKG tracings can vary widely.

QRS interval: the length of time associated with a complete QRS complex on an EKG tracing; normal measurement is less than 0.12 seconds.

radial pulse: the pulse located on the inside of the wrist, where the radial artery runs just beneath the skin.

rapid ventricular response: contractions of the ventricles in an atrial fibrillation rhythm at a rate of 100 BPM or greater.

regularly irregular rhythm: a general category of heart rhythm in which QRS complexes may or may not look alike but are irregular in a clear, repeating pattern.

regular rhythm: a general category of heart rhythm in which QRS complexes occur in a pattern that looks the same each time and repeats with consistent timing (for example, every 0.8 seconds).

regurgitation: leaking of blood back into the chamber from which it is being pumped; also called *backflow*.

repolarization: an electrical change in the heart in which the voltage of the cells becomes more negative and the cells relax.

respiration: the process of inhaling air into the lungs and exhaling air out of the lungs.

retrograde: moving backward; in cardiology, an impulse that travels backward compared to the usual cardiac conduction path.

rhythm strip: in electrocardiography, a 12-second recording of the activity in lead II on an EKG tracing.

R-on-T phenomenon: a situation in which the QRS complex of a premature ventricular complex falls on the T wave of the previous beat; may lead to ventricular tachycardia or ventricular fibrillation.

R-R interval: on an EKG tracing, the interval between the R wave of one complex and the R wave of the next complex.

scope of practice: a description of the duties a healthcare worker is expected and legally allowed to perform.

second-degree heart block Mobitz type I: a heart block rhythm in which the PR intervals of conducted beats get longer and longer until a beat is totally blocked, and then the pattern resumes; also called *Wenckebach*.

second-degree heart block Mobitz type II: a heart block rhythm in which there is usually a fixed number of blocked P waves for every conducted beat; the relationship between P waves and QRS complexes is expressed as a ratio (e.g., 2:1, 3:1).

segment: on an EKG tracing, the isoelectric area between two waves.

septum: in cardiology, the wall dividing the right and left sides of the heart.

single-chamber pacemaker: an artificial pacemaker that stimulates one area of the heart, either the atria or the ventricles.

sinoatrial node: part of the electrical conduction system of the heart, located in the upper part of the right atrium and acting as the primary pacemaker of the heart, with an intrinsic rate of 60–100 BPM; also called the *SA node* or *sinus node*.

sinus arrest: a sinus rhythm resulting when the SA node does not initiate an impulse, causing pauses in the heart's electrical activity; similar to *sinoatrial block* but with a greater time between complexes. Also called *sinus pause*.

sinus arrhythmia: a sinus rhythm in which all characteristics are normal except for rhythm regularity; R-R intervals are irregular and usually vary with the patient's breathing.

sinus bradycardia: a slow sinus rhythm with normal characteristics but with a rate below 60 BPM.

sinus rhythm: a cardiac rhythm originating in the sinus (SA) node.

sinus tachycardia: a fast sinus rhythm with normal characteristics but with a rate of 100–160 BPM.

6-second method: a method used to determine heart rate from an EKG tracing that involves identifying a six-second section of the EKG and counting the number of QRS complexes in that section, then multiplying by 10.

small block method: a method used to determine heart rate from an EKG tracing that involves counting the small blocks between two consecutive R waves and dividing that number into 1500, which is the number of small blocks representing the passage of one minute; also called the *1500 method*.

soft skills: skills that are not related to the performance of a specific task but which affect how a person performs her job, such as attention to detail and use of tact.

somatic nervous system: the division of the peripheral nervous system that controls voluntary actions.

somatic tremor: an EKG artifact usually caused by patient tremors or shivering.

sphygmomanometer: a device that measures blood pressure.

sputum: mucus coughed up from the lungs.

standard gain: 10 millimeters per millivolt, the most commonly used setting for the height of tracings on an EKG machine (a one-millivolt signal will create a mark 10 millimeters high).

Standard Precautions: a method of infection prevention in which all blood, body fluids, nonintact skin, and mucous membranes are treated as if they were infected with an infectious disease.

stimuli: changes that can cause a response in the body (singular is *stimulus*).

stress loop: a loop in the lead wire close to electrodes used in ambulatory monitoring; designed to reduce tension on the electrodes caused by the patient's movements.

stress test: an EKG application used to evaluate how the heart functions under controlled stress created either by exercise or medications (pharmacologic stress test); also called *exercise stress test*, *exercise tolerance test*, or *treadmill test*.

ST segment: on an EKG tracing, the segment from the J point (the end of QRS) to the beginning of the T wave.

ST segment depression: an abnormal EKG feature in which the ST segment is at least one millimeter (one small block) below the isoelectric line; can be associated with ischemia.

ST segment elevation myocardial infarction (STEMI): a type of heart attack marked on an EKG tracing by an ST segment elevated at least one millimeter (one small block) above the isoelectric line.

stylus: the part of the EKG machine that creates marks on the EKG paper.

subjective information: information that a person cannot or did not observe, but is based on something reported to the person that may or may not be true; also called *symptoms*.

superior vena cava: one of the largest veins in the body; returns oxygen-depleted blood from the upper body to the heart.

supine: a body position in which a person lies flat on his back.

supraventricular tachycardia: either a general term for all tachycardias (fast rhythms) that begin with impulses generated above the ventricles, or a specific dysrhythmia marked by a very fast rate, P waves that are difficult or impossible to distinguish, and narrow QRS complexes; also called *narrow complex tachycardia*.

sustained rhythm: a rhythm that is always present.

sympathetic nervous system: part of the autonomic nervous system that works to increase heart rate; can be associated with fear or threat, as in the fight-or-flight response.

sympathy: the expression of concern for a person's feelings or situation.

symptomatic: experiencing symptoms.

systemic circuit: the circulation of blood between the heart and the rest of the body (except the lungs).

systole: the phase in which the heart is at work, contracting and pushing blood out of the left ventricle.

systolic: blood pressure reading associated with the phase in which the ventricles are contracting; the top, larger number in the blood pressure measurement.

tachycardia: rapid heart rate.

tachypnea: rapid breathing.

telemetry: an application of EKG technology that allows continual monitoring of a patient's heart rate and rhythm; often used in an emergency room or hospital setting.

telemetry pack: a device attached to a patient to monitor heart rate and rhythm on an ongoing basis; also called a *telemetry unit*.

third-degree heart block: a potentially lethal heart block rhythm in which all impulses from the SA node are blocked; there is no relationship between the activity of the atria and the activity of the ventricles, and cardiac output is severely compromised.

thrombocytes: part of the formed elements of blood that play a role in blood clotting; also called *platelets*.

thrombus: a blood clot or collection of plaque formed within a blood vessel.

torsades de pointes: a variation of polymorphic ventricular tachycardia in which the QRS complex seems to "twist" from one side of the isoelectric line to the other.

trachea: the tube that goes from the larynx to the bronchi, allowing air to pass to the lungs; also called *windpipe*.

transient ischemic attack (TIA): a warning sign of a CVA/stroke resulting from a temporary lack of oxygen in the brain; symptoms may last up to 24 hours.

transient rhythm: a rhythm that comes and goes.

Transmission-Based Precautions: a method of infection prevention used when caring for persons who are infected or may be infected with certain infectious diseases.

tricuspid valve: the heart valve located between the right atrium and the right ventricle; also called the *right atrioventricular valve*.

trigeminy: a word used to describe premature ventricular complexes that occur every third beat.

T wave: an EKG wave that follows the QRS complex and corresponds to the relaxation of the ventricles.

T wave inversion: a situation in which the T wave deflects downward from the isoelectric line rather than upward; can be associated with ischemia, especially when paired with ST segment depression.

12-lead EKG: a common type of electrocardiogram that records the electrical activity of the heart in 12 different directions (leads).

underlying rhythm: the basic rhythm of a patient's heart, separate from any abnormal beats or complexes.

unifocal: in electrocardiography, originating from a single irritable site in the heart's conduction system, as in *unifocal premature ventricular contractions.*

unipolar leads: in electocardiography, leads that measure voltage at an electrically positive pole in comparison to a neutral reference point.

unstable angina: chest pain that occurs at rest and/or in the absence of stress; can be a warning sign for myocardial infarction.

vagal maneuver: action taken to stimulate the vagal nerve and slow the heart rate; may be recommended by a healthcare provider to stop certain dysrhythmias.

veins: blood vessels that carry blood toward the heart.

ventricles: the two lower chambers of the heart.

ventricular escape beat: a type of escape beat that occurs when the SA node and other potential pacemakers above the bundle branches fail to initiate an impulse.

ventricular fibrillation: a ventricular rhythm in which multiple sites in the ventricles are firing at a very fast rate. There is no organization to the impulses and therefore no organized contraction of the heart muscle; considered a lethal dysrhythmia and requires immediate intervention with a defibrillator; also called *VF* or *V-fib.*

ventricular rate: the rate at which the ventricles are contracting; in normal rhythms it is the same as the atrial rate.

ventricular rhythm: a cardiac rhythm originating in the ventricles rather than in the SA node; marked on an EKG tracing by a widened QRS complex.

ventricular tachycardia: a ventricular rhythm consisting of three or more premature ventricular complexes in a row; can be very dangerous if it lasts for more than a minute.

vital signs: measurements that monitor the functioning of the vital organs of the body; temperature, pulse, respiration, and blood pressure are included.

voltage: a difference in electrical charge.

wandering atrial pacemaker: an atrial rhythm that occurs when impulses arise from multiple areas, including the atria, the AV node, and the SA node; also called *multiformed atrial rhythm.*

wandering baseline: an EKG artifact in which the normally flat baseline moves up and down across the tracing.

wave: on an EKG tracing, movement upward or downward from the isoelectric line; a positive wave moves upward and a negative wave moves downward.

Wilson's central terminal: the center of Einthoven's triangle; acts as an electrically neutral point of reference for the precordial (chest) leads.

Index

aberrant (conduction path)	**124**
abbreviations	**8**
abrading	**70**
accelerated idioventricular rhythm	**121**
accelerated junctional rhythm	**113**
acute care	**2**
adaptations, see also specific conditions requiring adaptations	**68**, 72–75
AED, see *automated external defibrillator*	
AFib, see *atrial fibrillation*	
age-predicted maximal heart rate	**63**
agonal rhythm	**121**, 155
alternating current interference, see *electrical interference*	
alveoli	**34**, 39, 43
ambulatory care	**1, 2**
ambulatory monitor	**50**, 65–66
American Heart Association (AHA)	**7**, 11, 159
amputation, EKG adaptations in response to	72, **74**
anatomical terms	**32**–33
for parts of the body	32
lines of reference	32
of direction	32
anatomy	**31**, 32–40
angina	**42**, 160
aphasia	**46**
aorta	**34**, 36, 37, 38
aortic valve	**37**, 38
apex	**22**, 33
apical pulse	**22**, 23
apnea	**23**
arrhythmia, see *dysrhythmia*	
arteriosclerosis	**41**, 42
artery	**34**, 36, 37, 41–42
artifact, see also specific types of artifact	**55**, 68
artificial pacemaker	**142**
and electrode placement for EKG testing	73
complications	143–144
dual-chamber	**142**
fixed-rate	**142**
pacemaker spikes, illustrated	142–143
single-chamber	**142**
aspirin	**160**
asystole	**124**, 125, 155
atria	**37**, 48, 78
atrial fibrillation	**105**, 107
atrial flutter	**105**, 106
atrial kick	**113**
atrial rate	84, 106
atrial tachycardia	**103**
atrioventricular (AV) junction	**78**
atrioventricular node	**78**, 79, 94
augmented limb leads	**52**
auscultation	**21**
procedure for counting pulse by	23
automated external defibrillator (AED)	**126**, 158–159
autonomic nervous system (ANS)	**35**
AV block, see *heart block*	
AV bundle, see *bundle of His*	
backflow, see *regurgitation (cardiac)*	
bag valve mask (BVM)	**157**
baseline (as related to EKG, see *isoelectric line*)	
as related to vital signs	12, 29
Basic Life Support (BLS)	**7**, 11
bicuspid valve	**37**, 38
bigeminy	**119**
bipolar lead	**52**, 143
blocked beat	**132**, 133, 134
blood	33–34
blood clot, see also *deep vein thrombosis* and *pulmonary embolism*	**41**
blood oxygen, see *oxygen saturation*	
blood pressure	**24**
normal range, adult	12
normal range, pediatric	27
procedures for measuring	25–27
body systems	**31**
cardiovascular	31, 33–34, 35, 35–39
endocrine	31
gastrointestinal	31
integumentary	31
lymphatic	31
musculoskeletal	31
nervous	33, 37
reproductive	31
respiratory	33, 35, 38–39
urinary	31
body temperature, see *temperature*	
brachial pulse	**21**
bradycardia, see also specific types of bradycardia	95–96
breast implants, EKG adaptations in response to	73
broken recording	**71**, 75
bronchi	**34**
bronchiole	**34**
bundle branch block (BBB)	**122**
bundle branches	**78**, 79, 94
bundle of His	**78**, 79, 94
calibration mark	**56**
calipers	**85**, 87
capillaries	**34**, 38–39
cardiac arrest	**42**, 153, 158
cardiac catheterization	**146**
cardiac conduction system, see also entries for specific parts of the system	77, **78**, 79, 94
cardiac output	**42**, 77
symptoms of low	42
cardiac rhythm, see also specific rhythm entries	**82**, 94–151
artificially paced	142–143
atrial	101–107
heart block	132–135
identification of	94–96
junctional	111–114
naming of	96
sinus	96–99
ventricular	118–126
cardiologist	**1**
cardiomyopathy	**43**
cardiopulmonary resuscitation (CPR)	**7**, 158
cardiovascular system	
function of	33–34, 35, 36–39
parts of	33–34
carotid pulse	**21**, 156
Centers for Disease Control and Prevention (CDC)	**15**
central nervous system	**35**
cerebrovascular accident (CVA)	**46**
emergency response to	159
certification	**6**, 7

Index

chain of command — 8
chain of infection — 13–14
chambers of the heart — 36–38
Cheyne-Stokes — 24
circulatory system, see *cardiovascular system*
clinical experience — 6
code — 153
code of ethics — **5**, 9
code team — 153
communication
    verbal and nonverbal — 4–5
    with other members of care team — 7–8
complex (EKG) — 80
conducted beat — **132**, 133
conduction path — 124
confidentiality — 9, 10, 66–67
congenital defect — 45
congestive heart failure — **43**, 44
consciousness, level of — 12, 28–29
contiguous leads — 146
continuing education — 6, 7
continuous monitoring — 49, 51, 53, 57
controlled atrial fibrillation, see *atrial fibrillation*
coronary arteries — 34, 35, **36**, 38, 41–42
COVID-19 — 16, 17, 47
CPR, see *cardiopulmonary resuscitation*
crash cart — 63
cyanosis — 21, **39**, 152
deep vein thrombosis (DVT) — 45
defibrillation — **126**, 158–159
deoxygenated blood, see *oxygen-depleted blood*
depolarization — 48, 79, 81, 94
developmental disability
    and patient care — 59
dextrocardia — **72**, 74
diastole — 37
diastolic (blood pressure) — 12, **24**, 27
documentation — 66–67
dyspnea — 23
dysrhythmia, see also entries for specific dysrhythmias — 95
echocardiogram — 49

ectopic focus — 98
edema
    peripheral — 43
    pulmonary — 43
Einthoven's triangle — 52
EKG cable, see *lead wire*
EKG lead, see *lead*
EKG machine
    setup and operation — 48–49, 55–57
    troubleshooting — 75
EKG paper — 56
    and measuring time on EKGs — 82
EKG strip, see *EKG tracing*
EKG technician
    role of — 1–2
    scope of practice — 2, 79
EKG tests, see also specific test names
    described — 1, 51
    and pediatric patients — 59
EKG tracing — 48
    measuring waves and intervals on — 85–89
electrical activity of the heart — 77–81
electrical conduction system, see *cardiac conduction system*
electrical interference — **70**, 71
electrocardiogram (EKG), see also various entries under *EKG* — 1, 48
electrode cable, see *lead wire*
electrodes — 48
    names and standard colors — 55
    placement for 3-lead testing — 54
    placement for 5-lead testing — 54
    placement for 12-lead testing — 54
electronic health records (EHR) — 11, 66
embolus — 41, 45, 46
emergency, see also entries for specific emergencies — 152–153
    calling 911 — 153, 155, 156
    caring for conscious patient — 156
    caring for unconscious patient — 156–157
    during EKG testing — 59, 152–155
    response to nonmedical emergency — 160–162
empathy — 5
endocardium — 35
epicardium — 35
erythrocytes — **33**, 34

escape beat — **94**, 120
escape pacemaker — 134
escape rhythm — 94
ethics — 5, 9
event monitor — 50
exchange sites — 38
exercise stress test, see *stress test*
failure to capture — 143, 144
failure to sense — 143, 144
1500 method, see *small block method*
first-degree heart block — 132
flatline, see *asystole*
flutter waves, see *F waves*
formed elements — **33**, 34
Fowler's position — 30
F waves — 105, **106**
gain control — **56**, 57
gloves
    procedure for doffing — 16
    procedure for donning — 16
hand hygiene — **14**, 15
hard skills — 3
Health Information Technology for Economic and Clinical Health Act (HITECH) — 11, 67
Health Insurance Portability and Accountability Act (HIPAA) — 10–11, 67
heart
    chambers — 36–38
    disease, see also specific illnesses — 41–47
    electrical activity — 77–81
    location in chest — 33
    major blood vessels — 36
    mechanical activity — 36–38, 81
    movement of blood through — 36–38
    rhythm, see *cardiac rhythm*
    valves — 36–38, 44–45
heart block, see also specific types of blocks — **95**, 132–135
heart rate — 82
    methods for calculating — 83–84
heart rhythm — 82
    regular — 84
    irregular — 84, 85–86
hemiparesis — 46
hemiplegia — 48
hemoglobin — 34

Index

history, medical	2, 156	
Holter monitor, see also *ambulatory monitor*	**50**	
homeostasis	**31**	
hypertension	12, **24**, 27, 46–47	
hypoxia	**28**, 39	
identification		
of healthcare worker to patient	12	
of patient	58	
idioventricular rhythm	**121**, 125	
infection prevention	13, 14–19	
and EKG testing	68–69	
inferior vena cava	**36**	
injury, EKG adaptations in response to	72	
inpatient treatment	**2**	
in-service education, see *continuing education*		
interval	**80**	
intrinsic rate	**78**, 79	
irregular (heart rhythm)	**84**, 85–86	
ischemia	**41**, 42, 146, 153	
isoelectric line	69, **79**, 80	
Joint Commission	11	
junctional escape beat	**112**	
junctional escape rhythm	**112**, 113, 114	
junctional rhythm, see *junctional escape rhythm*		
junctional tachycardia	**113**, 114	
large block method	**83**, 84	
larynx	**34**	
lead (for pads placed on patient, see *electrodes*)	**48**	
areas of the heart examined by each	53–55	
groups, see also specific lead groups	51–53	
lead wire	**48**, 49	
left atrioventricular valve, see *bicuspid valve*		
lethal cardiac rhythms		
emergency response to	152–153	
illustrated	154–155	
listed	153	
leukocytes	**33**, 34	
liability	**8**	
licensure	**6**	

limb lead reversal	54, 95	
limb leads	**52**	
lungs	34, 38–39	
mastectomy, EKG adaptations in response to	73, 75	
measurement, see *EKG tracing, measuring waves and intervals on*		
mechanical activity of the heart	36–38, 81	
medication		
and patient medical history	2	
used in cardiac emergency	159–160	
metabolism	**31**	
methicillin-resistant *Staphylococcus aureus* (MRSA)	**18**, 68–69	
microorganism	**13**	
mitral valve, see *bicuspid valve*		
mobile cardiac telemetry	**50**	
monomorphic ventricular tachycardia, see *ventricular tachycardia*		
morphology	**79**	
multifocal	96, **119**	
multifocal atrial tachycardia	**103**, 104, 107	
multiformed atrial rhythm, see *wandering atrial pacemaker*		
myocardial infarction (MI)	**2**, 41–43	
emergency response to	152–153, 159–160	
myocardium	**35**, 36	
nervous system, see also entries for specific divisions, e.g., *autonomic nervous system*	**35**	
nitroglycerin	160	
non-ST segment elevation myocardial infarction (NSTEMI)	**146**, 153	
normal sinus rhythm	**80**, 96	
nuclear stress test	**62**	
objective information	**12**	
occlude	**45**	
Occupational Safety and Health Administration (OSHA)	**15**, 18–19	
orthopnea	**23**, 74–75	
outpatient treatment	**1**, 2	
oxygen (as medication)	159–160	
oxygenated blood, see *oxygen-rich blood*		

oxygen-depleted blood	**34**, 36, 40	
oxygen-rich blood	**34**, 36, 40	
oxygen saturation	**27**	
procedure for measuring	28	
pacemaker	**78**	
artificial (see also *artificial pacemaker*)	142–144	
ectopic	95	
escape	**134**	
pacemaker spikes	142	
atrial, illustrated	142	
dual chamber, illustrated	143	
ventricular, illustrated	143	
pain	12, 28–29	
palpation	**21**	
procedure for measuring pulse by	22–23	
palpitations	**45**	
parasympathetic nervous system	**35**, 98–99	
pathogen	**13**, 68–69	
pediatric patients		
and EKG testing	59	
electrode placement adaptation	73, 75	
vital signs ranges	27	
peripheral edema, see *edema*		
peripheral nervous system	**35**	
personal protective equipment (PPE)	**16**	
donning and doffing a full set	17	
pharynx	**34**	
physiology	**31**	
picket fence waves, see *F waves*		
plaque	**41**, 45	
plasma	**33**	
policy	**9**	
polymorphic ventricular tachycardia, see *ventricular tachycardia*		
posterior EKG	73–74, 75	
precordial leads	**52**, 56	
pregnancy, EKG adaptations in response to	74, 75	
prejudice	**4**	
premature atrial complex (PAC)	**102**, 106	
premature junctional complex (PJC)	**112**	
premature ventricular complex (PVC)	**118**, 119, 124	

Index

PR interval	**81**
measurement of	87
procedure	**9**
protected health information (PHI)	**10**, 11, 66–67
pulmonary circuit	**38**
pulmonary edema, see *edema*	
pulmonary embolism (PE)	**46**
pulmonary semilunar valve, see *pulmonary valve*	
pulmonary system, see *respiratory system*	
pulmonary valve	**37**, 38
pulse	**21**
normal range, adult	12
normal range, pediatric	27
points on the body	21–22
procedures for measuring	22–24
pulseless electrical activity	**125**, 155
pulse oximeter	**27**, 28
Purkinje fibers	**78**, 79, 94
P wave	**81**, 86
QRS complex	**81**, 88
QRS interval	81, 82, **88**
QT interval	**82**
radial pulse	**21**, 24
rapid ventricular response	**105**
record-keeping, see *documentation*	
regular (heart rhythm)	**84**
regularity (heart rhythm)	84–86
regurgitation (cardiac)	**44**, 45
repolarization	**48**, 79, 81
respiration	**23**
normal range, adult	12
normal range, pediatric	27
procedure for measuring	24
respiratory rate, see *respiration*	
respiratory system	31, **34**
in relation to cardiovascular system	38–39
retrograde	**111**
rhythm interpretation	82–96
6 steps	82–83
rhythm strip, see also *EKG tracing*	**51**
right atrioventricular valve, see *tricuspid valve*	
R-on-T phenomenon	**124**
R-R interval	**81**, 82, 85
SA node, see *sinoatrial node*	
sawtooth waves, see *F waves*	
scope of practice	**2**, 79
second-degree heart block, Mobitz type I	**132**, 133
second-degree heart block, Mobitz type II	**132**, 133
segment	**79**, 80, 81
semi-Fowler's position	**30**, 78
septum	**37**
sinoatrial (SA) node	**78**, 79, 94
sinus arrest	**98**, 99
sinus arrhythmia	97, **98**, 99
sinus bradycardia	97, **98**, 99
sinus pause, see *sinus arrest*	
sinus tachycardia	**97**, 99
6-second method	**83**
60-cycle interference, see *electrical interference*	
skin condition	21
small block method	**84**
soft skills	3, **4–6**
somatic nervous system	**35**
somatic tremor	**69**, 71
sputum	**44**
standard gain	**56**
Standard Precautions	**15**, 16, 59, 68
stress loop	**65**
stress test	51, **63–64**
stroke, see *cerebrovascular accident (CVA)*	
ST segment	**81**, 82
depression	**146**, 154
elevation	**146**, 154
stylus	**56**
subjective information	**12**
superior vena cava	**36**
supine position	**30**
supraventricular tachycardia	**104**
sustained rhythm	**107**
sympathetic nervous system	35, **78**
sympathy	**5**
symptomatic	**99**
syncope, vasovagal	**157**
systemic circuit	**38**
systole	**37**
systolic pressure	12, **24**, 27
tachycardia, see also specific types of tachycardia	**27**, 96
tachypnea	**24**
target heart rate, see also *age-predicted maximal heart rate*	**63**
telemetry	**50**
telemetry pack	50, **61**
procedure for applying	61–62
temperature	
normal ranges, adult and pediatric	12
procedures for measuring	20–21
sites for measuring	19
third-degree heart block	**134**, 135, 155
300 method, see *large block method*	
thrombocytes	**33**, 34
thrombus, see *blood clot*	
torsades de pointes, see *ventricular tachycardia*	
trachea	**34**
transient ischemic attack (TIA)	**159**
transient rhythm	**107**
Transmission-Based Precautions	**15**
Airborne Precautions	17
and EKG testing	68
Contact Precautions	18
Droplet Precautions	17–18
tricuspid valve	**37**, 78
trigeminy	**119**
troubleshooting	55, **75**
T wave	80, **81**
T wave inversion	**146**
12-lead EKG	51, **60–61**
uncontrolled atrial fibrillation, see *atrial fibrillation*	
underlying rhythm	**95**
unifocal	**119**, 120
unipolar lead	**52**, 143
U wave	**80**
vagal maneuver	**107**
vagal tone	**99**
vagus nerve	98–99
valves of the heart, see *heart*	
veins	**34**, 36
ventricle	37, **38–39**
ventricular escape beat	**120**, 125

ventricular escape rhythm, see *idioventricular rhythm*	
ventricular fibrillation (V-fib)	**124**, 126, 154, 158
ventricular rate	84, 106
ventricular tachycardia	**122**, 123
monomorphic	**122**, 123
polymorpic	**122**, 123
torsades de pointes	**122**, 123
vital signs	**12**
blood pressure	25–27
normal ranges, adult	12
normal ranges, pediatric	27
pulse	21–23
respiration	23–24
temperature	19–21
voltage	**49**
wandering atrial pacemaker	**102**, 103, 107
wandering baseline	**69**, 70, 71
wave	**79**, 80, 81
Wenckebach heart block, see *second-degree heart block, Mobitz type I*	
Wilson's central terminal	**52**